PSYCHIATRY
Self Assessment and Review

• TAYLOR
• TASMAN
• KAY
• LIEBERMAN

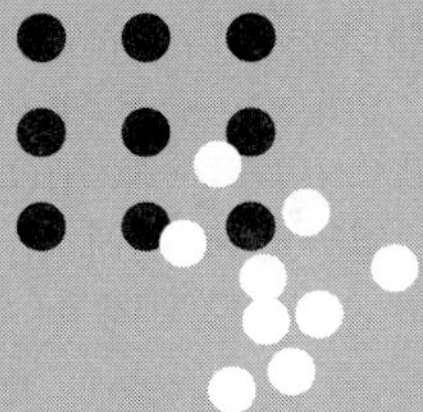

PSYCHIATRY

Self Assessment and Review

David H. Taylor, MD
Assistant Professor
Department of Psychiatry and Behavioral Sciences
University of Louisville School of Medicine
Louisville, Kentucky

Allan Tasman, MD
Professor and Chairman
Department of Psychiatry and Behavioral Sciences
University of Louisville School of Medicine
Louisville, Kentucky

In Consultation with:

Jerald Kay, MD
Professor and Chair
Department of Psychiatry
Wright State University School of Medicine
Dayton, Ohio

Jeffrey A. Lieberman, MD
Director of Psychiatric Research
Hillside Hospital
Long Island Jewish Medical Center
Albert Einstein College of Medicine
Glen Oaks, New York

W.B. SAUNDERS COMPANY
A Division of Harcourt Brace & Company
Philadelphia London Toronto Montreal Sydney Tokyo

W.B. SAUNDERS COMPANY
A Division of Harcourt Brace & Company

The Curtis Center
Independence Square West
Philadelphia, Pennsylvania 19106

Library of Congress Cataloging-in-Publication Data

Psychiatry : self assessment and review / David H. Taylor, Allan Tasman ; in consultation with Jerald Kay, Jeffrey A. Lieberman.

p. cm.

ISBN 0–7216–5242–5

1. Psychiatry—Programmed instruction. I. Taylor, David H. [DNLM: 1. Mental Disorders—therapy—programmed instruction. 2. Psychiatry—programmed instruction. 3. Psychotherapy—programmed instruction. WM 18.2 P9737 1997]

RC454.P79 1997
616.89′0076—dc20

DNLM/DLC 96-29396

PSYCHIATRY: SELF ASSESSMENT AND REVIEW ISBN 0–7216–5242–5

Printed in the United States of America

Last digit is the print number: 9 8 7 6 5 4 3 2 1

To Janet, Virgil, and Mabel

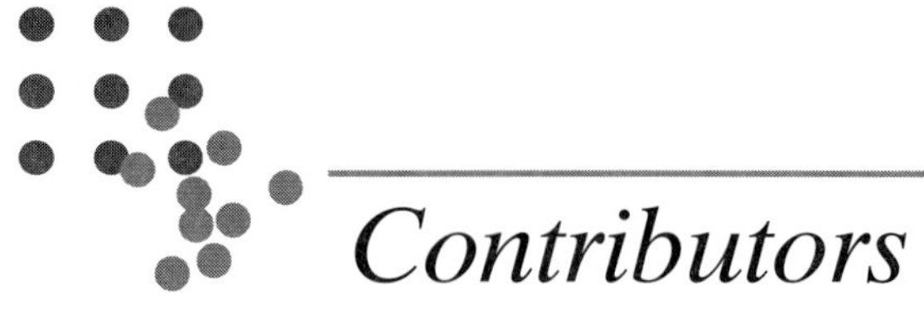

Contributors

Martin M. Antony, PhD
Assistant Professor, Department of Psychiatry, University of Toronto; Psychologist, Anxiety Disorders Clinic, Clarke Institute of Psychiatry, Toronto, Ontario, Canada

Thomas F. Babor, PhD, MPH
Professor, Department of Psychiatry, University of Connecticut, Farmington, CT

David H. Barlow, PhD
Professor and Director of Clinical Programs, Center for Anxiety and Related DIsorders, Boston University, Boston, MA

Mark S. Bauer, MD
Associate Professor, Department of Psychiatry and Human Behavior, Borwn University Program in Medicine; Chief, Mental Health and Behavioral Sciences Service, Veterans Affairs Medical Center, Providence, RI

William R. Beardslee, MD
George P. Gardner/Olga M. Monks Professor of Child Psychiatry, Harvard Medical School; Psychiatrist-in-Chief and Chairman, Department of Psychiatry, Children's Hospital, Boston, MA

David Bienenfeld, MD
Associate Professor, Vice Chair, and Director of Residency Training, Department of Psychiatry, Wright State University, Dayton, OH

Robert J. Boland, MD
Assistant Professor, Department of Psychiatry and Human Behavior, Borwn University, Providence, RI

Neil W. Boris, MD
Assistant Professor, Division of Infant, Child and Adolescent Psychiatry, Louisiana State University School of Medicine, New Orleans, LA; Clinical Assistant Professor, Departments of Pediatrics and Psychiatry and Human Behavior, Brown University School of Medicine, Providence, RI

Olga Brawman-Mintzer, MD
Assistant Professor, Department of Psychiatry and Behavioral Sciences, Medical University of South Carolina, Charleston, SC

Alan Breier, MD
Chief, Section on Clinical Studies, Experimental Therapeutics Branch, National Institute of Mental Health, National Institutes of Health, Bethesda, MD

Evelyn Bromet, PhD
Professor of Psychiatry and Behavioral Science, School of Medicine, State University of New York at Stony Brook, Stony Brook, NY

Deborah L. Cabaniss, MD
Assistant Clinical Professor of Psychiatry, Columbia University College of Physicians and Surgeons, New York, NY

Kenneth Certa, MD
Clinical Assistant Professor of Psychiatry, Jefferson Medical College; Director, Psychiatric Emergency Services, Thomas Jefferson University Hospital, Philadelphia, PA

Irene Chatoor, MD
Professor of Psychiatry and Behavioral Sciences, The George Washington University School of Medicine; Director of Infant Psychiatry, Children's Hospital National Medical Center, Washington, DC

John F. Clarkin, PhD
Professor of Clinical Psychology and Psychiatry, Cornell University Medical College, New York, NY; Director of Psychology, New York Hospital–Cornell Medical Center, Westchester Division, White Plains, NY

Keith H. Claypoole, PhD
Assistant Professor, Department of Psychiatry and Behavioral Science, University of Washington School of Medicine; Director, Neuropsychological Assessment Service, University of Washington Hospital, Seattle, WA

Robert B. Clyman, MD
Assistant Professor, Departments of Psychiatry, Behavioral Sciences, and Pediatrics, The George Washington University Medical Center; Research Scientist and Director, Developmental Psychiatry, Children's Hospital National Medical Center, Washington, DC

Patrick W. Corrigan, PsyD
Associate Professor of Psychiatry, The University of Chicago, Pritzker School of Medicine; Director, University of Chicago Center for Psychiatric Rehabilitation, Chicago, IL

Francine Cournos, MD
Professor of Clinical Psychiatry, Columbia University College of Physicians and Surgeons; Director, Washington Heights Community Service, New York State Psychiatric Institute, New York, NY

Linda W. Craighead, PhD
Associate Professor, Department of Psychology, University of Colorado, Boulder, Boulder, CO

W. Edward Craighead, PhD
Professor, Department of Psychology, University of Colorado, Boulder, Boulder, CO

Pedro L. Delgado, MD
Associate Professor of Psychiatry, Director of Research, and Associate Head, Department of Psychiatry, University of Arizona College of Medicine, Tucson, AZ

Joel E. Dimsdale, MD
Professor of Psychiatry and Director, Program in Consultation Psychiatry and Behavioral Medicine, University of California, San Diego, School of Medicine, La Jolla, CA

Ken Duckworth, MD
Instructor in Psychiatry, Harvard Medical School; Medical Director, Continuing Care Service, Massachusetts Mental Health Center, Boston, MA

Jane L. Elsen, MD
Assistant Professor, Department of Psychiatry and Human Behavior, Brown University Program in Medicine; Director, Obsessive-Compulsive Disorder Clinic, Butler Hospital, Providence, RI

Richard S. Epstein, MD
Clinical Professor, Uniformed Services University of the Health Sciences, F. Edward Hébert School of Medicine, Bethesda, MD; Clinical Professor, Georgetown University School of Medicine, Washington, DC

Eugene W. Farber, PhD
Assistant Professor, Department of Psychiatry and Behavioral Sciences, Emory University School of Medicine; Clinical Psychologist, Grady Health System, Atlanta, GA

Susan J. Fiester, MD
Private practice, Chevy Chase, MD

Michael B. First, MD
Assistant Professor of Clinical Psychiatry, Columbia University, New York, NY; Editor, DSM-IV Text and Criteria, American Psychiatric Association, Washington, DC

Allen Frances, MD
Chairman, Department of Psychiatry and Behavioral Sciences, Duke University Medical Center, Durham, NC

Gregory Franchini, MD
Assistant Professor, Director of Medical Student Education in Psychiatry, Department of Psychiatry, University of New Mexico School of Medicine, Albuquerque, NM

Robert L. Frierson, MD
Professor of Psychiatry and Director of Consultation/Liaison Psychiatry, University of Louisville School of Medicine; Psychiatrist, Jefferson Alcohol and Drug Abuse Center, Louisville, KY

Robert M. Galatzer-Levy, MD
Lecturer, University of Chicago, Pritzker School of Medicine; Training and Supervising Analyst, Child and Adolescent Supervising Analyst, Institute for Psychoanalysis, Chicago, IL

Alan J. Gelenberg, MD
Professor and Head, Department of Psychiatry, University of Arizona College of Medicine, Tucson, AZ

Stephen M. Goldfinger, MD
Assistant Professor of Psychiatry, Harvard Medical School; Senior Psychiatrist, Massachusetts Department of Mental Health, Boston, MA

Robert S. Goldman, PhD
Staff, Albert Einstein College of Medicine, Bronx, NY;
Chief, Neuropsychology Laboratory, Hillside Hospital, Glen Oaks, NY

Reed D. Goldstein, PhD
Clinical Associate, Department of Psychiatry, University of Pennsylvania School of Medicine; Research Associate, Dave Garroway Laboratory for the Study of Depression, Pennsylvania Hospital; Clinical Consultant, Psychology Department, Institute of Pennsylvania Hospital, Philadelphia, PA

Jackie Gollan, MS
Graduate Student, Department of Psychiatry, Center for Clinical Research, University of Washington, Seattle, WA

Eric Gortner, PhD
Graduate Student, Department of Psychiatry, Center for Clinical Research, University of Washington, Seattle, WA

Michael D. Greenberg, MA
Graduate Student, Department of Psychology, Duke University, Durham, NC

Laurence L. Greenhill, MD
Associate Professor of Clinical Psychiatry, Columbia University College of Physicians and Surgeons; Research Psychiatrist II and Medical Director, Disruptive Behavior Disorders Clinic, New York State Psychiatric Institute, New York, NY

Roland R. Griffiths, PhD
Professor, Department of Psychiatry and Behavioral Sciences and Neuroscience, Johns Hopkins University School of Medicine, Baltimore, MD

Amanda J. Gruber, MD
Instructor, Department of Psychiatry, Harvard Medical School, Boston MA; Assistant Psychiatrist, McLean Hospital, Belmont, MA

Alan M. Gruenberg, MD
Professor, Jefferson Medical College; Director, Dave Garroway Laboratory for the Study of Depression, Pennsylvania Hospital; Senior Attending Psychiatrist, Institute of Pennsylvania Hospital, Philadelphia, PA; Lecturer, Yale University School of Medicine, New Haven, CT

Barry Gurland, FRCP, FRC, Psyc
Sidney Katz Professor of Psychiatry, Columbia University College of Physicians and Surgeons; Director, Stroud Center, New York State Psychiatric Institute, New York, NY

Jeffrey M. Halperin, PhD
Professor, Department of Psychology, Queens College of the City University of New York, Flushing, NY; Professorial Lecturer, Department of Psychiatry, Mt. Sinai School of Medicine, New York, NY

Alexis D. Henry, ScD, OTR
Assistant Professor, Occupational Therapy Department, Worcester State College, Worcester, MA

Michael E. Henry, MD
Clinical Instructor, Department of Psychiatry, Harvard Medical School, Boston, MA; Director of Electroconvulsive Therapy, McLean Hospital, Belmont, MA

Ralph E. Hoffman, MD
Associate Professor of Psychiatry, Yale University School of Medicine; Attending Psychiatrist and Director, Center for Biocognitive Studies, Yale Psychiatric Institute, New Haven, CT

Michael F. Hogan, PhD
Associate Clinical Professor, Department of Psychiatry, Ohio State University College of Medicine, Columbus, OH

Heather Stone Hopkins, MD
Associate Editor, University of Arizona Health Science Center, Department of Psychiatry, Tucson, AZ

Stephen S. Ilardi, PhD
Instructor, University of Colorado, Boulder, Boulder, CO

Lawrence B. Inderbitzin, MD
Professor of Psychiatry and Behavioral Sciences, Emory University School of Medicine; Training and Supervising Analyst, Emory University

Psychoanalytic Institute; Director of Clinical Psychiatric Services, Grady Health System, Atlanta, GA

Neil Jacobson, PhD
Professor of Psychology, University of Washington, Seattle, WA

Dilip V. Jeste, MD
Professor of Psychiatry and Neurosciences, University of California, San Diego; Director, Geriatric Psychiatry, Clinical Research Center, San Diego VA Medical Center, San Diego, CA

Michael Kahn, MD
Instructor, Department of Psychiatry, Harvard Medical School; Medical Director, Deaconess/DMH Inpatient Unit, New England Deaconess Hospital, Massachusetts Department of Mental Health, Boston, MA

Marshall B. Kapp, JD, MPH
Professor, Departments of Psychiatry and Community Health, and Director, Office of Geriatric Medicine and Gerontology, Wright State University School of Medicine, Dayton, OH

Nadine J. Kaslow, PhD
Associate Professor, Department of Psychiatry and Behavioral Sciences, Emory University School of Medicine; Chief Psychologist, Department of Psychiatry, Grady Health System, Atlanta, GA

Samuel J. Keith, MD
Professor of Psychiatry and Psychology and Chairman, Department of Psychiatry, University of New Mexico School of Medicine, Albuquerque, NM

Martin B. Keller, MD
Mary E. Zucker Professor and Chairman, Department of Psychiatry and Human Behavior, Brown University Program in Medicine; Psychiatrist-in-Chief, Butler Hospital and Women and Infants Hospital; Executive Psychiatrist-in-Chief, Veterans Administration Medical Center, Emma Pendleton Bradley Hospital, Miriam Hospital, Rhode Island Hospital, and Roger Williams General Hospital, Providence, RI; Executive Psychiatrist-in-Chief, Memorial Hospital (Pawtucket), Pawtucket, RI

William M. Klykylo, MD
Associate Professor and Director, Division of Child and Adolescent Psychiatry, Wright State University School of Medicine, Dayton, OH

Robert Kohn, MD
Assistant Professor, Department of Psychiatry and Human Behavior, Brown University School of Medicine, and Butler Hospital, Providence, RI

Alex Kopelowicz, MD
Assistant Professor of Psychiatry, UCLA Neuropsychiatric Institute and Hospital, Los Angeles, CA; Medical Director, San Fernando Mental Health Center, Mission Hills, CA

Harold S. Koplewicz, MD
Professor, New York University; Vice Chairman for Child and Adolescent Psychiatry, New York University Medical Center, New York, NY

Thomas R. Kosten, MD
Professor of Psychiatry and Director, Division of Substance Abuse, Yale University School of Medicine, New Haven, CT

Henry R. Kranzler, MD
Associate Professor of Psychiatry, University of Connecticut School of Medicine, Farmington, CT

Stanley Kutcher, MD
Professor and Head, Department of Psychiatry, Dalhousie University; Psychiatrist-in-Chief, Queen Elizabeth II Health Sciences Center, Halifax, Nova Scotia, Canada

Lucy LaFarge, MD
Assistant Clinical Professor of Psychiatry, Columbia University College of Physicians and Surgeons, and Training and Supervising Analyst, Columbia University Psychoanalytic Center, New York, NY

Harriet P. Lefley, PhD
Professor of Psychiatry and Behavioral Sciences, University of Miami School of Medicine, Miami, FL

James L. Levenson, MD
Professor of Psychiatry, Medicine, and Surgery, Chairman, Division of Consultation/Liaison Psychiatry, Vice Chairman, Department of Psychiatry, Virginia Commonwealth University Medical College of Virginia, Richmond, VA

Stephen B. Levine, MD
Clinical Professor of Psychiatry, Case Western Reserve University School of Medicine, Cleveland, OH; Co-Director, Center for Marital and Sexual Health, Inc., Beachwood, OH

Steven T. Levy, MD
Bernard C. Holland Professor and Vice Chairman, Department of Psychiatry and Behavioral Sciences, Emory University School of Medicine; Director, Emory University Psychoanalytic Institute; Chief of Psychiatry, Grady Health System, Atlanta, GA

Robert Paul Liberman, MD
Professor of Psychiatry, UCLA School of Medicine, UCLA Neuropsychiatric Institute, and UCLA Hospital; Director, Clinical Research Center for Schizophrenia and Psychiatric Rehabilitation, West Los Angeles Veterans Administration Medical Center, Los Angeles, CA, and Camarillo State Hospital, Camarillo, CA

Walter Ling, MD
Professor and Chief of Substance Abuse Program, Department of Psychiatry and Biobehavioral Sciences, UCLA School of Medicine; Associate Chief of Psychiatry for Substance Abuse, West Los Angeles Veterans Administartion Medical Center; Director, Los Angeles Addiction Treatment Research Center; Medical Director, The Matrix Center, Inc., Health Care Delivery Services, Friends Medical Science Research, Los Angeles, CA

Joyce H. Lowinson, MD
Professor of Epidemiology and Social Medicine and Special Assistant (for Substance Abuse) to the Dean, Albert Einstein College of Medicine of Yeshiva University, Bronx, NY

Christopher P. Lucas, MB ChB, MRC Psych, M Med Sc
Assistant Professor of Child Psychiatry, Columbia University College of Physicians and Surgeons; Director, Suicide Disorders Clinic, Department of Pediatric Psychiatry, Columbia Presbyterian Medical Center, New York, NY

R. Bruce Lydiard, PhD, MD
Professor of Psychiatry, Department of Psychiatry and Behavioral Sciences, Medical University of South Carolina, Charleston, SC

José R. Maldonado, MD
Assistant Professor of Psychiatry and Behavioral Sciences, Stanford University School of Medicine; Section Chief, Medical Psychiatry, Medical Director, Consultation/Liaison Psychiatry, and Chief, Medical

Psychotherapy Clinic, Stanford University Medical Center, Stanford, CA

John S. March, MD, MPH
Director, Pediatric Anxiety Disorders Program, Duke University Medical Center, Durham, NC

Stephen R. Marder, MD
Professor and Vice Chair, Department of Psychiatry, UCLA School of Medicine; Chief, Psychiatry Service, West Los Angeles Veterans Administration Medical Center, Los Angeles, CA

John C. Markowitz, MD
Associate Professor of Clinical Psychiatry, Cornell University Medical College; Associate Attending Psychiatrist, The New York Hospital, New York, NY

Ronald L. Martin, MD
Professor and Chair, Department of Psychiatry and Behavioral Sciences, University of Kansas School of Medicine—Wichita, Wichita, KS

Kristin Matler-Sharma, PhD
Staff Psychologist, Rusk Institute of Rehabilitation Medicine, New York University Medical Center, New York, NY

Elinore F. McCance, MD, PhD
Assistant Professor, Division of Substance Abuse, Department of Psychiatry, Yale University School of Medicine, New Haven, CT

Thomas H. McGlashan, MD
Professor of Psychiatry, Yale University School of Medicine; Chief Executive Officer, Yale Psychiatric Institute, New Haven, CT

G. Darlene Warrick McLaughlin, MD
Assistant Professor of Clinical Psychiatry, University of Texas Southwestern Medical School at Dallas; Director of Clinical Program Development and Attending Psychiatrist, Mental Health Connections, Dallas, TX

Laura F. McNicholas, MD, PhD
Assistant Professor, Department of Psychiatry, University of Pennsylvania School of Medicine, and Veterans Administration Medical Center, Philadelphia, PA

Arthur T. Meyerson, MD
Professor and Vice Chair, Department of Psychiatry, University of Medicine and Dentistry of New Jersey; Clinical Director, UMDNJ Behavioral Health Care Programs of Newark, Newark, NJ

David J. Miklowitz, PhD
Associate Professor of Psychology, University of Colorado, Boulder, Boulder, CO

Paul C. Mohl, MD
Professor of Psychiatry and Director of Residency Training, University of Texas Southwestern Medical Center at Dallas, Dallas, TX

Pamela Moore, MD
Assistant Professor, University of Connecticut Health Center School of Medicine; Assistant Professor, Inpatient Unit Attending, John Dempsey Hospital, Farmington, CT

Richard F. Morrissey, PhD
Assistant Professor of Psychiatry, Albert Einstein College of Medicine, Bronx, NY; Coordinator of Psychological Services, Division of Child and Adolescent Psychiatry, Long Island Jewish Medical Center, New Hyde Park, NY

Loren R. Mosher, MD
Clinical Professor of Psychiatry, Uniformed Services University of the Health Sciences, Bethesda, MD; Chief Medical Director, Psychiatry, Montgomery Country Department of Human Services, Rockville, MD

David A. Mrazek, MD, FRC Psych
Professor of Psychiatry, Behavioral Sciences, and Pediatrics, The George Washington University School of Medicine; Professor and Chairman of Psychiatry and Behavioral Sciences and Director, Neuroscience Center, Children's Research Institute, Children's Hospital National Medical Center, Washington, DC

Jeff J. Mulchahey, MBA, PhD
Assistant Professor, Department of Psychiatry and Behavioral Sciences, Emory University School of Medicine, Atlanta, GA

Philip R. Muskin, MD
Associate Professor of Clinical Psychiatry and Collaborating Psychoanalyst, Psychiatric Center for Training and Research, Columbia University; Associate Chief of Service, Consultation/Liaison Psychiatry, Columbia-Presbyterian Medical Center, New York, NY

David Naimark, MD
Geriatric Psychiatry Fellow, San Diego Veterans Administration Medical Center, University of California, San Diego, School of Medicine, La Jolla, CA

Jeffrey H. Newcorn, MD
Associate Professor of Psychiatry and Pediatrics and Director, Division of Child and Adolescent Psychiatry, Mount Sinai School of Medicine of the City University of New York, New York, NY

John M. Oldham, MD
Professor and Vice Chairman, Department of Psychiatry, Columbia University College of Physicians and Surgeons; Director, New York State Psychiatric Institute, New York, NY

Michael J. Owens, PhD
Assistant Professor, Department of Psychiatry and Behavioral Sciences, Laboratory of Neuropsycho-pharmacology, Emory University School of Medicine, Atlanta, GA

Michele T. Pato, MD
Associate Professor and Director of Residency Training in Psychiatry, State University of New York at Buffalo; Medical Director, Outpatient Services, Department of Psychiatry, Buffalo General Hospital/Community Mental Health Center, Buffalo, NY

Katharine A. Phillips, MD
Assistant Professor, Department of Psychiatry and Human Behavior, Brown University School of Medicine; Chief of Outpatient Service and Director, Body Dysmorphic Disorder Program, Butler Hospital, Providence, RI

Debra A. Pinals, MD
Clinical Instructor, Harvard Medical School, Boston, MA;
Charles C. Gaughan Fellow in Forensic Psychiatry, Bridgewater State Hospital, Bridgewater, MA

Harold Alan Pincus, MD
Deputy Medical Director and Director, Office of Research, American Psychiatric Association, Washington, DC; Clinical Professor, Department of Psychiatry and Behavioral Sciences, George Washington University School of Medicine, Washington, DC;
Adjunct Professor of Psychiatry and Behavioral Sciences, Duke University Medical Center, Durham, NC;

Clinical Professor of Psychiatry, Uniformed Services University of the Health Sciences, Bethesda, MD

Paul M. Plotsky, PhD
Professor and Director, Stress Neurobiology Laboratory, Emory University School of Medicine, Atlanta, GA

Harrison G. Pope, Jr., MD
Associate Professor of Psychiatry, Harvard Medical School, Boston MA; Psychiatrist, McLean Hospital, Belmont, MA

Mark A. Riddle, MD
Director, Division of Child and Adolescent Psychiatry, Johns Hopkins University School of Medicine, Baltimore, MD

Priscilla Ridgway, MSW
Research Associate, Office of Social Policy Analysis, University of Kansas School of Social Welfare, Lawrence, KS

Arthur Rifkin, MD
Professor of Psychiatry, Albert Einstein College of Medicine, Bronx, NY; Attending Psychiatrist, Hillside Hospital, Long Island Jewish Medical Center, Glen Oaks, NY

Ellen A. Rosenblatt, MD
Clinical Assistant Professor of Psychiatry, Case Western Reserve University School of Medicine, Cleveland, OH; Director, The Program for Women, Center for Marital and Sexual Health, Inc., Beachwood, OH

Neil Rosenberg, MD
Colorado Neurological Institute, Englewood, CO

Matthew V. Rudorfer, MD
Assistant Chief, Clinical Treatment Research Branch, Division of Clinical and Treatment Research, National Institute of Mental Health, National Institutes of Health, Rockville, MD

Harold A. Sackeim, PhD
Professor of Clinical Psychology in Psychiatry, Columbia University College of Physicians and Surgeons; Chief, Department of Biological Psychiatry, New York State Psychiatric Institute, New York, NY

Cynthia J. Sanderson, PhD
Director, Personality Disorders Program, Department of Psychiatry, New York Hospital–Cornell Medical Center, Westchester, Division, White Plains, NY

Lon S. Schneider, MD
Associate Professor of Psychiatry, Neurology, and Gerontology, Department of Psychiatry and the Behavioral Sciences, University of Southern California School of Medicine, Los Angeles, CA

John E. Schowalter, MD
Albert Solnit Professor of Child Psychiatry and Pediatrics, Yale University Child Study Center; Associate Chief, Department of Child Psychiatry, Yale–New Haven Medical Center, New Haven, CT

Judith L. Schreiber, MSW
Private practice, San Diego, CA

David Shaffer, FRCP, FRC Psych
Irving Philips Professor of Child Psychiatry, Columbia University, College of Physicians and Surgeons; Director, Division of Child and Adolescent Psychiatry, Columbia Presbyterian Medical Center, New York, NY

Theodore Shapiro, MD
Professor of Psychiatry and Psychiatry in Pediatrics, Cornell University Medical College; Director, Child and Adolescent Psychiatry, Payne Whitney Clinic, New York Hospital, New York, NY

Vanshdeep Sharma, MD
Department of Psychiatry, Mt. Sinai Medical Center, New York, NY

Charles W. Sharp, PhD
Associate Director, Special Programs, National Institute on Drug Abuse, National Institutes of Health, Rockville, MD

M. Katherine Shear, MD
Associate Professor of Psychiatry, University of Pittsburgh School of Medicine; Director, Anxiety Disorders Prevention Program, Western Psychiatric Institute and Clinic, Pittsburgh, PA

Edward K. Silberman, MD
Clinical Professor of Psychiatry and Director of Residency Education, Jefferson Medical College, Philadelphia, PA

J. Arturo Silva, MD
Associate Professor of Psychiatry, University of Texas Health Care Center at San Antonio; Staff Psychiatrist, Audie Murphy Veterans Administration Medical Center, San Antonio, TX

Larry B. Silver, MD
Clinical Professor of Psychiatry and Director of Training in Child and Adolescent Psychiatry, Georgetown University School of Medicine, Washington, DC

Daphne Simeon, MD
Assistant Professor of Clinical Psychiatry, Mount Sinai School of Medicine of the City University of New York, New York, NY

Malini Singh, PhD
Staff Psychologist, St. Vincent's Hospital and Medical Center, New York, NY

Andrew E. Skodol, MD
Professor of Clinical Psychiatry, Columbia University College of Physicians and Surgeons; Research Psychiatrist, New York State Psychiatric Institute, New York, NY

Mark A. Slater, PhD
Assistant Clinical Professor of Psychiatry, University of California, San Diego, School of Medicine, La Jolla, CA; Vice President, Research, Sharp Healthcare, San Diego, CA

Irma C. Smet, PhD
Staff Neuropsychologist, University of Michigan Medical Center, Ann Arbor, MI

David E. Smith, MD
Associate Clinical Professor, Clinical Toxicology and Occupational Health, University of California, San Francisco Medical Center; Founder, President, and Medical Director, Haight-Ashbury Free Clinics, Inc., San Francisco; President, American Society of Addiction Medicine, Chevy Chase, MD; Research Director, MPI Treatment Services, Inc., Oakland, CA

Janet L. Sobell, PhD
Assistant Professor of Epidemiology and Psychiatry, Mayo Clinic/ Foundation, Rochester, NY

Phyllis Solomon, PhD
Professor of Social Work and Social Work in Psychiatry, University of Pennsylvania School of Social Work, Philadelphia, PA

Steve S. Sommer, MD, PhD
Professor of Molecular Biology, Mayo Clinic/Foundation, Rochester, MN

David Spiegel, MD
Professor of Psychiatry and Behavioral Sciences, Stanford University School of Medicine; Attending Psychiatrist, Stanford University Hospital, Stanford, CA

Walter N. Stone, MD
Professor of Psychiatry, University of Cincinnati College of Medicine, Cincinnati, OH

Steven C. Stout, BA
Medical Scientist Training Program, Emory University School of Medicine, Atlanta, GA

Eric C. Strain, MD
Associate Professor, Department of Psychiatry and Behavioral Sciences, Johns Hopkins University School of Medicine, Baltimore, MD

James J. Strain, MD
Professor of Psychiatry and Director, Division of Behavioral Medicine and Consultation Psychiatry, Mount Sinai School of Medicine of the City University of New York, New York, NY

Gordon Strauss, MD
Professor and Director, Residency Education Department of Psychiatry and Behavioral Science, University of Louisville School of Medicine; Staff Psychiatrist, Louisville Veterans Administration Medical Center, Louisville, KY

Loree Sutton, MD
Assistant Professor, Department of Psychiatry, Uniformed Services University of the Health Sciences, F. Edward Hébert School of Medicine, Bethesda, MD

Holly A. Swartz, MD
Instructor, Department of Psychiatry, Cornell University Medical College; Clinical Affiliate in Psychiatry, The New York Hospital, New York, NY

Ludwik S. Szymanski, MD
Assistant Professor of Psychiatry, Harvard Medical School; Director of Psychiatry, Institute for Community Inclusion, Children's Hospital, Boston, MA

Pierre N. Tariot, MD
Department of Psychiatry, University of Rochester School of Medicine, Monroe Community Hospital, Rochester, NY

Michael E. Thase, MD
Professor of Psychiatry, University of Pittsburgh School of Medicine; Director, Mood Disorders Module, and Associate Director, Clinical Research Center, University of Pittsburgh Medical Center, Western Psychiatric Institute and Clinic, Pittsburgh, PA

Mauricio Tohen, MD, DrPH
Associate Professor of Psychiatry, Harvard Medical School; Associate Professor of Epidemiology, Harvard School of Public Health, Boston, MA

Kenneth E. Towbin, MD
Associate Professor of Psychiatry and Behavioral Science and Director of Residency Training in Psychiatry, Children's Hospital National Medical Center, The George Washington University School of Medicine, Washington, DC

Gary J. Tucker, MD
Professor and Chairman, Department of Psychiatry and Behavioral Sciences, University of Washington School of Medicine, Seattle, WA

George Vaillant, MD
Professor of Psychiatry, Harvard Medical School; Director of Research, Division of Psychiatry, Brigham and Women's Hospital, Boston, MA

Susan C. Vaughan, MD
Instructor in Clinical Psychiatry, Columbia University College of Physicians and Surgeons; Research Fellow in Affective and Anxiety Disorders, New York State Psychiatric Institute, New York, NY

John T. Walkup, MD
Associate Professor, Johns Hopkins University School of Medicine, Baltimore, MD

Charles J. Wallace, PhD, MBA
Associate Research Psychologist, UCLA Neuropsychiatric Institute and UCLA Hospital, Los Angeles, CA; Chief, Behavioral Analysis and Social Skills Laboratory, Clinical Research Center for the Study of Schizophrenia and Psychiatric Rehabilitation, Camarillo State Hospital, Camarillo, CA

B. Timothy Walsh, MD
William & Joy Ruane Professor of Clinical Psychiatry, Columbia University College of Physicians and Surgeons; Director, Eating Disorders Research Program, New York State Psychiatric Institute, New York, NY

Anne L. Weickgenant, PhD
Research Assistant, Veterans Administration Medical Center, San Diego, CA

Donald R. Wesson, MD
Associate Clinical Professor, Department of Psychiatry, University of California, San Francisco, School of Medicine, San Francisco, CA; Medical Director and Scientific Director, MPI Treatment Services, Summit Medical Center, Oakland, CA

Thomas A. Widiger, PhD
Professor, Department of Psychology, University of Kentucky, Lexington, KY

Maija Wilska, MD
Developmental Pediatrician and Chief Physician (Retired), Rinnekoti Central Institution for Mental Retardation Espoo, Finland

Ronald M. Winchel, MD
Assistant Professor of Clinical Psychiatry, Columbia University College of Physicians and Surgeons; Psychiatrist, New York State Psychiatric Institute, New York, NY

June Grant Wolf, PhD
Instructor in Psychology, Department of Psychiatry, Harvard Medical School; Director of Psychology, Massachusetts Mental Health Center, Boston, MA

George E. Woody, MD
Clinical Professor, Department of Psychiatry, University of Pennsylvania; Chief, Substance Abuse Treatment Unit, Veterans Administration Medical Center, Philadelphia, PA

Jesse H. Wright, MD, PhD
Professor of Psychiatry, Department of Psychiatry and Behavioral Sciences, University of Louisville School of Medicine; Medical Director, Norton Psychiatric Clinic, Louisville, KY

Yoram Yovell, MD
Assistant Professor of Clinical Psychiatry, Columbia University College of Physicians and Surgeons; Psychiatrist, New York State Psychiatric Institute, New York, NY

Sean H. Yutzy, MD
Assistant Professor of Psychiatry and Director of Forensic Services,

Washington University Medical School; Assistant Professor of Psychiatry, Barnes Hospital, St. Louis, MO

Richard B. Zimmer, MD
Assistant Clinical Professor of Psychiatry, Columbia University College of Physicians and Surgeons; Faculty, Columbia University Center for Psychoanalytic Training and Research, New York, NY

Stephen R. Zukin, MD
Director, Division of Clinical and Services Research, National Institute on Drug Abuse, National Institutes of Health, Rockville, MD; Professor of Psychiatry and Neuroscience, Albert Einstein College of Medicine of Yeshiva University, Bronx, NY

Ilana Zylberman, MD
Assistant Professor of Psychiatry, Mount Sinai School of Medicine of the City University of New York; Attending Psychiatrist, Mount Sinai Medical Center, New York, NY

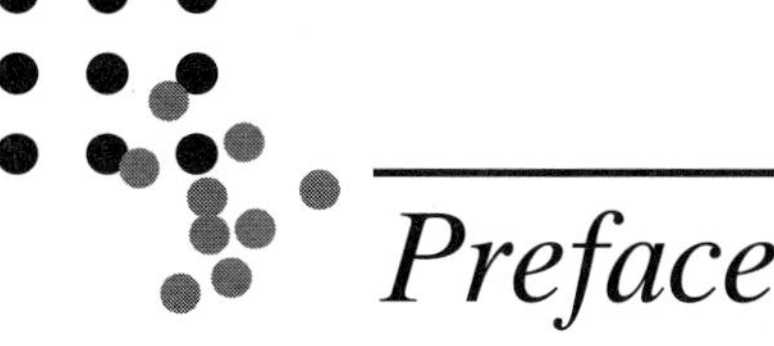

Preface

Psychiatry: Self Assessment and Review is designed to serve as a companion to the main text. It was prepared with the aim of helping the reader to test his or her knowledge of psychiatry. In the spirit of the textbook, the goal is to present questions that are intellectually challenging and that reflect the most advanced knowledge in the field at the time of publication. Most of the questions included herein have been prepared by the contributors to *Psychiatry* and thus reflect the comprehensive understanding that only these scholars, each of whom is a leader in their field, can provide. Each question is referenced to the specific page in the main text on which it is based. In addition, every question is followed by a detailed rationale for the correct answer. The questions are all in the multiple choice format currently used in the American Board of Psychiatry and Neurology, Part I: Examination. It is our hope that this review book will aid psychiatric residents, psychiatric fellows, psychiatrists, primary care physicians, and allied mental health specialists in a careful and comprehensive review of the discipline either for the purpose of self-assessment or board preparation.

This book could not have been written without the dedication and assistance of a number of individuals. Ms. Joan Lucas, Ms. Rozalyn Buckhalter at the University of Louisville, and Ms. Joanie Milnes at W.B. Saunders all made the project happen. Ms. Megan Hester made an extraordinary effort in all phases of the book, from administrative to creative, without which this book would never have been completed.

David H. Taylor, M.D.
Allan Tasman, M.D.
Jerald Kay, M.D.
Jeffrey A. Lieberman, M.D.

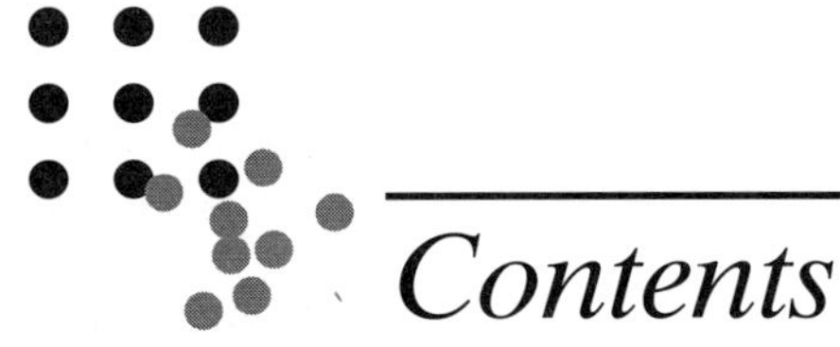

Contents

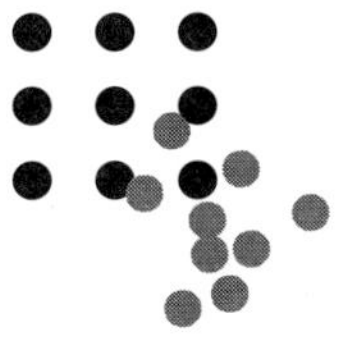

SECTION I

Section Editor: Robert J. Ursano

Approaches to the Patient

CHAPTER

1 Listening to the Patient

Paul C. Mohl • G. Darlene Warrick McLaughlin

1. The skill of accurate listening requires

A. use of the tools of asking, looking, and testing
B. imagination
C. a sense of humor
D. shared meanings of words, metaphors, and similes
E. all of the above

Discussion: Listening is a basic medical activity. In psychiatry, it is central and underpins all other skills in alliance building, diagnosis, and communication. It is a complex process that has been described in a variety of different theoretical ways historically.

Pages 3–4, Table 1–1 •

Answer E

2. The basic attitude of listening

A. assumes that occasionally one finds bad historians
B. requires that the listener block his or her own inner experience and center on the patient
C. places the listener in the active role of controlling the interview
D. assumes that the answer is always inside the patient
E. requires certainty on the part of the listener

Discussion: Good listening assumes that there are no bad historians. The listener must be sensitive to who the patient-storyteller is and not just what is wrong with him or her. Another assumption is that feeling confused and uncertain is part of careful listening.

Page 8, Table 1–3 •

Answer D

3. Keys to the accurate diagnosis of depression include all of the following **except**

A. never forgetting that depression, like almost all other psychiatric symptoms, is exclusively an inner experience
B. keeping in mind that many patients do not acknowledge depression
C. being aware that the patient's label of herself or himself may be different from sad, guilty, or down on oneself
D. basically simply reporting that one is depressed

Discussion: The diagnosis of a condition such as depression requires careful screening and inquiry. A distinction is made between symptomatic and narrative-experiential listening. Furthermore, the listener needs to pay attention to the quality of the person's behavior and interactions. The simple report of depression is in fact insufficient.

Pages 4, 8 •

Answer D

4. Listening is different from hearing. It includes the following:

A. seeing—movements, gestures, facial expressions
B. integration of changes in mode and dissonances between sensory modes
C. the biology of empathy
D. flexible processing of the data presented
E. all of the above

Discussion: Listening includes all of the above but of course also involves careful hearing of changes in inflection, tone, and stream of associations. Darwin first observed that there appeared to be a biogrammar of primary emotions that all humans possess and express in fixed patterns. The observation of such patterns needs to be integrated with all other heard information.

Page 5 •

Answer E

5. Blocks to good listening include

A. certain similarities between listener and patient
B. special meanings to certain words and expressions
C. external distractions
D. differences in regional dialect
E. all of the above

Discussion: Good listening is a challenge because there are often many factors that prevent one from doing it properly. In addition to the above, these include external forces, such as a need for control on an inpatient unit; countertransference phenomena; and differences in socioeconomic class between psychiatrist and patient.

Page 6, Table 1–2 •

Answer E

6. In family therapy:

A. The listener is an intruder who forces an imbalance in the family system.
B. The content of the session is patient centered and controlled by the family system.
C. The listening stance is one of positive regard and empathy.
D. The psychiatrist focuses attention on the patient's inner world of experience.
E. The psychiatrist concentrates on feelings, affect, and stream of association.

Discussion: Different clinical traditions in psychotherapy have influenced the ways in which the therapist's listening is characterized. The stance of the therapist in a family systems approach involves sitting midway among the pressures and forces emanating from each individual seeking to jiggle the system so that all must adapt differently. The therapist is thus a neutral intruder.

Page 10, Table 1–4 •

Answer A

7. The patient's use of figures of speech

A. purposely confuses and frustrates the listener by keeping the patient's true meanings hidden and undiscoverable
B. tells a deeper story offering a new level of understanding of the patient
C. is of little help in uncovering the patient's inner experience of himself or herself and his or her world
D. makes it difficult to concentrate on the objective signs and symptoms necessary for accurate diagnosis
E. has little connection with the patient's stream of associations

Discussion: Figures of speech, which include analogies, similes, and metaphors, are important windows to the inner world of the patient. All language is symbolic. Differences in meaning make the interpretation of special uses of language, such as figures of speech, complex but crucial in the assessment of a patient in psychotherapy.

Page 3–4 •

Answer B

8. When a psychiatrist finds herself or himself expressing thoughts and feelings in ways that may be different from her or his usual repertoire in the course of treating a patient:

A. The psychiatrist should be on guard that the patient has a hidden agenda.
B. The psychiatrist should be attentive to the possibility that such phenomena as countertransference or projective identification may be at work and that she or he may be changed in the process.
C. The psychiatrist should terminate the therapy with that particular patient.
D. The psychiatrist is having a bad day and unable to filter out her or his own inner experience.
E. The psychiatrist is losing necessary control in the therapeutic dyad.

Discussion: A key skill in careful listening is listening to oneself and paying attention to the variety of reactions to patients, especially those who are often difficult to listen to or be with. To recognize common human drives in oneself and in a patient will help further one's understanding of a patient.

Page 11, Figure 1–2 •

Answer B

CHAPTER

2 Psychiatric Interview: Settings and Techniques

Edward K. Silberman • Kenneth Certa

1. Which one of the following is true about the psychiatric assessment interview?

A. It is best performed from the point of view of a single, consistent theoretical perspective.
B. It is essentially complete when enough information has been gathered to make a diagnosis.
C. The patient's style of communication is an important source of information.
D. The interview should be structured according to a fixed succession of topics.
E. The interview adds little to the assessment when the results of laboratory tests, brain imaging, and psychological testing are available.

Discussion: The psychiatric interview is the principal means of assessment in clinical psychiatry. There are no other currently available procedures that can be as informative as observing, listening to, and interacting with the patient. How a patient communicates, interacts, and conducts himself or herself is important.

Page 19 •

Answer C

2. Which of the following would be **least** essential to a core database for all patients?

A. current symptoms
B. summary of developmental milestones
C. psychiatric disorders in first- and second-degree relatives
D. history of substance abuse
E. current cognitive functioning

Discussion: In an interview, a core database is gathered. This can be either a minimal amount of essential information or an expanded data set. Extrinsic and diagnostic factors affect the amount and type of data that it is possible or necessary to gather. Completeness is probably impossible, and some areas, such as developmental milestones, are potentially expansive.

Pages 23, 24, Table 2–4 •

Answer B

3. All of the following are true about transference **except**

A. It may enhance rapport with the interviewer.
B. It may diminish rapport with the interviewer.
C. It is specific to certain psychiatric disorders.
D. It may be an unconscious continuation of childhood perceptions and attitudes.
E. It is a source of information about the patient.

Discussion: Emotionally based biases of the patient are commonly referred to as transference. These include a wide variety of preconceptions, expectations, and tendencies toward distortion, which have their origin in childhood interactions with important individuals such as parents. Such transferential biases may be positive or negative and may be present even before the start of an interview. Transference is a quality that people have in their relationships and is therefore not limited to certain psychiatric disorders.

Page 27 •

Answer C

4. Which of the following is true about interviewing technique?

A. An active, fact-gathering style tends to interfere with patients' ability to express feelings.
B. Delusional patients should be confronted with the falsity of their ideas.
C. Yes-no and symptom-checklist–type questions are confusing to cognitively impaired or disorganized patients and should be avoided with them.

D. Asking *why* questions is a useful facilitative technique.
E. It is usually best to begin an interview with open-ended questions.

Discussion: A psychiatric interview has an opening, middle, and closing phase. In the opening phase, the use of open-ended questions is usually helpful in eliciting the patient's own experience. More directive approaches and closer questioning may be more appropriate as the interview proceeds.

Pages 29–30 •

Answer E

For each numbered item, select the lettered heading most closely associated with it. Each letter may be selected once, more than once, or not at all.

5. Match the intervention with the description.

____ 1. highly directive intervention	A. changing the topic
____ 2. nondirective intervention	B. avoidance of anxiety-provoking material
____ 3. supportive intervention	C. compound questions
____ 4. obstructive intervention	D. clarification

Discussion: There are four dimensions of interviewing style: degree of directiveness, degree of emotional support, degree of fact versus feeling orientation, and degree of feedback to the patient. Directiveness in the interview ensures that the necessary areas of information are covered and supplies whatever cognitive support the patient needs in discussing them. Patients vary in their need for emotional support. Obstruction involves impeding the flow of information with compound or vague questions as well as ones that begin with *why.*

Pages 31–33, Tables 2–6, 2–7, 2–8, 2–9 •

Answers 1, A; 2, D; 3, B; 4, C

6. Which of the following is true about the mental status examination?

A. "Inappropriate affect" refers to expressions of emotion that are not socially acceptable.
B. The performance of "serial sevens" is primarily a test of the patient's numerical calculating ability.
C. Most of the mental status examination is performed informally as an integral part of interacting with the patient.
D. Direct questions about suicidal intent are to be avoided, because they may stimulate suicidal behavior in suggestible patients.
E. Mood is judged primarily by the patient's facial expression and tone of voice.

Discussion: The mental status examination is largely conducted by careful observation that coincides with the conduct of the interview.

Pages 26–27, Table 2–5 •

Answer C

7. Which of the following is **not true** about difficult interviewing situations?

A. A patient's hostility is best dealt with by ignoring it.
B. It is generally unhelpful to try to talk psychotic patients out of delusional ideas.
C. Providing for physical control of an agitated patient is a prerequisite for performing an interview with such a patient.
D. Interviews with cognitively impaired patients are likely to generate more information about mental status than about history.
E. In dealing with a seductive patient, the interviewer must be accepting of the patient's feelings while making it clear that they cannot be acted on.

Discussion: Hostility in an interview is a special challenge because it threatens the formation or maintenance of a therapeutic alliance. Hostility is best acknowledged and then analyzed as much as possible to allow the interview to proceed. Ignoring or responding in kind is generally not helpful because the alliance of two people working together to solve the problems of one of them is undermined.

Page 34 •

Answer A

CHAPTER

3 Physician-Patient Relationship

David Taylor

1. The physician-patient relationship is one that
A. is entirely based in reality
B. is scientifically well understood
C. has a fantasy-based component
D. is always a support to the patient

Discussion: The physician-patient relationship is composed of both a reality-based component (working alliance) and a fantasy-based component (transference) derived from the patient's patterns of interpersonal behavior learned in childhood. Either or both of these may maximize or limit the patient's sense of reassurance, available information, feelings of comfort, or sense of hope.

Page 41 •

Answer C

2. Rapport, an essential part of a physician-patient relationship, has all of the following components **except**
A. empathy
B. acknowledgment of pain and suffering
C. joint process of discovery
D. projective identification

Discussion: Rapport is something that must be nurtured early in a treatment relationship. It is based on both the patient's and physician's shared recognition of the patient's pain. The ability to empathize, especially with those who are suicidal or are in intense conflict with family or caregivers, is the sine qua non of a treatment based on rapport. The psychiatrist who early on demonstrates an understanding of the patient's situation and fears is well positioned to help his or her patient. Projective identification is a complex defense mechanism that usually undermines treatment.

Pages 41–42 •

Answer D

3. Which of the following might increase the likelihood of countertransference responses in the physician?
A. death of her or his father
B. pregnancy
C. personal illness
D. anxiety over boards
E. all of the above

Discussion: Countertransference usually takes one of two forms; concordant countertransference, when one empathizes with the patient's position; or complementary countertransference, when one empathizes with an important figure from the patient's past. Typical countertransferences may involve wishes to save or rescue a patient or unrecognized feelings of deprivation leading to unspoken wishes for a patient to quit treatment. Major developmental events in a physician's life can influence his or her perceptions of patients.

Page 43, Table 3–2 •

Answer E

4. Defense mechanisms can be characterized in which of the following ways?
A. They are seen only in unstable and ill persons.
B. They are entirely unconscious.
C. They are a style of cognition.
D. They are rarely disruptive to a patient.

Discussion: All people, including patients, employ mechanisms of defense to protect themselves from the painful awareness of feelings and memories that can provoke overwhelming anxiety. Defense mechanisms are specific cognitive processes, ways of thinking, that the mind employs to avoid painful feelings. These are often characteristic of the person and form a style of cognition. On the basis of the degree to which they lead to distortion of reality and interpersonal disruption, defense mechanisms may be more or less mature.

Page 44, Table 3–3 •

Answer C

5. The physician-patient relationship includes all of the following **except**

A. One person is seen as the expert.
B. One person is the help seeker.
C. Hope is a primary motivator of the relationship.
D. A firm directive stance is the norm.

Discussion: The physician-patient relationship is based on specific roles and motivations. A physician requires a genuine interest in people and a desire to help.

Page 4 •

Answer D

6. Managed care can deeply affect the physician-patient relationship in all of the following ways **except** by

A. discontinuity of care
B. erosion of confidentiality
C. increased autonomy of the physician
D. shrinkage of the types of reimbursable services

Discussion: Managed care, broadly defined as any care of patients that is not determined solely by the provider, currently focuses on the economic aspects of delivering medical care, with little attention thus far to its potential effects on the physician-patient relationship. Autonomy of both the patient and physician is diminished by managed care.

Page 46 •

Answer C

For each numbered item, select the lettered heading most closely associated with it. Each letter may be selected once, more than once, or not at all.

7. Match the term with the definition.

____ 1. working relationship
____ 2. therapeutic alliance
____ 3. transference
____ 4. countertransference
____ 5. nonspecific aspects of cure

A. placebo effect
B. the physician's unique reaction to a patient based on his or her developmental experience
C. reality-based component of the physician-patient relationship
D. response of the patient to the physician as if the physician were a person from the patient's past
E. defense mechanism

Discussion: See text for further explanation. See also Chapter 71 on individual psychoanalytic psychotherapy.

Chapter 4 •

Answers 1, C; 2, C; 3, D; 4, B; 5, A

CHAPTER

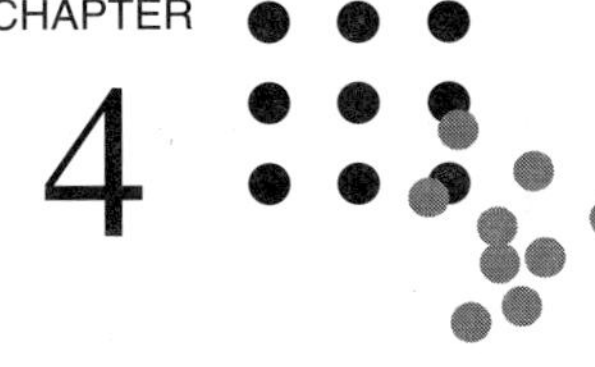

4 Professional Ethics and Boundaries of the Clinical Relationship

Richard S. Epstein

1. The essential features of all health care professions include all of the following characteristics **except**

A. adherence to a canon of ethics
B. specialized training
C. commitment to cost containment on behalf of third-party payers
D. technical expertise

Discussion: The modern concept of a professional is that such a person is assumed to be a learned person who has acquired special knowledge, adds to the welfare of the community, and abides by a code of ethics. The last commitment must take precedence over monetary compensation.

Page 50 •

Answer C

2. A comprehensive review of the literature on psychotherapy outcome shows the following factors to be present in all successful treatment methods **except**

A. The therapist employs a psychodynamic approach.
B. The therapist establishes an emotionally arousing, trusting, and confidential relationship.
C. The therapist gives a plausible explanation for the patient's problems along with a coherent treatment method for solving them.
D. Both therapist and patient work together in a collaborative endeavor they believe will be effective.

Discussion: Frank and Frank conducted an extensive review of the literature concerning psychotherapy outcome. Treatment efficacy, regardless of modality, depended on the ability of the therapist to form a structured, mutually trusting, confidential, and emotionally arousing relationship.

Page 52, Table 4–4 •

Answer A

3. The ethical principles of beneficence, nonmalfeasance, and confidentiality include all of the following behaviors **except**

A. dedicating one's efforts primarily for the patient's well-being
B. refraining from recommending treatment to the patient that his or her insurance company believes is too costly
C. avoiding any action that would be unnecessarily harmful to a patient
D. considering a patient's communication a sacred trust that must not be divulged without proper legal authorization

Discussion: The six core principles of modern medical ethics include beneficence, nonmalfeasance, confidentiality, autonomy, justice, and veracity. The first three are included in the Hippocratic Oath. The principle of beneficence might apply when there are concerns about the financial burden of treatment on the patient but not with regard to his or her insurance company.

Pages 50–51, Table 4–1 •

Answer B

4. A coherent psychiatric treatment frame includes all of the following **except**

A. The therapist provides a reasonably stable treatment setting.
B. The therapist guarantees to resolve the patient's problems.
C. The therapist protects herself or himself from being exploited by the patient.
D. The therapist avoids burdening the patient with unnecessary personal disclosures.

Discussion: The purpose of a therapeutic frame is to protect the patient's safety and to promote recovery. It is the therapist's responsibility to construct and maintain it.

Pages 51, 53 •

Answer B

5. A coherent treatment frame is necessary for the following reasons:

A. to increase the likelihood of successful treatment
B. to promote the patient's sense of autonomy
C. to protect the patient from being victimized
D. to maintain the patient's confidentiality
E. all of the above

Discussion: The treatment frame enables the patient to maintain a feeling of trust and connectedness while learning to deal with the unrealistic nature of his or her expectations. The frame is composed of various boundary factors that include acting in a reliable way, showing respect for the patient's autonomy by explaining the risks and benefits of treatment, maintaining confidentiality, avoiding exploitation of the patient's sexual feelings, and resisting the patient's manipulative efforts.

Pages 53–54, Table 4–5 •

Answer E

6. Elements common to all boundary violations include all the following **except**

A. double-binding messages by the clinician
B. an insistence on the clinician's part that the patient maintain secrecy about their relationship's becoming more like a friendship
C. the clinician's placing the patient in a situation of reversed roles by expecting gratification from the patient, beyond the financial compensation for treatment
D. the clinician's failing to give advice to the patient's family at the family's request

Discussion: In boundary violations, there are several common themes. These include efforts on the part of the clinician to reverse roles with the patient, to intimidate the patient to maintain secrecy, to place the patient in a double bind, and to indulge professional privilege. This last often reveals that the therapist believes that he or she is entitled to have his or her way with the patient.

Pages 52–53 •

Answer D

7. The boundary issue of stability entails the following responsibilities on the practitioner's part:

A. striving for a predictable time and place for treatment
B. avoiding socializing with patients
C. beginning and ending sessions punctually
D. offering appropriate psychotropic medication
E. both A and C

Discussion: Configuring a stable and consistent treatment setting is analogous to the "holding environment" provided by parents in early childhood. Consistency, concern, and respect for the patient are all elements of a stable treatment setting.

Page 54 •

Answer E

8. Examples of potentially damaging dual-relationship behavior on the psychiatrist's part include:

A. A psychiatrist owns a flower shop three blocks from her or his office.
B. A psychiatrist treats his or her brother-in-law for depression by prescribing fluoxetine for him.
C. A psychiatrist in a remote rural area administers brief crisis intervention with her neighbor and then refers the neighbor to another psychiatrist in a town 20 miles away.
D. A psychiatrist who is seeing a patient regularly in psychotherapy agrees to testify in court to render an opinion about the cause of the patient's posttraumatic stress disorder.
E. Both B and D are correct.

Discussion: Psychiatrists should avoid treatment situations that place them in a conflict between therapeutic responsibility to patients and third parties. Examples of this include treating friends and relatives or testifying as a forensic witness for current psychotherapy patients. There are risks even to seemingly benign common practices, such as accepting a referral from a current or former patient.

Page 55 •

Answer E

9. The following clinical attitudes or behaviors tend to strengthen the treatment framework by enhancing the patient's autonomy:

A. The psychiatrist explains the risks, potential benefits, and alternative treatment options regarding the recommended treatment plan to the patient.
B. The psychiatrist gives a patient advice about nonurgent major life decisions.
C. The psychiatrist tells the patient the rationale for the treatment and fosters the patient's participation in the treatment process.
D. The psychiatrist disapproves when the patient wants to terminate treatment after being

asymptomatic for 8 months and informs her that she is making a "flight into health."
E. Both A and C are correct.

Discussion: Encouraging autonomy can be done as above and in some instances can be accomplished paradoxically by assuming responsibility for the safety of a suicidal patient. Such a maneuver models autonomy. There are numerous ways to interfere with autonomy, such as using power over patients for gratification or retaliation.

Page 55 •

Answer E

10. Maintaining treatment boundaries through the use of the principle of abstinence entails all of the following activities **except**

A. refraining from embracing or caressing patients
B. refraining from socializing with patients outside of the therapy setting
C. encouraging patients to refrain from acting on their impulses
D. engaging in romantic behavior with former patients only if one has waited a period of at least 2 years after termination of treatment with the patient

Discussion: Abstinence means that psychiatrists should discourage direct forms of pleasure such as touching or sexuality in the course of their interactions with patients. This requires not using patients for gratification and is analogous to the incest taboo in most cultures.

Pages 56–57 •

Answer D

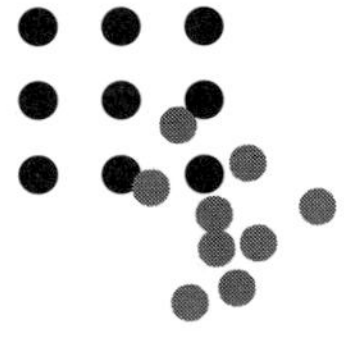

SECTION **II**

Section Editor: David A. Mrazek

A Developmental Perspective on Normal Domains of Mental and Behavioral Function

CHAPTER

5 A Psychiatric Perspective on Human Development

David A. Mrazek

1. For decades, there has been extensive study to determine the relative influences of genes and environment on human development. Which of the following statements *best* summarizes contemporary beliefs about the "nature versus nurture" debate?

A. Children's personalities are shaped by their environments in the first 5 years of life.
B. Genes determine the course, pace, and nature of human development.
C. Genetic endowment and environmental experience interact to shape the course of human development.
D. In most areas of human development, a child's genes will be expressed regardless of the nature of environmental exposure.

Discussion: Modern evidence supports the transactional model of human development, which states that genes and experiences interact to determine the outcome of development. Evidence is becoming more explicit in supporting the position that experience and the environment regulate gene expression at the molecular level.

Pages 63–64 •

Answer C

For each numbered item, select the lettered heading most closely associated with it. Each letter may be selected once, more than once, or not at all.

2. Match the following periods of life with the biological development that generally occurs during that time.

____ 1. integrative capacities peak	A. preschool
____ 2. Puberty	B. adulthood
____ 3. visual cortex reaches peak synaptic density	C. infancy
____ 4. maximal brain weight is first achieved	D. adolescence
____ 5. pattern of temperament can be identified	E. school age
____ 6. biological rhythms become established	
____ 7. growth spurt	

Discussion: See Chapter 5 text for a fuller correlation of the timing of biological development.

Pages 64–66, Figure 5–1 •

Answers 1, B; 2, D; 3, C; 4, D; 5, A; 6, C; 7, D

3. Which of the following statements about risk and protective factors is true?

A. The overall risk for developmental psychopathology increases with the number of risk factors to which the child has been exposed.
B. Resiliency in childhood is rare in disadvantaged children.
C. Most individuals are unable to handle any risk factors unless each risk is offset by a corresponding protective factor.
D. Risk and protective factors interact during the first years of life and cease to be relevant by adolescence.

Discussion: One strategy that has been used to determine a rough overall risk for developmental psychopathology is to sum the specific factors with which a child must deal to create an adversity index.

Pages 70–73, Figure 5–6 •

Answer A

4. Which of the statements about autism is true?

A. Autism provides an example of a disease that is always expressed early in life.

B. Autistic children experience difficulties, developmental delays, and communication problems from birth.
C. Environmental factors and experience have a major influence on the onset of autism.
D. Modern treatments have proved highly effective in treating autism.

Discussion: Autistic children appear normal at birth and during their first months of life but always begin to express autistic symptoms before 30 months.

Pages 72–73 •

Answer A

5. Which of the following is **not** an example of a risk factor?
A. alleles that convey a specific disadvantage
B. intense anxiety
C. poverty
D. minority status
E. nationality

Discussion: Nationality is generally not considered a risk factor.

Pages 70–72 •

Answer E

6. Which of the following statements about moral development is true?
A. By the second year of life, the emergence of embarrassment and shame in children provides evidence of the development of a moral code.
B. Adults tend to adhere to strict and absolute moral codes.
C. During the preschool years, the individual's capacity for abstract reasoning allows him or her to meet the expectations of others and to accept the maintenance of societal norms and rules.
D. Kohlberg's stages of conventional morality (stages 3, 4, 5, and 6) progress in a sequential manner through adolescence and adulthood.
E. The final stages of moral development include the acceptance of the conviction that man-made laws should supersede moral justice.

Discussion: Although the newborn lives in a world that is free of moral structure, children in the second year of life begin to experience "moral emotions." These emotions (such as embarrassment, guilt, and shame) are early evidence of a code of moral behavior. By 36 months, children demonstrate internalization of parental standards.

Pages 68–69, Figure 5–5 •

Answer A

7. Which of the following statements about social development is true?
A. Infants are socially interactive from the first days of life.
B. It is during adolescence that the role of peers in social development first becomes significant.
C. Erikson described the central objective of adulthood as the establishment of identity.
D. It is within the first weeks of life that infants develop separation protest and a negative reaction to the approach of a stranger.
E. Cultural context rarely influences the nature of social interaction until adolescence.

Discussion: In the past, it was believed that the first 2 months of life were a time of passivity and inactivity. However, infants have been shown to be socially interactive from the first days of life.

Page 68, Figure 5–4 •

Answer A

8. Which of the following statements about emotional development is true?
A. It is during the second year of life that children are first able to communicate their feelings and emotions.
B. Children generally experience the full range of adult emotions during infancy.
C. There is a dramatic increase in suicidality during adolescence.
D. The "rapprochement crisis," which occurs as the infant becomes aware of his or her separateness from the primary attachment object, generally occurs during the fifth year of life.
E. During adolescence, children begin to understand the relationship between emotion and behavior.

Discussion: The increase in suicidality that occurs during adolescence can be partly attributed to increased cognitive ability. During adolescence, there is greater reflection on the "existential crisis" that is experienced from a more complex vantage point. Adolescents also experience a greater frequency of affective disorder and anxiety.

Pages 67–68, Figure 5–3 •

Answer C

9. The preoperational stage of cognitive development is characterized by which of the following phenomena?

A. magical thinking
B. development of metacognitive capacity
C. explosive language development
D. transductive reasoning
E. answers A, C, and D

Discussion: The preoperational stage of development, which occurs by the third year of life, is characterized by magical thinking, explosive language development, and transductive reasoning. The development of metacognitive capacity occurs during adolescence (during *formal operations*) and refers to the ability to reflect on cognition as a process.

Page 66 •

Answer E

For each numbered item, select the lettered heading most closely associated with it. Each letter may be selected once, more than once, or not at all.

10. Match each of the following cognitive abilities to the stage of cognitive development during which it **first** appears.

____ 1. ability to consider the perspectives of others	A. preoperational
____ 2. ability to engage in recursive thinking	B. operational
____ 3. ability to understand reversibilities including inversion, reciprocity, and symmetry	C. formal operations
____ 4. ability to engage in logical dialogue	
____ 5. ability to attribute causality based on temporal or spatial juxtaposition	

Discussion: Piaget established the field of cognitive development, and his stage theory of evolution of cognitive processes has dominated the field. By the third year of life, children usually enter the preoperational stage of development; by age 6 or 7 years, they enter the stage of operational thinking. The stage of formal operations, which is characterized by the ability to manipulate ideas and concepts, is generally reached during adolescence but is never reached by some adults.

Page 66, Figure 5–2 •

Answers 1, B; 2, C; 3, C; 4, B; 5, A

11. Which of the following statements about Piaget's concept of decalage is true?

A. Decalage refers to an unevenness in development.
B. The concept of decalage adequately describes a disruption in the normal evolution of parallel development of specific cognitive abilities but is inadequate for explaining such problems in moral or emotional development.
C. Developmental delay can be defined as the multilineal progression of development without decalage.
D. A decalage between cognitive development and moral judgment is associated with adaptive behavior.

Discussion: Decalage refers to an unevenness of development in any area and specifically includes emotional, cognitive, and moral development.

Page 73 •

Answer A

12. Which of the following statements about the concept of "lines of development" is true?

A. Anna Freud popularized the concept of parallel and interacting lines of development.
B. Piaget's concept of decalage suggests that the basic theory supporting lines of development is flawed.
C. Curvilinear lines of development measure deviations in function.
D. It is impossible to reconcile the stage model and the longitudinal lines of development model in the study of human development.

Discussion: Anna Freud popularized the idea of parallel yet interacting lines of development. Whereas some of her original nine lines of development as described in her monograph on adolescence have since been abandoned, the underlying principles of lines of development have proved valuable.

Page 64 •

Answer A

CHAPTER

6 Infant Development: The First 3 Years of Life

Megan Hester • David Taylor

1. All of the following are true about the transactional model of development in the first 3 years of life **except**

A. Genetic and environmental regulators of an individual's behavior transact continually over time, mutually influencing one another.
B. The transactional model is able to predict particular sets of risks and protective factors.
C. The transactional model is the most widely accepted description of the developmental process.
D. The transactional model was proposed by Sameroff and Chandler.

Discussion: The transactional model of development is currently the most widely accepted description of the developmental process. However, whereas the transactional model does take both genetic and environmental factors into account, it is not able to predict a particular set of risks or protective factors.

Page 78 •

Answer B

2. In the first 2 months of life:

A. Newborns are able to preferentially distinguish between their mother's voice and another female's voice.
B. Infants are unable to communicate in understandable ways.
C. Infants are able to display a whole range of emotions including anger, distress, contentment, joy, and fear.
D. Temperament is developed in reaction to the environment only.

Discussion: In the first 2 months of life, newborns are able to distinguish between their mother's voice and the voice of another female. In fact, infants seem to prefer the pitch ranges of female voices over male voices. However, infants are able to communicate in many ways, such as through crying, quieting, cuddling, looking, and occasional vocalizations. Although able to communicate, infants in the first 2 months seem to display only two emotions—distress and contentment. Meaningful differences in temperament appear difficult to discern within the first 2 months of life. However, all major theories of temperament suggest that temperamental dispositions are rooted in biological differences.

Pages 82–84 •

Answer A

3. Between 2 and 3 months of age, infants demonstrate

A. enhanced classical conditioning
B. operant conditioning
C. habituation
D. none of the above
E. all of the above

Discussion: At 2 to 3 months of age, infants develop greatly enhanced cognitive abilities. They demonstrate classical conditioning, operant conditioning, and habituation at this time.

Page 85 •

Answer E

4. All of the following are true about the 7- to 9-month transition **except**

A. A new rise in glucose metabolism in the frontal lobes occurs at the time of the 7- to 9-month transition.
B. Infants demonstrate object permanence.
C. Infants are able to "pretend play."
D. Emotions begin to be used instrumentally for the first time.
E. Infants begin to behave not only as if they understand others but also as if they anticipate that others will understand them.

Discussion: During this period of 7 to 9 months, major developmental transitions occur. It has been one of the best studied transitions and has been termed the "onset of focused attachment" or the "discovery of intersubjectivity." Fischer and Rose have suggested that changes that occur biologically may account for developmental changes during this period. Accordingly, there is a new rise in glucose metabolism in the frontal lobes as well as changes in the electroencephalogram's frequency and coherence, which suggest more sophisticated coordination of pathways. Also, during this transition, infants demonstrate object permanence, and emotions are used to "get what they want." In addition, infants begin to behave as if they understand others and anticipate that others will understand them. However, infants are not truly able to pretend play until after the 18- to 20-month transition.

Pages 86–88 •

Answer C

5. *Symbolic representation* refers to

A. the qualitative change that underlies the child's remarkable advances in language, cognition, affect, and social functioning
B. a variety of changes in behavior that seem to indicate that infants now understand that their own inner experience—their thoughts, feelings, and desires—can be appreciated by and shared with others
C. the emergence of behaviors that reflect an innate motivational system in human infants
D. the infant's use of cues from others to resolve affective uncertainty

Discussion: Symbolic representation refers to the qualitative change that underlies the child's remarkable advances in language, cognition, affect, and social functioning. Symbolic representation, unlike the other answers, occurs in the 18- to 20-month transition. Answer B refers to intersubjectivity, which occurs in the 7- to 9-month transition. Answer C refers to mastery motivation, which also occurs in the 7- to 9-month transition. Social referencing is what answer D refers to, and this occurs in the 7- to 9-month transition as well.

Page 88 •

Answer A

6. In the transition from 18 to 20 months, children are in which one of the following stages defined by Piaget?

A. operational
B. preoperational
C. concrete
D. sensorimotor
E. formal operations

Discussion: In the 18- to 20-month transition, children move into Piaget's preoperational stage. Judgments that children make are limited to their perceptions of objects and events, and difficulty occurs when they try to attend to more than one perceptual attribute at a time. Egocentrism is also a part of the preoperational stage, and toddlers may have trouble differentiating between subjective experiences and objective reality. In addition, Piaget noted that toddlers use transductive reasoning.

Page 89 •

Answer B

7. Kagan and colleagues have suggested in regard to temperament identified after the 18- to 20-month transition:

A. Behavioral inhibition to the unfamiliar characterizes about 10% of middle-class African-American 2-year-olds.
B. Infants of adults with panic disorder exhibit a high frequency of behavioral inhibition.
C. Behavioral inhibition is a heritable trait, mediated through the central and peripheral nervous systems.
D. Answers A and B
E. Answers B and C

Discussion: Kagan and colleagues have suggested that behavioral inhibition is a measurable and reliably identifiable trait that is inherited. Supporting this assertion, they demonstrated the stability of the trait in a 4-year period and found the trait to be associated with physiological activation of the hypothalamic-pituitary-adrenal axis, the reticular activating system, and the sympathetic arm of the central nervous system. Infants of adults with panic disorder exhibit a high frequency of behavioral inhibition. Kagan and colleagues have suggested that behavioral inhibition to the unfamiliar characterizes 10% of middle-class white 2-year-olds and is counterbalanced by a roughly equal number of children deemed uninhibited.

Page 89 •

Answer E

CHAPTER

7 Preschool Development

Robert B. Clyman

1. Modern theories of development indicate:

A. Difficulties in one domain of early development essentially guarantee subsequent problems in that domain later in life.
B. In general, development proceeds at the same rate in all domains of development.
C. Parents who assist their children to acquire the next level of developmental skills are working in the so-called zone of proximal development.
D. Erik Erikson suggested that a principal development issue for preschoolers is the development of autonomy.
E. Transactional developmental models emphasize that parents and children each influence the other, ensuring continuities in the child's developmental course.

Discussion: The concept of a zone of proximal development was put forward by Vygotsky. Difficulties in one domain of early development do not guarantee subsequent problems in that domain later in life. There are often different rates of development in different domains, such as emotional or language development. The principal eriksonian task for preschoolers is initiative versus guilt. Transactional models do specify that parents and children each influence the other, but these processes yield both continuities and discontinuities in development.

Pages 101–102 •

Answer C

2. Which of the following is true about biological-neurological development in the preschool period?

A. The difference between siblings is due to their different genetic inheritances.
B. Behavioral genetics studies often offer good evidence of environmental influence on the development of a psychiatric disorder.
C. Most cortical neurons have not formed until the end of gestation.
D. Substantial cortical migration occurs during infancy.
E. Infants' brains weigh 90% of adults' brains.

Discussion: The difference between siblings is often explained by the effects of the "non-shared environment," by which parents influence their children differently. Behavioral genetics studies often offer the best evidence of environmental influence on the development of a psychiatric disorder by estimating the proportion of variance explainable by the contribution of the genes. Most cortical neurons have formed and migrated by 18 weeks of gestation. Infants' brains weigh approximately one third of adults' brains.

Pages 102–104, Figure 7–1 •

Answer B

3. Which of the following additional statements is true about biological-neurological development in the preschool period?

A. The pruning of synapses in the frontal cortex begins in infancy.
B. Preschoolers cannot recover any language function after damage to their dominant hemisphere.
C. Autism is a disorder predominantly caused by the influence of the psychosocial environment.
D. Mapping the human genome will contribute to gene therapy for psychiatric disorders but will not contribute to the development of psychosocial interventions to prevent psychiatric disorders.
E. Neural networks that are activated are more likely to survive the pruning of synapses.

Discussion: Neural networks that are activated by experience are more likely to survive the pruning of synapses. The pruning of synapses in the frontal cortex begins by age 7 years. Preschoolers can recover some language function after damage to their dominant hemisphere. Twin data indicate a principal role for genes in the etiology of autism. Mapping the human genome will contribute to gene therapy for psychiatric disorders and to the development of psychosocial interventions to prevent psychiatric disorders by enabling us to identify children at risk for disorders that also require environmental influences for the disorder to develop.

Pages 102–104 •

Answer E

4. Which of the following statements about cognitive development is true?

A. The end of the preoperational stage is marked by the development of recall.
B. Animism is a characteristic of the preoperational stage.
C. The preoperational stage is characterized by conservation.
D. Preschool children demonstrate egocentrism with both emotional and spacial tasks.
E. Children's performance on piagetian tasks does not change when more familiar task materials are used.

Discussion: Animism is a characteristic of the preoperational stage. The onset, not the end, of the preoperational stage is marked by the development of recall. Acquisition of conservation marks the beginning of the operational stage. Preschool children demonstrate egocentrism with spatial tasks but can show empathy by 18 to 24 months, indicating some absence of emotional egocentrism. Children's performance on piagetian tasks is sensitive to a range of variables, and in general, children perform at a higher level when more familiar task materials are used.

Pages 104–106, Figure 7–3 •

Answer B

5. Language development is characterized by which of the following?

A. Children learn correct grammar primarily by having adults point out their errors and correcting them.
B. The two-word phase typically begins by the third year of life.
C. Psychiatrists should be concerned about a relationship disturbance if young toddlers use "mommy" to refer in general to women.
D. Although mothers talk an equal amount to girls and boys, girls are more advanced in their language development in this period.
E. Children learn that questions can be indirect commands (e.g., Is that door shut?) by the end of the preschool period.

Discussion: Children learn correct grammar primarily by listening to adults use language, not by being corrected. The two-word phase typically begins by the third year of life. Toddlers often overgeneralize the use of words, referring to an overinclusive set of referents until they understand exactly what the word refers to. Mothers talk more to girls than to boys, and girls are more advanced in their language development in this period. Children learn that questions can be indirect commands (e.g., Is that door shut?) as early as 2 years of age.

Pages 106–107 •

Answer B

6. Which of the following statements about emotional and social cognitive development is **not true?**

A. Emotions can have a beneficial, adaptive effect on children's behavior.
B. Social referencing refers to the use of another person's emotional signals to determine a course of action.
C. Toddlers can discriminate facial expressions of emotion.
D. Children can typically evaluate others' goals and beliefs beginning in the second grade.
E. Emotional and cognitive development interact during preschool development.

Discussion: By 4 to 5 years of age, children can evaluate others' goals and beliefs.

Page 107, Figure 7–4 •

Answer D

7. Which of the following is a true statement about emotional development?

A. Peers and siblings play an increasingly important role in the development of emotion language as the preschool period progresses.
B. The presence of object constancy protects the young child from the development of avoidant personality disorder later in life.
C. Internal working models are thought to develop from the infant's early fantasies about the attachment relationship with his or her caregivers.
D. Object constancy refers to the continuous presence of one caregiver in the young child's life.
E. The Oedipus complex refers to thoughts, feelings, and fantasies about one's parents that are derived from the child's experiences within the family.

Discussion: Inadequate development of object constancy is hypothesized to be linked to the development of borderline personality disorder later in life. Internal working models are thought to develop from the infant's attachment relationship with his or her caregivers, not from his or her fantasies about the relationship. Object constancy refers to the capacity to calm yourself, self-soothe, and modulate anxiety in response to separation from the primary caregiver. The Oedipus complex refers to thoughts, feelings, and fantasies about one's parents. There is only a limited relationship between actual experiences and one's oedipal fantasies, according to psychoanalytic theory.

Page 108 •

Answer A

8. Which one of the following statements about sociocultural influences on preschoolers' development is true?

A. Offering toddlers simple choices, such as choosing the shirt they wish to wear, typically overwhelms them, impairing their later ability to make choices.
B. Research indicates that permissive parents have children who are loving and regulate their frustration well.
C. Children who show sibling rivalry are rarely cooperative in their play with them.
D. Gender differences in children's play become evident by the end of the preschool years.
E. Gender segregation is evident in all cultures.

Discussion: Offering toddlers simple choices, such as choosing the shirt they wish to wear, adaptively supports their later ability to make choices. Research indicates that permissive parents have children who do not regulate their frustration well but rather have behavior problems. Children who show sibling rivalry are often also cooperative in their play with their siblings. Gender differences in children's play become evident by age 2 years. Gender segregation, in which children prefer to play with same-sex partners, is evident in all cultures that have been studied.

Pages 108–110 •

Answer E

9. The following are correct statements about moral development in the preschool period **except**

A. Parental modeling and instruction influence children's moral development.
B. Children normatively develop empathy by the end of the second year of life.
C. Children's capacity for empathy shows heritability.
D. Toddlers show anxiety when viewing flawed objects, suggesting the development of internalized standards.
E. Children act in accordance with parental rules only by struggling with the conflict between their own and their parents' wishes.

Discussion: Children act in accordance with parental rules both with and without a sense of conflict. For example, they will feel pride on meeting a parental standard.

Pages 110–112 •

Answer E

10. Which of the following statements about moral development in the preschool period is true?

A. Moral emotions include fear, shame, and guilt.
B. Moral emotions involve characteristic facial expressions of emotion.
C. All moral emotions involve an internalized voice, which reminds the child that she or he is transgressing against a rule.
D. Moral emotions develop out of shared experiences with important others.
E. Preschoolers will follow parental rules only when their caregivers are present.

Discussion: Moral emotions include shame, pride, and guilt, but fear is a darwinian or "basic" emotion. Moral emotions do not involve characteristic facial expressions of emotion. Whereas guilt appears to evoke an internalized voice articulating a moral rule, shame evokes a sense of a disapproving look at oneself. They do develop out of shared experiences with important others. Although toddlers often observe parental rules only when their caregivers are present, preschoolers have increasingly internalized rules and act in concert with them in the absence of caregivers.

Page 111 •

Answer D

CHAPTER

8 School-Age Development

Theodore Shapiro

1. The period of the school-age child was called latency by Freud because a hiatus was seen in

A. cognitive development
B. psychosexual instinctual forces
C. polymorphous perverse activity
D. object relations

Discussion: Different observers, with different theoretical constructs, have described this period, and the labels applied reflect a particular theoretical view. Latency suggests that early infantile sexuality was repressed and remained latent until puberty. The term middle childhood advocated by Chess and Thomas has the advantage of being atheoretical.

Page 116 •

Answer B

2. The concept of the difficult child in latency derives from which of the following frames of reference?

A. dimensional psychopathology
B. DSM-IV
C. temperamental studies
D. developmental psychopathology

Discussion: Longitudinal studies of development have characterized patterns of behavioral difficulties in middle childhood. Chess and Thomas described difficult children who express early behaviors that predict later school problems, social difficulties, and psychiatric disorders. Temperamentally, such children showed slower adaptability to new situations and intense negative reactions to stimuli.

Pages 117–118, 120 •

Answer C

3. When 3-year-olds were tracked into middle childhood, those who showed the most pathology

A. had enuresis
B. were polysymptomatic
C. had speech disorders
D. showed separation anxiety

Discussion: Polysymptomatic 3-year-olds were found to show persistent trouble when they were followed up at 7 and 9 years old. Kagan has shown that early behavioral and emotional inhibition often evolves in middle childhood as anxiety disorders that match parental anxiety.

Pages 117–118, 119–120 •

Answer B

4. Age 7 years is most significant to any study of middle childhood because

A. cognitive structures emerge
B. the Oedipus complex has passed
C. superego is now operative
D. biological and psychological studies suggest discontinuity

Discussion: This period is characterized by its discontinuity from early childhood. This is a period of new capacities and new opportunities to learn. Across cultures, there are new social roles, and biologically there are discontinuities in development.

Pages 116, 118 •

Answer D

5. Erikson calls middle childhood the age of industry because

A. children were apprenticed at that age
B. cross-cultural studies show entry into work tasks
C. children become devoted to tasks and learning
D. play is diminished

Discussion: Erikson provided ego dimensions to Freud's developmental model. He noted that children at this age tend to become persistent and task oriented. Historically, this was considered the age of reason, and children were considered capable of swearing oaths and being apprenticed to a trade.

Pages 116–117 •

Answer C

6. Among neurodevelopmental facts that recommend the idea of discontinuity during latency are

A. changes in level of norepinephrine
B. shift in focus from limbic to cerebral dominance
C. onset of dendritic pruning
D. increases in γ-aminobutyric acid metabolism

Discussion: Children of this age have achieved a distinct set of neurological milestones. These include visual-motor and intersensory integration, increased cortical thickness, and accelerated change in pyramidal cell shape and size. Hippocampal maturity is related to the emergence of declarative memory. There is decreased brain plasticity, and dendritic pruning begins in succeeding years.

Page 118, Figure 8–2 •

Answer C

7. Prepubertal depression during latency is characterized by

A. recurrent course
B. transient disability
C. masked depression
D. conduct disorder

Discussion: Whereas epidemiological studies show that depression is not highly prevalent in middle childhood, it is now clear that major depressive disorders do occur, with a rising rate of emotional disorders in early adolescence and a steep continuing rise of incidence into late adolescence. Moreover, prepubertal depression is followed by recurring depression within 7 years in 80% of those afflicted.

Page 120 •

Answer A

8. The social matrix of latency adds to all the following behaviors **except**

A. exclusive clubs
B. close attention to fairness
C. chumships between sexes
D. diligence in tasks

Discussion: Children of this age make clubs, mimicking parental social groups. Many behaviors of middle childhood can be construed as new aspects of the socialization process that is fostered by schooling, community involvement, and the move away from the family. The unisex friendships of this period lead to a number of avoidant practices that emerge in groups.

Pages 120–122 •

Answer C

9. Piagetian cognitive psychology indicates that middle childhood is marked by new abilities to

A. decenter spatially
B. count with one-to-one correspondence
C. formulate sentences of greater than seven words
D. reason from abstract to particular

Discussion: The transition to an operational intelligence represents a major development in children of this age. Children are no longer egocentric and can literally and figuratively imagine another's perspective. They are also able to appreciate conservation of volume and number.

Page 119 •

Answer A

10. Moral judgments are thought to be possible during latency for all the following proposed reasons **except**

A. Superego is formed as a legacy of the passing Oedipus complex.
B. Children can now see another's point of view.
C. The age of reason permits moral judgment.
D. Children of this age can decenter.

Discussion: The preconventional stage of moral development has an emphasis on avoiding punishments and getting rewards. According to Kohlberg, the successive conventional and postconventional stages emphasize social conformity and moral principles, respectively. Clearly emotional and cognitive lines of development influence the moral capacities of school-age children.

Pages 121–122, Table 8–1, Figure 8–5 •

Answer C

CHAPTER

9 Adolescent Development

John E. Schowalter • Kenneth Towbin

1. Puberty is a developmental phase rooted in

A. sociology
B. religion
C. psychology
D. biology

Discussion: Although the phase of adolescence has broad biopsychosocial roots, puberty is defined biologically.

Page 127 •

Answer D

2. Adolescence as defined today was influenced most by the

A. Vietnam war
B. automobile
C. industrial revolution
D. Magna Carta

Discussion: After the industrial revolution, teenagers most often needed to learn skills to join the adult workplace. Machines also reduced the size of the work force needed.

Page 128 •

Answer C

3. An ego defense mechanism that typically begins during adolescence is

A. denial
B. intellectualization
C. repression
D. suppression

Discussion: With the attainment of more education and some formal operational thought, it is possible for adolescents to use intellectualization. The other defense mechanisms are already used commonly in earlier childhood.

Page 128 •

Answer B

4. Adolescents are typically viewed by society as relatively mature during times of

A. high unemployment
B. industrialization
C. war
D. job specialization

Discussion: Society views adolescents as most mature when they are needed to fight, but not when they are an economic danger to take scarce adult jobs.

Page 138 •

Answer C

5. Violence is the major cause of death for adolescents. The highest death rate is from

A. African-American male homicides
B. African-American male suicides
C. Anglo male homicides
D. Anglo male suicides

Discussion: Homicides account for more than half of African-American males' deaths between ages 15 and 24 years.

Page 139 •

Answer A

6. Which statement best describes the relationship between puberty and adolescence?

A. Puberty and adolescence are related to one another through the capability to marry.
B. Puberty defines the social criteria society uses for adolescence.
C. Puberty and adolescence are entirely separate designations for biological and social conditions, respectively.
D. Puberty determines when society begins to deem one an adolescent.
E. All adolescents have reached puberty.

Discussion: Adolescence is a term connoting a biopsychosocial stage of development. Adolescence is related to but not identical with puberty. Biological changes define puberty. Puberty originates from the Latin *puber,* which refers to "being of marriageable age." The biological changes are the most rapid and striking of the physical changes the body experiences after infancy.

Page 130 •

Answer C

7. Which of the following statements about puberty is **not true?**

A. On average, girls begin puberty about 2 years before boys.
B. Initiation and sustaining of the adolescent growth spurt depend on both circulating growth hormone and gonadotropin levels.
C. Staging male sexual development relies on penile length, testicular size, and pubic hair growth.
D. In girls, puberty usually begins with breast development, but first appearance of pubic hair is not pathological.
E. In boys, the appearance of facial hair is closely linked to pubic hair growth.

Discussion: Male axillary and facial hair growth is affected by testosterone and is not tightly linked to the appearance of other sexual features. In nearly all boys, the onset of puberty begins with testicular enlargement. In girls, puberty usually commences with breast development, although the onset of pubic hair growth may be noted first in about 15% of girls.

Pages 130–134 •

Answer E

8. Which statement about adolescent cognitive development is **not true?**

A. In comparison to school-age children, adolescents are far better able to manipulate ideas that are separate from their subjective experience.
B. Adolescence is when metacognitive functions first begin to emerge.
C. Recursive thinking, which develops during adolescence, refers to the ability to think about another person's thoughts about oneself.
D. Studies of cognitive development propose that adolescents are not more accomplished in making logical inferences but that they possess more knowledge and experience to guide them in making conclusions.
E. Adolescents possess superior skills in transfer processing, which means they can place new ideas and information into the context of knowledge that has already been mastered.

Discussion: Metacognition refers to "any knowledge or cognitive activity that takes as its objects or regulates any aspect of any cognitive enterprise." It is also characterized as executive control or process. The ability to think about thinking means that the adolescent can consider his or her own thinking styles, aptitudes, and limitations. Some elements of metacognition begin to appear in childhood and are relatively well established in the latter part of childhood.

Pages 134–136 •

Answer B

9. Which of these statements is **not true** of the modern revision in our understanding of adolescent social development?

A. Peer relationships are equally important in both the older view and the more modern empirical view of social development.
B. Seeking the counsel of and maintaining warm emotional ties to one's parents is highly characteristic of well-adjusted, normal adolescents.
C. The incidence of sexual abuse declines as children reach adolescence.
D. A problem with the previous concepts of adolescent turmoil is that they were derived from subjects who were ascertained from clinical populations.
E. Early sexual activity, alcohol and drug use, early pregnancy, and sexually transmitted diseases are all highly intercorrelated.

Discussion: The overall incidence of family abuse and neglect is if anything higher for adolescents than it is for younger children. It is common for parental abuse or neglect to push adolescents into associations with bad peer influences.

Pages 138–141 •

Answer C

10. Which of these statements regarding adolescent risk and protective factors is **not true?**

A. In childhood, biological factors figure prominently; but in adolescence, interpersonal factors assume a progressively prominent role as risk factors.
B. Genetic endowment is a major risk or protective factor, but family and community living circumstances may be as highly influential.
C. The relationship between personality factors and community responses may create a feedback loop that promotes healthy or maladaptive behaviors.

D. The Kauai study suggested that actual jeopardy may be less influential than whether one has the feeling of being in charge of his or her life.
E. Relative to risk factors, there appears to be no particular advantages associated with being male or female.

Discussion: The potency of any particular stressor appears to vary with age and sex. Boys appear more vulnerable to both physical and psychosocial stressors from the prenatal period to about age 10 years; girls grow more vulnerable to stressors during their teens. In terms of protective factors, there are suggestions that sex factors may be relevant to resiliency. Females appear to posesss a wider range of coping skills than do males, particularly in forming relationships.

Pages 141–142 •

Answer E

11. Lower rates of condom use by teenage males is associated with

A. less education
B. minority status
C. drug use
D. poverty
E. all of the above

Discussion: Factors that have a negative impact on educational attainment or increase impulsivity are associated with a decrease in condom use.

Page 139 •

Answer E

12. The authoritative style of parental discipline is characterized by all of the following **except**

A. consistency
B. firmness
C. warmth
D. punitiveness

Discussion: Baumrind classified three types of parental discipline: permissiveness, authoritarian, and authoritative. The authoritative approach is most linked to a gain of social attributes.

Page 139 •

Answer D

13. Compared with later adolescent groups, early adolescent peer groups are typically

A. larger
B. loosely structured
C. broad in scope
D. same-gender

Discussion: Early adolescent groups tend to be smaller, narrow in focus, demanding of conformity, and of the same gender.

Pages 139–140 •

Answer D

CHAPTER

10 Adult Development

William R. Beardslee • George Vaillant

1. The single most difficult issue in studying development over time in adults is:

A. Development occurs only during certain periods in adulthood.
B. Development in adulthood occurs during a much longer time interval than in childhood.
C. Development does not occur in adulthood.

Discussion: A series of factors document that the study of development is difficult. The most central one, from the point of view of either the subjects or the researchers, is that individuals must be observed for a long time for important questions to be answered.

Page 145 •

Answer B

2. Central nervous system development occurs

A. only up until age 20 years
B. only up until age 30 years
C. only up until age 50 years, but some functions may decline after about age 20 years

Discussion: Complex associational skills may improve over time in adults; some simpler brain functions, such as sensation or reaction time, may decline.

Pages 146–147, Figure 10–1 •

Answer C

3. Which is correct about patterns of substance abuse or depression during the life span?

A. There is no pattern to the occurrence of either substance abuse or depression during the life span.
B. There is a definite pattern to the occurrence of either substance abuse or depression during the life span.
C. There is a definite pattern to the occurrence of depression only.

Discussion: It is evident that there are clear patterns in drug use across the life span. Most stimulant drug use occurs before age 20 years, and the use of sedative drugs increases after age 45 years. There are also developmental patterns in depression.

Pages 147–148 •

Answer B

4. There is empirical support for which developmental model of adulthood?

A. Erikson's stage sequential model of adult development
B. Kohlberg's sequences of moral development
C. neither A nor B
D. both A and B

Discussion: Empirical justification for the Erikson model has been found in three major longitudinal studies including the Grant Foundation study of Harvard men, the core city study of the men in Boston enrolled in the early 1930s, and the Terman study of women in northern California. Individuals reached different stages at different ages in a manner that was relatively independent of social class and education.

Pages 150–153 •

Answer D

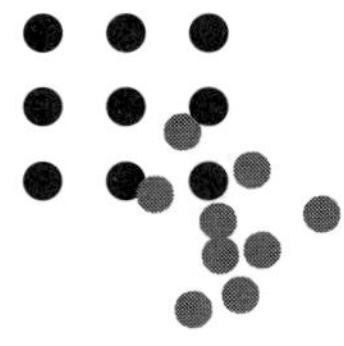

SECTION III

Section Editor: Charles B. Nemeroff

Scientific Foundations of Psychiatry

CHAPTER

11 Introduction

Charles B. Nemeroff

There are no questions for this chapter.

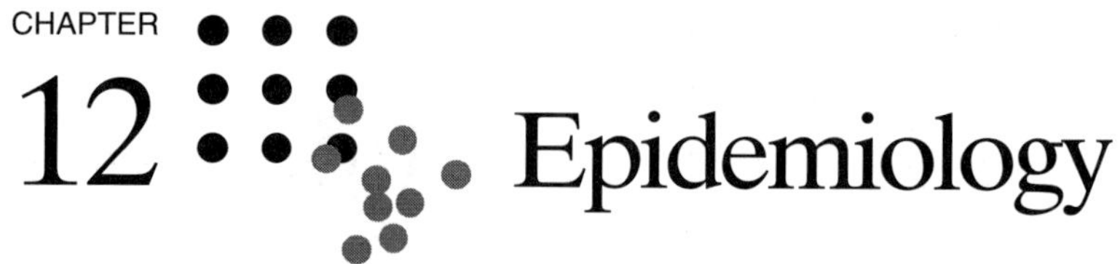

CHAPTER 12 Epidemiology

Mauricio Tohen • Evelyn Bromet

1. Which of the following is **not** a structured diagnostic interview?

A. Schedule for Affective Disorders and Schizophrenia
B. Diagnostic Interview for Genetic Studies
C. Global Assessment of Functioning Scale
D. Present State Examination
E. Diagnostic Interview Schedule

Discussion: Structured diagnostic interviews are used to systematically elicit criteria for objectively defined disorders. The Global Assessment of Functioning Scale measures degrees of impairment in ill individuals.

Pages 161–162 •

Answer C

2. A cumulative incidence rate

A. is an ideal measure for dynamic cohort studies
B. is an ideal measure for fixed cohort studies
C. uses person-time in the denominator
D. may include prevalent cases in the numerator
E. is the best measure for causation studies

Discussion: The cumulative incidence rate, or the incidence proportion rate, is the proportion of a population at risk that has a disease in a set period of time. Fixed cohorts (i.e., those in which no cases are lost in the period of time) are better suited for cumulative incidence rate measures than are dynamic cohorts, in which there is attrition. Prevalent cases are not included.

Page 163 •

Answer B

3. A confounding factor is

A. associated with exposure
B. associated with outcome
C. a source of bias
D. all of the above
E. none of the above

Discussion: Confounding bias is one of several threats to the validity of epidemiological studies. Others include selection bias and information bias. A confounding factor is an independent cause of a disease under investigation that is also associated with the pertinent exposure variable.

Page 167 •

Answer D

4. The following are examples of second-generation studies:

A. the Stirling County study
B. the Epidemiologic Catchment Area study
C. the National Comorbidity Survey
D. the McLean First-Episode Psychosis study
E. the Genetic Linkage study

Discussion: The Stirling County (Nova Scotia) study as well as the Midtown Manhattan study and the University of Michigan's National Study of Mental Health were all done in the 1950s and used symptom questionnaires, direct interviews, and supplemental data. These were an improvement on earlier surveys of the insane.

Page 168 •

Answer A

5. The Epidemiologic Catchment Area study (ECA)

A. included New York City
B. provided prevalence data for all DSM-III diagnoses
C. provided prevalence data for antisocial personality disorder
D. included communities in North America and Western Europe
E. used the Schedule for Affective Disorders and Schizophrenia as its diagnostic interview schedule

Discussion: The ECA study was conducted in the United States in the cities of New Haven (CT), Baltimore (MD), Raleigh-Durham (NC), St. Louis (MO), and Los Angeles (CA). The Diagnostic Interview Schedule was the instrument used.

Pages 169–173, Tables 12–3, 12–5, Figure 12–2 •

Answer C

6. The Epidemiologic Catchment Area study identified the following lifetime prevalence rates:

A. 1.5% for schizophrenia
B. 15% for major depression
C. 12.5% for phobia
D. 2% for dysthymia
E. A and C are correct

Discussion: The rates for major depression and dysthymia are 5.8% and 3.3%, respectively.

Pages 169–170, Table 12–3 •

Answer E

7. The National Comorbidity Survey

A. was conducted by investigators from the University of Michigan
B. used the Composite International Diagnostic Interview
C. was conducted after the Epidemiologic Catchment Area study
D. identified bipolar disorder as the Axis I disorder with the highest comorbid substance use disorders
E. all of the above

Discussion: See text for a full discussion.

Pages 173–174 •

Answer E

8. Prospective cohort studies

A. are a type of longitudinal study
B. classify individuals as exposed and non-exposed.
C. have feasibility as the main drawback
D. are less likely to suffer from bias
E. all of the above

Discussion: In prospective cohort studies, subjects are identified in terms of exposure or nonexposure status and observed for a period of time to determine the presence or absence of a health outcome. Examples of cohorts are birth cohorts, soldiers in battle, or university students (e.g., George Vaillant's study of Harvard students). These studies are expensive and difficult to conduct.

Page 166 •

Answer E

9. Case-control studies

A. are restrospective studies
B. may have recall bias
C. define control subjects as those individuals who would be classified as cases if they come up with a disease of interest
D. are ideal for rare diseases
E. all of the above

Discussion: Subjects are defined in terms of either having or not having a disease. Whereas health records can be used to verify the history of cases, control subjects may suffer from recall bias. These studies, which are simpler to do than prospective ones, are ideal for rare diseases such as anorexia nervosa.

Pages 165–166 •

Answer E

10. The following is an example of selection bias:

A. healthy worker effect
B. association to the exposure and the outcome
C. loss to fôllow-up
D. recall bias
E. control by blindness

Discussion: Selection bias occurs when the sampling procedure is influenced a priori by the disease or exposure. For instance, studies of employed populations are limited by the healthy worker effect because disabled or affected individuals may not be in the cohort. Other examples are of self-selection bias among people volunteering to participate in a study. Blinding is an attempt to control for information bias. Confounding bias is discussed in the answer to question 3.

Pages 166–167 •

Answer A

CHAPTER

13 Genetics

Janet L. Sobell • Steve S. Sommer

1. The majority of common human diseases are the result of

A. single-gene mendelian inheritance
B. mitochondrial transmission
C. autosomal recessive transmission
D. multifactorial causes

Discussion: There are several thousand single-gene disorders, some of which are autosomal recessive, yet overall they affect approximately 125 per 10,000 live births. Mitochondrial genes are a rare cause of disease. Most diseases are caused by the action of several genes and environmental factors.

Pages 182–186 •

Answer D

2. Which is an example of a molecular genetic research strategy?

A. linkage analysis
B. marker-based association studies
C. candidate gene–based association studies
D. all of the above

Discussion: These studies, which all examine the molecular DNA genotype, are distinct from pedigree, family, twin, and adoption studies. These other studies also look for patterns of transmission of illness.

Pages 186–190, Figure 13–4 •

Answer D

3. A centimorgan is

A. the midpoint of a human chromosome
B. the number of base pairs in a gene
C. a unit of measure of recombination frequency
D. the amount of DNA needed for analysis

Discussion: One centimorgan (cM) is equal to a 1% chance that a marker at one genetic locus will be separated from a marker at a second locus because of crossing over in a single generation; 1 cM is about 1 million base pairs.

Pages 189, 201 •

Answer C

4. Genetic association studies

A. are similar to epidemiological case-control studies
B. do not require related individuals
C. consider genotype to be a risk factor
D. can include linkage disequilibrium studies
E. all of the above

Discussion: The chapter text characterizes this and other types of genetic studies.

Pages 193, 200 •

Answer E

5. Anticipation

A. can be assessed only by careful clinical evaluation of affected individuals in multiple generations
B. involves trinucleotide repeat expansion
C. is observed in psychiatric disease
D. has not been observed in psychiatric disease
E. A, B, and C are correct

Discussion: Anticipation is observed when a disease has increasingly severe phenotype or earlier age at onset in successive generations. However, in psychiatric disorders, it is often difficult to distinguish true anticipation from ascertainment bias. The phenomenon of anticipation is due to expansion of trinucleotide repeat DNA sequences in unstable alleles. Once a threshold level of expansion is reached, the disease phenotype occurs. The unstable expanded allele is likely to expand further in a subsequent meiosis, producing more severe disease by more fully disrupting gene function. Some evidence for anticipation has been reported in bipolar disorder and schizophrenia.

Pages 189–190 •

Answer E

6. Linkage analysis in psychiatric disease is a problem because

A. these are multifactorial diseases in which a major single gene may not be operating
B. boundaries of clinical illness vary
C. penetrance of susceptible genotypes is incomplete
D. biases are due to decreased reproduction by ill individuals
E. all of the above

Discussion: Other problems include assortative mating and difficulty in finding families with multiple affected individuals.

Pages 192–193, 201 •

Answer E

7. Which of the following statements are true?

A. One disease phenotype may have a variety of underlying single-gene causes.
B. Different mutations in the same gene may result in varied phenotypes.
C. The known trinucleotide repeat expansions that cause disease are located in protein coding sequences.
D. Answers A and B
E. Answers A and C

Discussion: Trinucleotide repeat expansions in the 5′ untranslated region of the *FMR1* gene and in the 3′ untranslated region of the myotonin protein kinase gene are responsible for fragile X and myotonic dystrophy, respectively.

Page 186, Table 13–3; Pages 189–190, Table 13–6 •

Answer D

8. Candidate gene association studies may be useful in examining genetic predisposition to multifactorial diseases. To succeed, these studies must match case patients and control subjects for

A. age
B. gender
C. ethnicity
D. all of the above

Discussion: If autosomal genes or gene regions are being analyzed and if the phenotype of interest is not related to age or gender, then only matching by ethnicity is essential to avoid spurious results. The use of parental controls (i.e., transmitted versus untransmitted alleles) is the best control for ethnicity.

Pages 193–195 •

Answer C

CHAPTER

14 Molecular and Neurobiological Mechanisms in the Treatment of Psychiatric Disorders

Michael J. Owens • Jeff J. Mulchahey • Steven C. Stout • Paul M. Plotsky

1. The following class of drug produces no effect on neurons in the absence of γ-aminobutyric acid (GABA), increases GABA-mediated chloride ion influx, and reduces the physiological and behavioral effects of diazepam:

A. barbiturate
B. benzodiazepine receptor antagonist
C. $GABA_A$ receptor antagonist
D. partial benzodiazepine receptor–positive allosteric modulator
E. partial benzodiazepine receptor–negative allosteric modulator

Discussion: Barbiturates at certain concentrations can increase chloride currents in the absence of GABA and potentiate the effects of diazepam. A benzodiazepine receptor antagonist such as flumazenil would produce no effect on GABA-mediated chloride ion influx. A $GABA_A$ receptor antagonist such as bicuculline would decrease GABA-mediated chloride influx. A full or partial benzodiazepine receptor–negative allosteric modulator (also called inverse agonist) would also decrease GABA-mediated chloride influx but by reducing the affinity of the GABA-binding site rather than by competing with GABA as bicuculline does.

Pages 238–241, Figures 14–13, 14–14, Table 14–11 •

Answer D

2. The following is a leading hypothesis for the antimanic mechanism of action of valproate but not of lithium or carbamazepine:

A. inhibition of phosphoinositide metabolism
B. increased levels of GABA by decreased enzymatic breakdown or increased synthesis
C. increased density of $GABA_B$ receptors
D. decreased membrane excitability by direct effect on voltage-gated ion channels
E. blockade of D_2 dopamine receptors

Discussion: The antimanic drugs' mechanisms of action are largely unresolved. Choice B is the best answer, although it is not known to what extent GABAergic mechanisms explain valproate's antimanic versus anticonvulsant efficacy. Inhibition of phosphoinositide metabolism is a leading hypothesis for lithium's mechanism of action. $GABA_B$ receptor mechanisms have been proposed for carbamazepine and other antimanic drugs but remain speculative. Direct membrane effects have been observed for both carbamazepine and other antimanic drugs but remain speculative. Direct membrane effects have been observed for both carbamazepine and valproate and are thought to be involved more in their anticonvulsant than antimanic efficacy. D_2 receptor antagonism is a property of antipsychotic rather than antimanic drugs.

Pages 241–242 •

Answer B

3. The following is a putative cognition-enhancing drug that inhibits acetylcholinesterase and may produce other neurotransmitter effects:

A. piracetam
B. tetrahydroaminoacridine
C. deprenyl
D. vinpocetine
E. scopolamine

Discussion: Deprenyl is a monoamine oxidase B inhibitor currently used for Parkinson's disease. Piracetam is a nootropic, and vinpocetine is a vinca alkaloid, both of which have several proposed mechanisms of action (see text); scopolamine is a muscarinic antagonist that produces learning deficits.

Pages 243–245 •

Answer A

4. The following experimental observation is **least** consistent with the hypothesis that long-term antidepressant treatment decreases functional noradrenergic neurotransmission:

A. somatodendritic α_2-receptor down-regulation in the locus coeruleus
B. β_1-receptor down-regulation in certain terminal fields
C. decreased spontaneous firing rates of locus coeruleus neurons after administration of monoamine oxidase inhibitors
D. decreased tyrosine hydroxylase expression in the locus coeruleus
E. desensitized norepinephrine receptor–coupled adenylate cyclase activity

Discussion: The choices are taken from actual data in the literature, although some published findings contradict certain of these data, and not all classes of antidepressants produce each effect. The balance of data support the hypothesis that despite an acute elevation of synaptic norepinephrine by tricyclic antidepressants, tricyclic and other antidepressants chronically inhibit functional noradrenergic neurotransmission. Tyrosine hydroxylase down-regulation in the locus coeruleus (D), a consistent finding, and decreased firing rate of locus coeruleus neurons in response to monoamine oxidase inhibitors (C) both support the hypothesis because most noradrenergic transmission in the central nervous system originates in the locus coeruleus. Down-regulation and desensitization of norepinephrine receptors in terminal fields (B and E) might serve as postsynaptic mechanisms for reducing functional noradrenergic signaling; if these effects occur along with a chronic reduction of norepinephrine release, this implies some mechanism other than homologous regulation of receptors by ligand concentration. A single, comprehensive explanation of these phenomena along with the role of chronic norepinephrine uptake inhibition by tricyclic agents has yet to be elucidated. Moreover, some findings, such as down-regulation (A) or desensitization of autoinhibitory somatodendritic α_2-receptors in the locus coeruleus, although not in direct contradiction to the hypothesis of reduced norepinephrine output, are at least a challenge to this hypothesis.

Pages 230–232, Figure 14–10 •

Answer A

5. Antidepressants appear to increase which of the following?

A. 5-HT_{1A} somatodendritic autoreceptor responsiveness
B. 5-HT_{1D} terminal autoreceptor responsiveness
C. serotonin nerve terminal α_2-receptor responsiveness
D. serotonin neuronal firing rate
E. net serotonin neurotransmission

Discussion: Various classes of antidepressants produce decreases in one or more of A through C as well as increases in postsynaptic 5-hydroxytryptamine (5-HT) receptor responsiveness. The net effect of each of these chronic antidepressant effects should be an increase in serotonin neurotransmission. It has been consistently shown that long-term antidepressant treatment does not produce a change in serotonin neuronal firing rate (D).

Pages 230–232, Table 14–10 •

Answer E

6. The following are characteristic of "atypical" antipsychotics such as clozapine **except** for

A. little or no induction of depolarization block in nigrostriatal neurons
B. preferential effects on mesolimbocortical dopamine neurons
C. higher affinity for several 5-HT receptor subtypes than typical antipsychotics
D. higher D_4/D_2 receptor affinity ratio than typical antipsychotics
E. little or no D_1 receptor affinity

Discussion: Numerous electrophysiological, neurochemical, and pharmacological distinctions typify most of the atypical antipsychotics (i.e., newer agents such as clozapine), which produce few extrapyramidal and other side effects compared with classic antipsychotics, such as haloperidol. In general, atypical drugs largely affect the mesolimbocortical dopamine neurons originating in the ventral tegmental area while sparing nigrostriatal neurons (A and B). One pharmacological basis for this phenomenon could be the weaker antagonism of D_2 receptors, thus producing a slower or milder effect. Alternatively, the greater affinity ratios of atypical drugs for D_4 receptors over D_2 (D) may underlie their efficacy. The higher affinity of many of the atypical drugs for several 5-HT receptors has also been noted (C); blockade of certain of these 5-HT receptors may dampen the dopamine effects. Atypical antipsychotics do bind to D_1 receptors (E).

Pages 232–234, Figure 14–11 •

Answer E

7. Which of the following is responsible for the hyperpolarization "overshoot" after an action potential?

A. potassium conductance
B. sodium conductance
C. chloride conductance
D. inactivated potassium channels
E. inactivated sodium channels

Discussion: Sodium conductance causes the upstroke, and potassium conductance causes the repolarization of an action potential. The hyperpolarization phase occurs because of a delayed closing of potassium channels (i.e., continued potassium conductance). Sodium channel inactivation is responsible both for the refractory period after an action potential and for the diminished responsiveness of neurons that are continuously depolarized. Chloride channels do not normally take part in an action potential.

Pages 211–212, Figures 14–1 and 14–2 •

Answer A

8. Which of the following is a possible correct sequence of events after binding of an agonist to a G protein–coupled receptor? (Multiple intermediate steps may be missing.)

A. dissociation of α-subunit from the $\beta\gamma$ subunit, exchange of GDP for GTP, activation of guanylate cyclase
B. receptor association with G protein heterotrimer, exchange of GDP for GTP, activation of adenylate cyclase, dissociation of receptor from G protein
C. dissociation of α-subunit from the $\beta\gamma$ subunit, activation of adenylate cyclase, hydrolysis of GTP to GDP, change in gene expression
D. dissociation of α-subunit from the $\beta\gamma$ subunit, hydrolysis of GTP to GDP, activation of adenylate cyclase, association of α-subunit with the $\beta\gamma$ subunit
E. receptor association with G protein, activation of adenylate cyclase, association of α-subunit with the $\beta\gamma$ subunit, exchange of GDP for GTP

Discussion: Binding of agonist to receptor changes the conformation of the receptor so that it associates with the G protein. Exchange of GDP for GTP allows GTP-bound α-subunit to dissociate (A and E are wrong). The α-subunit dissociates from the receptor and then produces catalytic effects such as activation of adenylate cyclase (B is wrong). Intrinsic GTPase activity of the α-subunit hydrolyzes GTP, rendering the α-subunit inactive and terminating this step of the cascade (D is wrong). α-GDP reassociates with the $\beta\gamma$ subunit, and the cycle is complete; however, downstream effects of the second messenger, such as changes in gene expression, may occur later (C).

Pages 215–219, Figures 14–4, 14–5 (A) •

Answer C

9. Both ligand-gated ion channels and G protein–coupled receptors are known to exist for each of the following neurotransmitters **except**

A. acetylcholine
B. GABA
C. glutamate
D. norepinephrine
E. serotonin

Discussion: Ligand-gated ion channels include nicotinic acetylcholine, $GABA_A$, ionotropic glutamate (AMPA, kainate, and NMDA types), and 5-HT_3 receptors. G protein–coupled receptors include muscarinic acetylcholine, $GABA_B$, metabotropic glutamate, and most serotonin receptors. The multiple α- and β-subtypes of adrenergic receptors that have been defined are all G protein–coupled receptors.

Page 215 •

Answer D

10. Nitric oxide directly produces which of the following effects?

A. activation of guanylate cyclase
B. activation of adenylate cyclase
C. inhibition of adenylate cyclase
D. stimulation of phospholipase C
E. stimulation of protein kinase C

Discussion: Nitric oxide permeates the plasma membrane and activates soluble guanylate cyclase. Choices B through D are among the results of G protein–mediated signal transduction. Protein kinase C is sensitive to inositol triphosphate and calcium ion concentrations.

Pages 227–228 •

Answer A

11. Known functions of steroids in the central nervous system include each of the following **except**

A. modulation of hypothalamic peptide synthesis or release
B. modulation of NMDA receptors
C. modulation of $GABA_A$ receptors
D. activation of G proteins by binding to a plasma membrane receptor

E. activation of DNA transcription by binding to an intracellular receptor

Discussion: Peripherally synthesized steroid hormones are known to modulate hypothalamic releasing hormone production; for example, gonadal steroids inhibit gonadotropin-releasing hormone production (A). Various neurosteroids, such as alloTHDOC, enhance $GABA_A$ receptor opening through a nonbenzodiazepine receptor mechanism (B). Similarly, pregnenolone sulfate modulates NMDA receptors (C). In general, however, most steroids such as steroid hormones diffuse into the cell and bind to intracellular receptors that also have DNA binding sites (E). A plasma membrane receptor that activates a G protein has not been discovered for steroids.

Pages 226–227 •

Answer D

12. Which statement is true regarding opiates and the locus coeruleus?

A. Opiates acutely increase the firing rate of locus coeruleus noradrenergic neurons.
B. Opiates chronically increase cAMP concentrations in locus coeruleus noradrenergic neurons.
C. Opiates chronically increase expression of adenylate cyclase mRNA and protein in locus coeruleus noradrenergic neurons.
D. Opiate withdrawal is marked by a depletion of cAMP and a diminished locus coeruleus firing rate.
E. The locus coeruleus, along with the nucleus accumbens, mediates the rewarding and reinforcing aspects of psychological dependence to opiates.

Discussion: Acutely, opiates decrease cAMP concentrations and consequently inhibit locus coeruleus noradrenergic firing rate. Chronic adaptation to opiates includes an unregulated (i.e., extrasensitive) cAMP pathway, including G proteins, adenylate cyclase, and cAMP-dependent protein kinase. During withdrawal, there is a marked increase in locus coeruleus noradrenergic firing owing to the absence of inhibitory opiate input and the unregulated cAMP pathway. The locus coeruleus is thought to mediate mostly physical dependence; the mesolimbocortical system (e.g., nucleus accumbens, E) is more involved with the reinforcing properties of drug addiction.

Page 246 •

Answer C

CHAPTER

15 Pathophysiological Basis of Psychiatric Disorders: Focus on Mood Disorders and Schizophrenia

David Taylor

1. Evidence for the role of corticotropin-releasing factor (CRF) in the pathophysiological mechanism of depression is drawn from which of the following observations?

A. CRF concentrations are elevated in the cerebrospinal fluid (CSF) of drug-free patients with major depression.
B. CRF concentrations are elevated in the CSF of treated patients with major depression.
C. Diminished CRF concentrations in the CSF of patients with major depression are observed regardless of treatment status.
D. The response to the dexamethasone suppression test (DST) is nonsuppression in depressed patients.
E. Adrenal cortex atrophy is observed in postmortem examination of suicide victims.

Discussion: Involvement of CRF in the pathophysiological mechanism of depression is suggested by *elevated* CRF concentrations in CSF, which have been documented in multiple studies of drug-free patients with major depression as well as in suicide victims, although not all studies agree. There is virtually universal agreement that CRF CSF concentrations are elevated in depressed DST nonsuppressors. The DST findings are not evidence of CRF hypersecretion. Aside from CSF analysis, the hypothalamic-pituitary axis can be assessed by the administration of CRF intravenously. Elevations of CRF concentrations in the CSF are believed to be due to central CRF hypersecretion. Reduction of CRF concentrations in CSF have been reported in healthy volunteer subjects after administration of desipramine.

Pages 259–261, Table 15–1, Figure 15–1 •

Answer A

2. Studies of the hypothalamic-pituitary-thyroid (HPT) axis in depressed individuals have found that

A. nocturnal plasma thyroid-stimulating hormone (TSH) levels are elevated
B. bipolar depressed patients have different TSH responses to thyrotropin-releasing hormone (TRH) stimulation than do unipolar depressed patients
C. hypothyroidism is invariably present in severe depressions
D. the pituitary gland is diminished in size in part owing to changes in the HPT axis
E. all of the above

Discussion: Hypothyroidism has long been associated with the finding of a depressed mood. Elevated TRH has been observed in the CSF of depressed patients, as has an increased pituitary gland size. The TSH response to TRH stimulation is blunted in hyperthyroidism and in some depressed individuals. This is thought to be due to diminished anterior pituitary responsiveness brought about by chronic TRH hypersecretion. This finding can be demonstrated in rats. Another assessment of the HPT axis involves sampling nocturnal TSH levels, which are found to be diminished in depressed individuals. Whereas most depressed patients have a blunted TSH response to TRH stimulation, about 15% have an opposite response. This may be due to the co-occurrence of hypothyroidism, which can cause an opposite TSH response. Bipolar patients also have an exaggerated TSH response, and there is a higher prevalence rate of hypothyroidism in rapid-cycling bipolar patients.

Pages 261–262, Table 15–2, 15–3, 15–4, Figure 15–2 •

Answer B

3. Which of the following statements about the role of serotonin (5-HT) in depression is true?

A. There are three main classes of 5-HT receptors, and all of them have been implicated in the pathophysiological mechanisms of depression.
B. The finding of low CSF 5-hydroxyindoleacetic acid (5-HIAA) levels is pathognomonic of depression.
C. The binding of [^{3}H]-imipramine to 5-HT transporters on platelet membranes is a biological marker of depression.
D. Fenfluramine challenge leads to a blunted prolactin response in depressed patients only.
E. There is no interaction between serotonin and the hypothalamic-pituitary-adrenal (HPA) axis as is seen with dopamine.

Discussion: Whereas there have been some findings to the contrary, the reduction in the number of platelet [^{3}H]-imipramine binding sites in depressed patients has been reported by several groups. [^{3}H]-paroxetine is an even more specific ligand for these transporters. There is a hypothesized interaction between serotonin and the HPA axis based in part on observations of elevated CSF 5-HIAA levels in psychotic depression. Low CSF 5-HIAA levels are therefore not pathognomonic of depression but have been observed in violent and impulsive individuals such as arsonists. Blunted prolactin response to fenfluramine is seen in depressed patients and in those with other illnesses.

Pages 266–267, Table 15–7 •

Answer C

4. The subgroup of patients with psychotic depression exhibit all of the following **except**

A. lower serum dopamine β-hydroxylase activity
B. higher plasma dopamine and homovanillic acid concentrations
C. higher platelet monoamine oxidase activity
D. DST nonsuppression
E. elevated γ-aminobutyric acid (GABA) CSF concentrations

Discussion: GABA levels are generally found to be reduced in depression, alcoholism, and mania. The group of patients with psychotic depression have all of the other findings in some studies. There is interest in the interaction between catecholamines and the HPA axis in this population.

Pages 268–269 •

Answer E

5. Which of the following is evidence of "hypofrontality" in schizophrenia?

A. lack of activation of the dorsolateral prefrontal cortex (DLPFC) in schizophrenic patients given an automated version of the Wisconsin Card Sorting Test (WCST) during xenon 133 regional cerebral blood flow measurement.
B. enlargement of the lateral ventricles
C. decreased neuronal diameter in the nucleus accumbens
D. all of the above
E. none of the above

Discussion: The concept of hypofrontality refers to observations of regional cerebral blood flow during the performance of cognitive tasks by schizophrenic patients. Whereas the other findings have been observed neuroradiologically and neuropathologically in the forebrains of schizophrenic patients, the diminished cerebral blood flow to the DLPFC is a measurement of functional physiological activity. In studies of monozygotic twins discordant for schizophrenia, diminished activation of the DLPFC during the WCST is invariably associated with illness, is not present in unaffected co-twins, is not affected by long-term neuroleptic exposure, and is correlated with diminished hippocampal volume in the affected twins.

Page 277 •

Answer A

6. In light of the structural brain abnormalities observed in schizophrenia, alterations in neurotransmitter function may be regarded as secondary to neuronal loss or altered neuronal development. This hypothesis is supported by which of the following observations?

A. In laboratory animals, cortical lesions can differentially affect dopamine neurotransmission in subcortical and in distant cortical areas.
B. Prefrontal regional cerebral blood flow in schizophrenics during cognitive tasks is correlated with CSF metabolites of dopamine.
C. Hippocampal size is correlated with activation of prefrontal cortical blood flow in schizophrenic patients.
D. A and C are correct.
E. All of the above are correct.

Discussion: All of the above statements can be made in support of the stated hypothesis as discussed in depth in the chapter. However, the possibility exists that primary dysfunction of dopaminergic or other neurotransmitter systems may underlie the schizophrenic syndrome. Future research with more rigorously defined postmortem samples will be necessary before one can reliably conclude that increased concentrations of dopamine, altered dopamine receptor function, or alterations in other neurotransmitters occur in schizophrenic patients independently of drug treatment artifacts and structural brain abnormalities.

Pages 272–281 •

Answer E

7. Which of the following homologous animal models of depression has **not** been examined for antidepressant response?

A. lesioning of the dorsomedial amygdala in dogs
B. isolation-separation–induced depression in monkeys
C. separation of Siberian hamsters
D. chronic mild stress model
E. uncontrollable shock model

Discussion: All of the above are homologous models that attempt to reproduce the syndrome of depression in animals. They therefore are distinct from animal assays, which are reproducible methods to test medication effects in ways that may not be at all related to the effects in humans. All of the above except the lesioning of the dorsomedial amygdala in dogs, which produces a remarkable depressive syndrome of lethargy, negativism, reluctance to eat, and saddened facial expression, have been studied for their response to antidepressant medications. In all those models, the animal's symptoms are reversible with medication.

Pages 286–291 •

Answer A

8. Which of the following statements about the prepulse inhibition (PPI) of the startle reflex is **not** true?

A. It is an animal behavior model of sensorimotor gating functions.
B. Rats and humans have parallel responses in terms of both gradation and threshold.
C. PPI (of an eye blink reflex) is absent or dramatically reduced in patients with schizophrenia compared with normal control subjects.
D. Antipsychotic drugs affect PPI in normally functioning animals.
E. PPI is inhibited by the administration of D_2 but not D_1 receptor agonists.

Discussion: An animal model of the information-processing–stimulus-filtering deficits of schizophrenia is represented by the inhibition of the startle reaction to an acoustic or tactile stimulus when the startling stimulus is preceded by a weak prestimulus (hence, prepulse inhibition, or PPI). All of the above statements about PPI are true except that as opposed to other models, such as latent inhibition of conditioned responses, PPI responses are affected by antipsychotics only in animals who already exhibit a deficit in the normal response. In this respect, the model more closely reflects the illness state of schizophrenia. Other illnesses, such as Huntington's disease, obsessive-compulsive disorder, and other psychoses, are associated with PPI deficits. Antipsychotic medications actually have a negligible effect on PPI in schizophrenic patients, which is a problem.

Pages 294–295 •

Answer D

CHAPTER

16 Cognitive Neuroscience

Robert S. Goldman • Irma C. Smet • Malini Singh

1. Which of the following neurotransmitters is thought to be involved in long-term potentiation?

A. serotonin
B. dopamine
C. GABA
D. glutamate

Discussion: Glutamate mediates long-term potentiation in the mammalian brain. Glutamate acts on the *N*-methyl-D-aspartate (NMDA) receptor to maintain neuronal firing. Studies in the hippocampus have suggested that long-term potentiation may represent a cellular mechanism of memory.

Page 317, Figure 16–4 •

Answer D

2. A type of aphasia that is characterized by normal fluency, impaired comprehension, and the presence of paraphasic speech is known as

A. Wernicke's aphasia
B. Broca's aphasia
C. alexia
D. agraphia

Discussion: Wernicke's aphasia is marked by normal fluency, impaired comprehension, and the presence of errors in speech known as paraphasias. Lesions to the posterior temporal cortex (auditory association cortex), typically in the left hemisphere, produce this type of syndrome.

Pages 327–329, Table 16–1, Figure 16–10 •

Answer A

3. After a brain injury, a normally placid individual becomes irritable, disinhibited, and episodically aggressive. Damage to which brain area is most likely to explain these behaviors?

A. premotor area
B. occipital lobe
C. prefrontal cortex
D. temporal lobe

Discussion: The behavioral syndrome depicted would most often be associated with damage to the prefrontal cortex, specifically to orbitomedial prefrontal cortex. Individuals with damage to this area often undergo changes in personality that are marked by behavioral disinhibition.

Page 335 •

Answer C

4. Which of the following technologies would be most useful to revealing the in vivo functional capacity of a particular brain region?

A. magnetic resonance imaging
B. positron emission tomography
C. single-unit recording
D. WADA Test

Discussion: Studies using positron emission tomography have proved useful in revealing the functional capacity of particular brain regions. Regional cerebral blood flow studies have examined the cognitive capacities of brain regions; receptor studies try to examine the role of particular neurotransmitters.

Pages 322–323 •

Answer B

5. A type of memory that involves the ability to hold brief amounts of information in the context of performing various cognitive tasks is known as

A. explicit memory
B. implicit memory
C. working memory
D. source memory

Discussion: Working memory refers to the ability to represent visual or auditory elements of stimuli for brief intervals while performing various cognitive operations. Working memory is thought to be mediated by the prefrontal cortex.

Pages 320–324 •

Answer C

6. You examine a new patient with Wernicke-Korsakoff's syndrome who tells an elaborate and somewhat coherent story about having met you in the past, all of which is untrue. This type of pathological memory is known as

A. contamination
B. confabulation
C. retrograde amnesia
D. anterograde amnesia

Discussion: Confabulation refers to a pathological symptom whereby a patient will fill gaps in memory with wholly untrue information, which may have the appearance of coherence. This is frequently seen with Korsakoff's syndrome and is associated with the frontal lobe impairment frequently seen in this disorder.

Pages 315–316, 318 •

Answer B

7. The role of reduced cholinergic activity has been found to be most relevant to which disorder?

A. Parkinson's disease
B. Huntington's disease
C. schizophrenia
D. Alzheimer's disease

Discussion: Dysfunction in the basal forebrain cholinergic system has been implicated in producing the impairment in memory functioning seen in Alzheimer's disease. The basal forebrain region sends cholinergic projections from the medial septal area to the hippocampus. The use of cholinergic agonists such as ergoloid mesylates (Hydergine) and tacrine hydrochloride (Cognex) has been seen as a partial strategy to stimulate memory functioning in Alzheimer's disease.

Pages 318–319, Figure 16–5 •

Answer D

8. A patient is known to have a lesion in the left inferior frontal area. What type of language deficit is often associated with damage to this region?

A. impaired fluency
B. impaired comprehension
C. alexia
D. agraphia

Discussion: Broca's area is situated in the inferior left frontal area. Damage to this region typically results in impaired fluency, impaired repetition, and usually intact comprehension of spoken and written material.

Page 327 •

Answer A

9. Which of the following neuropsychological tests has been widely used for the assessment of the integrity of frontal lobe functions?

A. Pursuit Rotor Task
B. Wepman Planning Inventory
C. Wisconsin Card Sorting Test
D. Boston Diagnostic Aphasia Examination

Discussion: The Wisconsin Card Sorting Test has been increasingly used to examine frontal lobe functions in humans. A series of positron emission tomography studies in normal individuals and various psychiatric and neurological populations have revealed that frontal regions are active during the performance of this task, which involves planning, set shifting, and error correction.

Page 337 •

Answer C

10. Amnesia typically does **not** involve impairment in which of the following cognitive operations?

A. anterograde memory
B. source memory
C. immediate memory
D. long-term memory

Discussion: Studies of human amnesias reveal that immediate memory is typically intact in amnesia. Anterograde memory and long-term memory, which are impaired in amnesia, refer to the ability to learn and retain new information. Source memory refers to the ability to recall the context in which information was learned, which is also impaired in amnesia.

Pages 315–316, 320 •

Answer C

CHAPTER

17 Cognitive Psychology: Basic Theory and Clinical Implications

W. Edward Craighead • Stephen S. Ilardi •
Michael D. Greenberg • Linda W. Craighead

1. Cognitive psychology is

A. the scientific study of human behavior
B. the study of *only* intellectual development in humans
C. the scientific study of human memory and mental processes
D. the scientific study of cognitive-behavioral therapy

Discussion: Cognitive psychology developed as a distinct subarea of the broader field of experimental psychology and separate from developmental psychology during the 1950s and 1960s. Ashcraft has defined it as the "scientific study of human memory and mental processes."

Page 350 •

Answer C

2. Problem solving refers to

A. use of modeling research with hyperactive children
B. the behaviorist's explanation of insight in psychodynamic psychotherapy
C. the clinical process of solving a specific problem in cognitive-behavioral therapy
D. the clinical use of cognitive psychology to teach patients to identify and solve problems as a part of more general self-control processes

Discussion: The clinical application of problem solving involves teaching the patient a general strategy to cope independently with problems as they arise. Problem solving is first modeled by the therapist, then the patient is coached through a number of current problem situations.

Pages 361–363 •

Answer D

3. A "schema" refers to

A. a term in learning theory that describes how classical conditioning occurs
B. a construct in cognitive psychology that is used to explain how long-term memory is organized
C. a process that has its impact on human functioning at a conscious or "aware" level
D. the cognitive processes of identifying and selecting the most salient pieces of information to be processed

Discussion: The term schema has never been formally defined and in vernacular usage has come to mean category or prototype. Schema theories generally postulate the existence of a set of memory structures that can selectively direct attention and can subsequently influence memory encoding through abstraction, interpretation, and integration.

Page 363 •

Answer B

4. Which of the following was **not** a major cause of the focus during the 1950s on cognitive processes in theory and research?

A. the development of the computer and its use as a model for information processing in humans
B. the application of principles of learning in behavior therapy
C. the development of complex theories of learning to explain human learning processes
D. the applied needs of World War II (e.g., person-machine interactions)

Discussion: Cognitive psychology grew out of the recognition of the limitations of a purely behavioral approach that could not explain complex human behaviors. The application of principles of learning in behavioral research proposed the acquisition of responses.

Pages 351–352 •

Answer B

5. The "cognitive revolution" during the 1950s and 1960s refers to

A. the application of principles of learning in cognitive-behavioral therapy
B. the focus on the study of mental processes primarily by experimental psychologists
C. the study of the structures of the brain as exemplified by the *structuralism* of Titchner
D. the theoretical developments of Piaget, especially his focus on stages of psychological development

Discussion: One of the major developments in experimental psychology of the 1940s was the formulation of sophisticated learning theories to explain the complex processes of human functioning and behavior acquisition.

Page 352 •

Answer B

6. Automatic cognitive processes

A. are characterized by compulsive repetition
B. occur in the absence of attentional focus
C. are best illustrated by the phenomenon of command auditory hallucinations
D. are unrelated to the phenomenon of parallel processing

Discussion: Some mental processes occur in the complete or partial absence of attentional focus. Such cognitive processes are often referred to as automatic, because they seem to operate without conscious awareness or involvement.

Pages 353–354 •

Answer B

7. Which of the following statements regarding "attention" is false?

A. Heightened emotional arousal is associated with a narrowing of attentional focus.
B. Anxious individuals give heightened attention to threat-related cues.
C. Borderline individuals appear to experience profound dysregulation in attentional control.
D. Mood-congruent attentional biases serve to reduce the intensity of negatively valenced mood states.

Discussion: Some automatic cognitive processes may be etiologically involved in certain forms of psychiatric illness. This malfunctioning can be observed in generalized anxiety disorder, major depression, attention-deficit/hyperactivity disorder, and borderline personality disorder. Individuals suffering from major depression are susceptible to a negativistic bias in cognitive processing, and these depressotypic negative thoughts are held to be centrally involved in the onset and maintenance of the depressive episode.

Pages 354–357, Table 17–2 •

Answer D

8. The mood-congruency effect refers to

A. the association, in depression, between symptoms of emotional distress and physical-neurochemical dysregulation
B. the association between depressive affect and some corresponding set of experimental stressors
C. the association between prevailing emotional state and facilitated recall of emotionally toned material, leading to bias in memory
D. the association between depression (impaired emotional functioning) and poorly structured encoding of new information (impaired cognitive functioning)

Discussion: The study of memory in depressed and nondepressed individuals suggests that not only is there a generic impairment of memory in depression but also an emotional bias termed the mood-congruency effect. Depressed individuals are negatively biased in their capacity to recall affectively toned materials.

Pages 358–359 •

Answer C

CHAPTER

18 Social Psychology: Theory, Research, and Mental Health Implications

Eugene W. Farber • Nadine J. Kaslow

1. From a social psychological perspective, the self is characterized best as a psychological phenomenon that

A. is influenced largely by temperament and mediates social relationships
B. is based largely on individuation processes and organizes inner experiences of social relationships
C. is defined by attributional processes and influenced by social dissonance processes
D. is socially defined and influenced by interpersonal context and social role expectations
E. is based on neurochemical processes that organize inner experiences into a sense of identity

Discussion: From a social psychological perspective, the self is presumed to be influenced by social relationships and the interpersonal context. There are several models in current social psychology that attempt to account for the functions of the self.

Pages 370–372, Table 18–1 •

Answer D

2. The social psychological process by which individuals formulate impressions of others is called

A. impression management
B. person perception
C. reactance
D. deindividuation
E. self-verification

Discussion: Person perception or social perception refers to the ways in which we formulate impressions of others. Research has found that people have a tendency to formulate viewpoints on human nature and behavior that influence their understanding of others and permit rapid evaluation of persons and interpersonal situations.

Pages 372–374 •

Answer B

3. The primary focus of attribution theory is on

A. explanations that individuals generate to account for events, outcomes, and behavior
B. enduring viewpoints consisting of cognitive, affective, and behavioral components
C. group polarization effects on socialization processes
D. central and peripheral routes involved in the persuasion process
E. the mechanisms by which groups formulate decisions regarding particular courses of action

Discussion: Attribution theory focuses on causal explanations generated by an individual to account for why a particular event or set of outcomes has occurred. There are three main sorts of attribution bias: the fundamental attribution error, actor-observer bias, and the self-serving (hedonic) attribution bias.

Pages 374–376, Tables 18–2, 18–3 •

Answer A

4. Cognitive dissonance theory is characterized best as an attitude theory focusing primarily on

A. learning and reinforcement principles
B. the role of personal needs and motives in attitude formation and change
C. heuristic-systematic processes
D. discrepancies between simultaneously held contradictory beliefs
E. behavioral intentions as they relate to the probability of acting in accord with attitudinal beliefs

Discussion: Cognitive dissonance theory holds that discrepancies between simultaneously held attitudinal cognitions (dissonance) produce psychological tension, requiring attitudinal changes to reestablish consistency (consonance).

Pages 376–377 •

Answer D

5. Which of the following is **not** a factor that increases the likelihood that an individual will engage in helping behavior?
   A. mood of the helper
   B. empathy for the person in need
   C. perception that the problem was caused by factors outside the control of the person in need
   D. the presence of multiple others at the scene in which help is required
   E. view of the person in need as similar to oneself.

Discussion: Altruism refers to instances in which there is no reproductive gain attributable to the helping behavior. Helping behaviors are shaped by all of the above. The bystander effect is a situational variable that has empirically been found to decrease the likelihood of an individual's offering help.

Pages 379–380, Table 18–7 •

Answer D

6. Which is **not** a factor that can contribute to the prevention of aggressive behavior?
   A. reduction of frustration levels
   B. reduction of empathy for potential targets of aggressive behavior
   C. reduction of the likelihood of deindividuation processes
   D. arrangement of situations such that the benefits of cooperation outweigh those of aggression
   E. teaching behavioral alternatives to aggressive responses

Discussion: The prevention of aggression can be accomplished by all of the above with the exception that it is important to decrease an individual's sense of deindividuation and enhance empathy for the potential victim. In addition, education about the uninhibiting effects of alcohol and drugs is a useful strategy.

Pages 384–386, Table 18–11 •

Answer B

7. Group decision-making can be influenced adversely by
   A. group comparison and group reflection processes
   B. social facilitation and social loafing processes
   C. group polarization and group-think processes
   D. social comparison and social judgment processes
   E. group cohesion and group retroflection

Discussion: Group decision-making is often more effective than individual efforts. This requires cooperative and collective work to complete the additive tasks. Group cohesion is enhanced by all of the above except polarization and group-think processes, which are deleterious to thoughtful and productive decisions.

Pages 387–388, Table 18–13 •

Answer C

8. The ______ approach to the study of psychological functioning seeks to identify universal psychological principles that are applicable across cultures; the ______ approach examines psychological phenomena identified as being different across cultures.
   A. ideographic; nomothetic
   B. nomothetic; ideographic
   C. global; indigenous
   D. etic; emic
   E. emic; etic

Discussion: In the study of culture and psychological functioning, the etic approach seeks to identify universal psychological principles applicable across different cultures. The emic approach seeks to examine psychological phenomena identified as being different across cultures.

Page 389, Table 18–14 •

Answer D

9. Positive health behaviors may be associated with
   A. high self-efficacy and optimistic attributional style
   B. high self-verification and low self-discrepancy
   C. high self-evaluation and low cognitive dissonance
   D. high heuristic processing and low actor-observer bias
   E. secure attachments and deindividuation

Discussion: A collection of attributional processes referred to as positive illusions are more likely to lead to good health habits than is a pessimistic attributional style, which can place young adults at increased risk for physical problems later in life.

Page 375 •

Answer A

10. According to the health belief model, which of the following does **not** influence responses to threats of illness?

A. sociocultural factors
B. perceptions of the extent to which the condition is threatening
C. the extent to which the fundamental attribution error is operative
D. expectations about the ability to minimize threats associated with the illness
E. personal environmental cues regarding appropriate courses of action

Discussion: According to the health belief model proposed to explain health-related behavior, individuals' decisions regarding their responses to threats of illness are influenced by sociocultural and demographic factors, perceptions of the threat of the condition, expectations regarding the ability to minimize such a threat, and personal and environmental cues regarding the appropriate courses of action.

Page 378 •

Answer C

CHAPTER

19 Psychoanalytic Theories

Steven T. Levy • Lawrence B. Inderbitzin
• Lucy LaFarge • Richard B. Zimmer
• Robert M. Galatzer-Levy

1. Psychoanalysis is

A. a clinical treatment method
B. a general theory of the mind
C. a research method to study mental life
D. all of the above

Discussion: Psychoanalysis is a clinical therapy for the treatment of the neuroses originally developed by Sigmund Freud. By extension, the term refers as well to a theory of psychopathology underlying the therapeutic practice; a general theory of the mind, based on the understanding arising from the clinical procedure; and a mode of research into mental life that is inherent in and inextricably intertwined with the clinical therapeutic process.

Page 396 •

Answer D

2. Freud's structural model of the mind

A. includes three mental agencies: id, ego, and superego
B. superseded his topographic model
C. neither A nor B
D. both A and B

Discussion: The initial foundation of psychoanalytic theory was the topographic model of the mind, which delineated three regions of the mind: the unconscious, preconscious, and conscious. In 1923, Freud revised this theoretical formulation to account for aspects of his developing understanding of the mind. This later concept of a tripartite division into id, ego, and superego is known as the structural model of the mind.

Pages 404–405, 406–407, Table 19–8, Figure 19–5 •

Answer D

3. Many early dissenting analysts diverged from Freud

A. around the issue of the importance of sexual etiology of neuroses
B. by emphasizing environmental issues as more important than innate, constitutional issues
C. neither A nor B
D. both A and B

Discussion: Early dissenting analysts diverged from Freud on the issue of the sexual etiology of the neuroses. Many of these analysts abandoned instinct theory altogether and emphasized the role of the environment in the genesis of personality and neurotic symptoms. Others retained a role for sexuality as one of the host of needs pressing for satisfaction and leading to potential conflict and symptom formation.

Page 409 •

Answer D

4. The concept of defense

A. was important in Freud's earliest theorizing
B. was studied and developed by Anna Freud, culminating in her 10 mechanisms of defense
C. has changed considerably but remains important in modern structural theory
D. all of the above

Discussion: Defense, a central ego concept, appears early (1894, 1896) in Freud's writings, referring there mainly to the avoidance of painful reality experiences encoded as memories, which leads to the damming up of affect and subsequent psychiatric illness. Ego psychology, which expanded the structural theory of the mind, focused on concepts such as reality testing, sublimation, altruism, modes of internalization, ideal formation, and self-esteem regulation. Anna Freud categorized and developed the first theory of mechanisms of defense. She outlined 10 mechanisms of defense.

Pages 412–414, Table 19–10 •

Answer D

5. Object relations theory

A. is a unitary theory
B. is based on the idea that the mind is composed of elements taken in from the outside
C. was not an aspect of Freud's theory
D. all of the above

Discussion: There is no unitary theory of object relations. Freud did define the term *object* in 1915 as "the thing in regard to which or through which the instinct is able to achieve its aim." Object relations theory can be defined as "a system of psychological explanation based on the premise that the mind is composed of elements taken in from the outside, primarily aspects of functioning of other persons. This occurs by means of the processes of internalization. This model of the mind explains mental functions in terms of relations between the various elements internalized" (Moore and Fine, 1990).

Page 420 •

Answer B

6. The integration of ego psychology and object relations

A. has been attempted by some analysts such as Kernberg
B. is impossible according to some analysts
C. both A and B
D. neither A nor B

Discussion: Both Edith Jacobson and Otto Kernberg have attempted to integrate ego psychology and object relations. Jacobson, for example, suggested that the early nucleus of what will eventually become the child's superego is the early "bad" internal object representation that is linked with punishing and prohibiting affect. Kernberg envisions the inner world of the borderline or psychotic patient as being populated by numerous unintegrated part self–part object dyads that are each linked by a predominant affect. These internal nuclei are kept separate by the defense of splitting. Thus, both these authors blend aspects of ego psychology with object relations.

Pages 425–427 •

Answer C

7. Erik Erikson

A. criticized Freud's epigenetic concepts
B. in emphasizing sociocultural factors disagreed with Freud on the importance of the individual's body experiences
C. concluded that his findings were incompatible with modern structural theory
D. none of the above

Discussion: Erikson did not criticize Freud's epigenetic concepts; instead, he incorporated this idea into his own epigenetic schema. Likewise, Erikson did not disagree with Freud on the importance of the individual's body experiences; instead, his theory was firmly rooted in the individual's experience of his or her body as demonstrated in his studies of children of the Sioux and Yurok cultures.

Pages 428–430, Table 19–12
See also Chapter 10 pages 150–153 •

Answer D

8. In modern structural theory

A. Freud's economic (energic) concepts remain central
B. the expanded components of conflict are central
C. the importance of anxiety and other affects is diminished
D. the concept of defense is limited to Anna Freud's 10 mechanisms of defense

Discussion: Modern structural theory, as developed by Arlow, Brenner, and others, embraces the presuppositions underlying Freud's structural hypothesis: that psychoanalysis is primarily a psychology of conflict. These theorists broadened the field of inquiry of the ego psychologists to include the id and superego in the understanding of conflict and compromise formation.

Pages 416–417 •

Answer B

9. Intersubjectivity in psychoanalysis

A. refers to the dynamic interplay between the analyst's and patient's subjective experience during psychoanalysis
B. is often contrasted with positivistic models and theories
C. refers to only "humanistic" therapeutic approach
D. both A and B

Discussion: Intersubjectivity in psychoanalysis refers to the dynamic interplay between the analyst's and the patient's subjective experiences in the clinical situation. Intersubjectivity embodies the notion that the very formation of the therapeutic process is derived from an inextricably intertwined mixture of the clinical participants' subjective reactions to one another. This is in contrast to a more positivist classical approach in which the observer's own subjectivity is factored out.

Pages 435–436 •

Answer A

10. Jacques Lacan, a French psychoanalyst, has suggested that

A. the unconscious is structured like a natural language
B. the Oedipus complex had been overemphasized
C. nonverbal communication is paramount
D. Freudian methods of dream interpretation are not therapeutic

Discussion: Lacan is a controversial psychoanalytic thinker who has helped shape modern psychoanalytic therapy by infusing it with novel linguistic theories. His focus is on verbal communication, and he conceives of the unconscious as a kind of discourse, a natural language. The lacanian analyst focuses on the relationship of signifiers and the underlying signified to understand the unconscious. The discourse of the unconscious refers to the main unconscious conflicts and fantasies described by Freud, centering on the unconscious.

Pages 440–441 •

Answer A

11. Countertransference is

A. simply the response to transference
B. the attempt by the therapist to counter his or her feelings
C. the attitudes and feelings of the therapist toward the patient
D. evident only in psychotherapeutic treatments

Discussion: Countertransference, which is part of all types of medical and psychological treatments, refers to the attitudes and feelings on the part of the psychiatrist or therapist. In a narrow sense, it is defined as a result of activation of wishes, fantasies, or conflicts from the psychiatrist's life. In a broader sense, it also includes reactions to the patient's projections or role enactments.

Page 444, Glossary •

Answer C

12. Adler's concept of the masculine protest

A. describes the central developmental role of rebellion in male development
B. describes the fundamental urge of both sexes to overcome the feeling of inferiority
C. was as central, in his theory, as the sexual instinct
D. was particularly useful in explaining neuroses that stem from a failure in development of social interest
E. was welcomed by Freud as a valuable extension of instinct theory

Discussion: Alfred Adler was the first among Freud's early followers to break with him. Their disagreement over the importance of sexuality in human motivation proved to be irreconcilable. Universal strivings for superiority were given direction by a personal goal or self-ideal that was outside of conscious awareness and organized all psychological processes. Adler believed that the psychology of the individual could not be considered separately from her or his relation to the social milieu.

Page 409 •

Answer B

13. Freud's concept of infantile sexuality was retained as of central importance in the theory of

A. Jung
B. Adler
C. Sullivan
D. Ferenczi
E. Rank

Discussion: Sandor Ferenczi, who never made a final break with Freud, based his work on Freud's central concepts, such as the importance of sexuality in motivation, psychic determinism, and centrality of the Oedipus complex. He emphasized the importance of introjection as a mechanism, the importance of aggression, and the role of a death instinct. He also believed that real trauma was a frequent cause of neurotic symptoms and character pathology.

Pages 410–411 •

Answer D

14. Jung's "collective unconscious" describes

A. a deep layer of the personality, incorporating inherited archetypes that predate individual development
B. a group of primitive archetypes that date from the earliest months of life
C. the phenomena that underlie group processes
D. unconscious archetypes that arise from universal childhood experiences
E. a group of primordial, archetypal fantasies that underlie experience but do not cause symptom or conflict

Discussion: Carl Jung felt that there was a more profound layer of unconscious conflict and transferences that were often apparent once more superficial neurotic conflicts were resolved. He saw these as inherited symbolic images that were often impersonal in character, arising from the collective unconscious. These archetypes, as he called them, resemble the phenomenon of narcissism.

Pages 409–410 •

Answer A

15. Birth trauma

A. is Rank's metaphor for the anxiety accompanying autonomy
B. is a theory built on Rank's observations of his patients' memories of the experience of birth
C. was felt by Rank to be as important as castration anxiety in explaining the dread of incest
D. was central to the theories of both Rank and Ferenczi
E. is a theory that asserts that all anxiety arises from the separation from the mother's womb at birth

Discussion: Otto Rank published *The Trauma of Birth* in 1924. In this work, he asserted that at the deepest level, all anxiety derived from the experience of separation from the haven of the mother's womb at birth. In his focus on the ambivalently held wish to return to the mother's womb, he deemphasized the role of the father in neurosogenesis and placed a greater importance on the mother. He thus shifted to a focus on preoedipal conflicts presaging later developments in psychoanalytic thinking.

Page 410 •

Answer E

16. Horney believed that penis envy

A. was not an important dynamic in female development
B. precluded the girl's attainment of an awareness of the vagina before puberty
C. gained its main power as a defense against the girl's oedipal attachment to her father
D. was most important in its primary form, which arose during the girl's phallic phase
E. gained its main power from the girl's perception of men's privileged status within society

Discussion: Karen Horney was critical of Freud's psychology of women. She contended that the girl's experience was uniquely feminine from the first and included an early awareness of the vagina. Although the girl did experience penis envy during the phallic phase, this primary penis envy was not the universally important experience that Freud had described. What analysts observed in adult women was secondary penis envy, a fantasy of masculinity that served as a defense against the girl's oedipal wish for her father's love.

Page 411 •

Answer C

17. Sullivan believed that the environment

A. imposed both interpersonal roles and the earliest experience of anxiety on the individual
B. imposed on the child the sexual feelings that Freud had considered manifestations of infantile sexuality
C. caused conflict and symptom formation by opposing the discharge of sexual and aggressive drives
D. led to the establishment of a self-system in early childhood, which was impervious to change at later stages of life
E. was less important than constitution in the etiology of neurosis

Discussion: Harry Stack Sullivan rejected the notion of infantile sexuality and emphasized the central role of environment on individual development. He characterized anxiety as exclusively interpersonal in origin. Later experiences triggered anxiety because they evoked the recollection of the contagious anxiety felt with early objects. Adolescence and adulthood were seen as crucial periods of growth and change.

Pages 411–412 •

Answer A

For each numbered item, select the lettered heading most closely associated with it. Each letter may be selected once, more than once, or not at all.

18. Match the term with the associated individual.

____ 1. will therapy	A. Jung
____ 2. analytical psychology	B. Horney
____ 3. self-system	C. Rank
____ 4. real self	D. Sullivan

Discussion: Each of these terms is associated with a particular alternative school.

Pages 409–412 •

Answers 1, C; 2, A; 3, D; 4, B

19. Match the technique with the associated alternative school.

____ 1. analyst builds relationship that anchors patient in reality
____ 2. analyst prohibits symptomatic acts and analyzes patient's reaction
____ 3. analyst demonstrates mistaken perceptions to be unrealistic and encourages development of social interest
____ 4. analyst explores both transferences built on experiences with real objects and transferences that stem from phylogenetic inheritance

A. analytical psychology
B. individual psychology
C. active therapy
D. interpersonal therapy of schizophrenia

Discussion: The theoreticians of the alternative schools were all of course practicing analysts and influential teachers. Naturally, their theoretical constructs both grew out of and influenced their clinical work.

Pages 409–412 •

Answers 1, D; 2, C; 3, B; 4, A

20. As used in self psychology, the term *empathy* refers to

A. the natural warm and positive feeling that human beings experience toward one another
B. the comprehension of complex psychological states as a whole of another person
C. the realization that all people experience intense sexual and aggressive drives, some of which are unconscious
D. the sharing of another's emotional pain
E. the process by which the patient unconsciously causes the therapist to experience the same painful affects as the patient

Discussion: Empathy, the fundamental mode of comprehension in self psychology, is the knowledge of others' complex experience as a whole. It is likened to vicarious introspection.

Page 431 •

Answer B

21. In self psychology, the term *self-object* refers to

A. the infant's lack of personal boundaries, which results in a psychological symbiosis with caregivers
B. a set of necessary interactions with caregivers that support the development of self
C. the experience, limited to early childhood, that others are needed to support the self
D. the pathological assumption that other people are psychologically exactly like oneself
E. the intrapsychic experience that the self is made vigorous and cohesive through relations with others

Discussion: Self-objects are intrapsychic experiences that are needed throughout the life course to support the experience that the self is vigorous and coherent over time and space.

Pages 431–432 •

Answer E

21. *Hypochondriacal symptoms* in disorders of the self are

A. concrete representations of the sense that something is gravely amiss with the self
B. attempts to manipulate others to gain needed attention
C. symbolic representations that the self has been invaded by evil self-objects
D. the result of parental overinvolvement with body functions at the expense of emotional responsiveness
E. the experience of buildup of excessive sexual energies in psychological representation of the organ about which the person is worried

Discussion: Hypochondriasis is one way in which feelings of emptiness, depletion, and incoherence can find vivid expression.

Pages 432–433 •

Answer A

23. Investigators have studied infant development in relationship to the ideas of self psychology.

A. These studies clearly confirm that the self in infancy develops through interactions with self-objects.
B. The findings of infant studies are inconsistent with self psychology.
C. The findings of infant studies are consistent with self psychology but do not support its theory fully.
D. The findings of infant research are inconsistent with self psychology but are irrelevant because they are so psychologically superficial.

E. The studies show that infant psychology is so primitive that meaningful psychological development does not begin until the oedipal period.

Discussion: Whereas many different types of study of infant development show the centrality of caretakers and caretaker function to the young child's emerging manifestations of self, the lack of access to the infant's internal psychological world makes it impossible for these studies to confirm or disconfirm central portions of the self psychology theory of development.

Page 431 •

Answer C

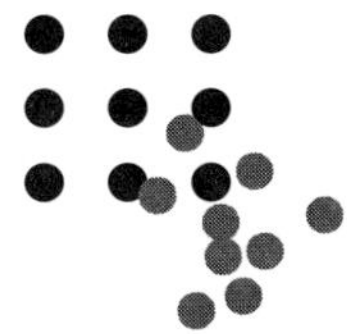

SECTION IV

Section Editor: Andrew E. Skodol

Manifestations of Psychiatric Illness

CHAPTER

20 Psychopathology Across the Life Cycle

Andrew E. Skodol • David Shaffer • Barry Gurland

1. The following is **not** true of psychopathology across the life cycle:

A. Behavioral disorders of childhood are associated with increased risk of behavioral disorders in adolescence.
B. The more severe the disorder in childhood or adolescence, the more likely it is to be persistent.
C. Mental disorders of adults rarely have an onset before age 20 years.
D. Mental disorders may be expressed differently at different ages.

Discussion: Epidemiological surveys of adults indicated that the age at onset of mental disorders for many patients was during adolescence, which reinforces the notion of persistence or progression of disorders across the life cycle.

Page 450 •

Answer C

For each numbered item, select the lettered heading most closely associated with it. Each letter may be selected once, more than once, or not at all.

2. Match the symptom with the associated type of problem.

____ 1. separation anxiety
____ 2. hyperactivity
____ 3. learning disorder
____ 4. enuresis

A. developmental problem of childhood
B. emotional problem of childhood
C. behavioral problem of childhood
D. childhood problem of physical functioning

Discussion: Developmental problems in childhood fall into five main types: intellectual, learning, motor skills, communication, and pervasive developmental disorders. Emotional problems of children involve anxiety and depression. Separation anxiety, selective mutism, social and specific phobias, generalized anxiety, obsessive-compulsive disorder, and posttraumatic stress disorder are emotional problems of childhood involving anxiety. Oppositional behavior, hyperactivity, and conduct disturbance are behavioral problems of childhood. Enuresis and encopresis are elimination problems; along with abnormal eating, sleeping, sexual, and motor behaviors, they are childhood problems in physical functioning.

Pages 450–456 •

Answers 1, B; 2, C; 3, A; 4, D

3. The following is a common disorder of childhood:

A. autistic disorder
B. major depressive disorder
C. conduct disorder
D. Tourette's disorder

Discussion: More than 5% of children may have conduct disorder. Autistic disorder and Tourette's disorder are rare, affecting fewer than 5 children in 10,000. Major depressive disorder is rare in childhood, occurring in about 1% to 2% of children.

Pages 453–456, Table 20–6 (p. 457) •

Answer C

4. The following disorder is more common among young girls than young boys:

A. reading disorder
B. separation anxiety disorder
C. oppositional defiant disorder
D. enuresis

Discussion: All childhood anxiety disorders are more common among girls than boys, except obsessive-compulsive disorder, which has an equal gender distribution. Most other childhood disorders including developmental disorders (reading disorder), behavioral disorders (oppositional defiant disorder), and elimination disorders (enuresis) are more common among boys than girls.

Pages 452–457, Table 20–6 •

Answer B

5. All of the following are characteristic of the development of adolescents **except**

A. attainment of sexual maturity
B. development of identity
C. development of values and morals
D. financial independence from family of origin

Discussion: Attainment of financial independence from the family of origin is rarely accomplished in modern Western societies before young adulthood.

Pages 456–460 •

Answer D

6. The following are all characteristic of adolescent depression **except:**

A. More girls are affected than boys.
B. Major depressive episodes rarely recur.
C. The outcome may be suicide.
D. Major depressive episodes are often accompanied by other mental disorders.

Discussion: Although 90% of adolescents with major depressive disorder should recover within 2 years, adolescents who have had an episode have an elevated risk of recurrence of mood disorders into young adulthood.

Pages 457–458 •

Answer B

7. An adolescent manifestation of the continuity of social anxiety across the life cycle is

A. social phobia
B. shy, inhibited temperament
C. alcohol abuse
D. avoidant personality disorder

Discussion: Shy, inhibited temperament during childhood predisposes to the development of social phobia during childhood or adolescence. Alcohol abuse is common in adolescence, but it is not a manifestation of social anxiety. Avoidant personality disorder may develop in adulthood if social anxiety becomes generalized into a pervasive, maladaptive style of avoidant behavior.

Page 458, Table 20–9 (p. 459) •

Answer A

8. The most common disorder of adolescence is

A. major depressive disorder
B. panic disorder
C. alcohol intoxication
D. bulimia nervosa

Discussion: Eighteen percent of 10th graders and 30% of 12th graders report that they have been intoxicated with alcohol in the past month. Major depressive disorder is common in adolescence but affects less than 10%. Although the most common age at onset for panic disorder is in adolescence, only about 1 in 200 adolescents will have panic disorder. The prevalence of bulimia nervosa is between 1% and 3% of adolescent and young adult women.

Pages 458–460, Table 20–10 •

Answer C

9. The following are all true of comorbidity in young adulthood **except:**

A. Comorbidity helps to account for the high prevalence of mental disorders in the United States.
B. Comorbidity may occur because one disorder develops as a complication of another.
C. Panic disorder, obsessive-compulsive disorder, eating disorders, substance-related disorders, and personality disorders are all frequently comorbid with major depressive disorder.
D. Comorbidity refers to the occurrence of independent psychopathological entities with distinctive etiologies, pathogenic mechanisms, or outcomes.

Discussion: Although comorbidity is common, whether comorbid "disorders" are actually independent entities remains to be determined.

Page 461 •

Answer D

For each numbered item, select the lettered heading most closely associated with it. Each letter may be selected once, more than once, or not at all.

10. Match the symptom with the disorder.

____ 1. instability of interpersonal relations and self-image, mood lability, and impulsivity	A. posttraumatic stress disorder
____ 2. isolation of memory and emotions from consciousness, disturbance in identity, and experiences of intense absorption	B. dissociative disorder
____ 3. reexperiencing, avoidance, and hyperarousal symptoms	C. bipolar II disorder
____ 4. hypomanic and major depressive episodes	D. borderline personality disorder

Discussion: Although these disorders may occur in association with one another, they can be distinguished by their core defining features.

Pages 462–464 •

Answers 1, D; 2, B; 3, A; 4, C

11. Good prognostic features in schizophrenia include **all but one** of the following:

A. good premorbid adjustment
B. acute onset
C. male gender
D. family history of mood disorder

Discussion: Female patients with schizophrenia have a better prognosis than do male patients.

Pages 465–466, Table 20–14 •

Answer C

12. Multiple cognitive deficits including memory impairment and aphasia, apraxia, agnosia, or disturbance in executive functioning due to a progressive degenerative central nervous system process are characteristic of

A. delirium
B. dementia of the Alzheimer's type
C. vascular dementia
D. depression-induced cognitive impairment

Discussion: The hallmark of delirium is a disturbance of consciousness, with reduced ability to focus, sustain, or shift attention. Although the clinical features of Alzheimer's dementia and vascular dementia may be the same, the former is due to a degenerative central nervous system process and the latter to cerebrovascular disease. Depression-induced cognitive impairment of "pseudodementia" is usually not as severe as a true dementia, is caused by depression, and is usually reversible with appropriate treatment of the depression.

Pages 469–470 •

Answer B

CHAPTER

21 Clinical Evaluation and Treatment Planning: A Multimodal Approach

Francine Cournos • Deborah L. Cabaniss

For each numbered item, select the lettered heading most closely associated with it. Each letter may be selected once, more than once, or not at all.

1. Match the description with the test.

____ 1. used as Axis V in DSM-IV diagnosis	A. Bender Gestalt Test
____ 2. part of the mental status examination	B. educational background
____ 3. screens for neuropsychiatric impairment	C. Global Assessment of Functioning Scale
____ 4. part of the personal history	D. Overt Aggression Scale
____ 5. used to establish psychiatric diagnosis	E. rate of speech
____ 6. part of the comprehensive treatment plan	F. rehabilitation assessment
	G. Structured Clinical Interview for DSM-IV (SCID)

Discussion: Each component of the psychiatric evaluation is well defined. Specialized psychological and neuropsychological tests are usually reserved for situations in which there is uncertainty as to a patient's diagnosis, cognitive capacity, or psychological functioning. The Bender Gestalt Test involves copying a set of diagrams and can be useful in assessing central nervous system impairment. Structured instruments and rating scales have been developed primarily for research in which investigators need to compare and quantify findings as well as measure response to interventions. Most practicing psychiatrists do not regularly use such scales, but some, such as the Global Assessment of Functioning Scale, have become part of routine practice.

Pages 479–480, 483–484, Table 21–10 •

Answers 1, C; 2, E; 3, A; 4, B; 5, G; 6, F

2. A test that can assess the metabolism of glucose in the brain is

A. computed tomography (CT)
B. lumbar puncture
C. magnetic resonance imaging (MRI)
D. positron emission tomography (PET)
E. serum blood glucose level

Discussion: PET scans are used only for research purposes at present. Compared with MRI and CT, which convey information only about brain structure, PET scanning allows the analysis of brain functioning that is represented on a visual image of actual brain structure. Multiple timed images are necessary in this technology. The injection of radio-labeled organic compounds and the tracking of their metabolism is the essential distinctive feature of PET and single-photon emission computed tomography (SPECT).

Pages 490–492 •

Answer D

3. A risk factor for human immunodeficiency virus (HIV) infection is

A. having vaginal intercourse without a condom
B. hugging a gay man who injected drugs
C. living in the same household as a patient with acquired immunodeficiency syndrome (AIDS)
D. receiving insect bites in a geographical area endemic for HIV
E. sharing food with an HIV-infected person

Discussion: Careful elicitation of the medical and substance abuse history involves a correct working understanding of modes of transmission of HIV. Misconceptions about the possibility of acquiring HIV by casual contact are the most common misunderstandings about infection. HIV either is involved as a cause of neuropsychiatric disorders or can co-occur with certain psychiatric disorders such as substance dependence.

Page 487, Table 21–5 (p. 480) •

Answer A

4. Completed suicide is associated with all of the following **except**

A. alcohol use
B. female gender
C. intractable pain
D. older age
E. recent psychiatric hospitalization

Discussion: Women attempt suicide more frequently than men do, but they complete suicide less often. There are certain demographic and epidemiologic risk factors for suicide. However, there is no substitute for a careful individualized assessment because of course any person can complete suicide regardless of risk factors. The most consistent predictor of future suicidal behavior is a prior history of such behavior.

Pages 492–493, Tables 21–18, 21–19 •

Answer B

5. Predictors of violence include all of the following **except**

A. delirium
B. history of head injury
C. male gender
D. older age
E. unemployment

Discussion: Unlike suicidal individuals, most people who commit violent acts have not been diagnosed with a mental illness. Most commonly, there are substance-related diagnoses. Conduct disorder and antisocial personality disorder involve violent behavior as a matter of definition. Young men are the group most often involved in violent acts. Past behavior is also the best predictor of future violence as with suicidal individuals.

Page 493, Table 21–20 (p. 494) •

Answer D

6. Abnormalities of speech, thinking, and perception are most pronounced in

A. borderline personality disorder
B. bulimia nervosa
C. Huntington's disease
D. major depression
E. schizophrenia

Discussion: Disturbances of speech, thinking, perception, and self-experience are common in psychotic states, which can be seen in patients with such diagnoses as schizophrenia and mania as well as in central nervous system dysfunction caused by substance use or a medical condition.

Page 495 •

Answer E

7. Abnormalities of consciousness and orientation would most often be found in

A. bipolar I disorder
B. delirium due to a general medical condition
C. depersonalization disorder
D. panic disorder with agoraphobia
E. schizophrenia

Discussion: The combination of disturbances of consciousness, orientation, and memory is most typically associated with delirium. Delirium is usually due to a general medical condition or a substance use disorder.

Page 494–495 •

Answer B

CHAPTER

22 Neuropsychological Testing

David Taylor

1. The finding of "organicity"

A. is a highly precise finding
B. does not fit current concepts in contemporary neuropsychology
C. reflects specific localizable manifestations of brain disease
D. is the result of thorough state-of-the-art neuropsychological testing
E. is not frequently associated with confounding factors

Discussion: The psychodiagnostic test batteries employed until the 1970s that psychiatrists would request attempted to determine the presence or absence of organicity on the basis of certain pathognomonic signs. Whereas there was some value in such a process clinically, it was limited on empirical and conceptual grounds. Many of the "organic" test impairments were associated with confounding irrelevant factors, such as poor motivation, low IQ, or psychosis. Many manifestations of brain damage, such as language deficits and memory problems, were not reflected on the single visual-motor test typically used to assess organicity. The basic assumption underlying the concept, i.e., that brain damage was unitary, was faulty. This concept has been gradually replaced by the neuropsychological approach.

Page 498 •

Answer B

2. All neuropsychological approaches assess some aspects of

A. intelligence, reasoning, and abstraction
B. attention, "executive," and self-control functions
C. learning and memory
D. language, perceptual, and constructional tasks
E. all of the above

Discussion: Comprehensive test batteries examine all of the above as well as subsets of the above categories. Sensory and motor function are also assessed. These tests are long because the human brain-behavior relationship is complex. Test data are interpreted in the context of many factors including the age, sex, education, and handedness of the patient. The neuropsychological evaluation covers the same functions as the mental status examination used by psychiatrists and neurologists but in a more elaborate, deep, and quantified manner.

Pages 499–500 •

Answer E

3. Reasons to consider neuropsychological evaluation for psychiatric patients include all of the following **except**

A. It is much less expensive than neuroimaging, such as magnetic resonance imaging.
B. It is less invasive than procedures such as computed tomography or magnetic resonance imaging with contrast or lumbar puncture.
C. It yields not only information about differential diagnosis but also a profile of adaptive strengths and weaknesses.
D. Disorders such as Alzheimer's disease do not have reliable and valid laboratory tests that aid in diagnosis.
E. Extremely subtle distinctions are possible to elucidate between overlapping clinical psychiatric syndromes.

Discussion: In considering neuropsychological testing referrals, one needs to consider alternative modalities of neurodiagnostic evaluation. Neuropsychological testing is labor-intensive and is therefore expensive. It is less invasive and therefore may be safer and less threatening to some patients. Overlapping syndromes such as schizophrenia and the schizophreniform psychoses associated with temporal lobe epilepsy can best be distinguished by neuropsychological testing.

Page 500, Tables 22–1, 22–4 (p. 499) •

Answer A

4. Reitan has articulated four types of analyses that neuropsychologist use to evaluate neuropsychological data. Which of the following is **not** one of these four basic principles?

A. level of performance
B. left-right comparisons
C. pathognomonic signs
D. differential patterns
E. process approach

Discussion: According to Reitan, the neuropsychologist evaluates level of performance, the absolute deviation and dispersion of individual test scores compared with normative expectancies; left-right comparisons made on sensory, perceptual, and motor performances; pathognomonic signs, special features of poor performance suggestive of discrete disorders; and differential patterns, large arrays of test profiles that are predictions of disease or damage. The process approach describes another tradition of test interpretation that includes all of the above.

Page 503 •

Answer E

5. Which of the following neuropsychological tests has been used to demonstrate that most patients with schizophrenia have cognitive deficits consistent with those seen in patients with frontal network dysfunction?

A. Boston Naming Test
B. Boston Diagnostic Aphasia Examination
C. Wisconsin Card Sorting Test
D. Mini-Mental State Examination
E. Wechsler Adult Intelligence Scale–Revised

Discussion: The Wisconsin Card Sorting Test, which assesses the capacity to shift set, has been used to demonstrate a pattern of cognitive deficits in schizophrenia that relate to impaired executive functioning.

Page 503 •

Answer C

CHAPTER

23 Consciousness, Orientation, and Memory

Keith H. Claypoole • Gary J. Tucker

1. Hypervigilance is a level of consciousness that

A. is frequently observed in psychiatric disorders, such as agitated depression, and paranoid conditions
B. has been characterized as a key component of posttraumatic stress disorder
C. may be induced by drugs such as amphetamines
D. all of the above
E. none of the above

Discussion: Hypervigilance is a level of consciousness in which response to stimuli is increased; an individual may respond in an almost random manner or be unable to focus attention.

Page 509, Table 23–2 (p. 510) •

Answer D

2. Partial alterations in consciousness are apparent in

A. catatonia and akinetic mutism or "locked-in" syndrome
B. dissociative identity and conversion disorders and hypnotic trances
C. memory disorders characterized by retrograde amnesia
D. mild to moderate levels of mental retardation
E. distinct neuropathological lesions in the central nervous system

Discussion: Partial alterations in consciousness may represent both normal and psychopathological conditions. Dissociative identity disorder, dissociative fugue, hypnotic trance, and conversion disorder would all be classified as partial alterations of consciousness, in which consciousness of the body or identity is separated from awareness but the remaining ability to relate to the world is intact.

Pages 510–511, Table 23–1 •

Answer B

3. The traditionally hypothesized model of memory as a temporally based storage system postulates three memory stages consisting of

A. short-term, long-term, and immediate memory
B. sensory memory, motor memory, and perspective memory
C. episodic memory, semantic memory, and procedural memory
D. registration, retention, and recall
E. sensory memory, short-term memory, and long-term memory

Discussion: In the temporally based storage model of memory, information is input primarily through visual or auditory systems, where it is briefly maintained for up to several seconds before being transferred to short-term memory storage. In short-term storage, elaboration strategies such as rehearsal increase the likelihood of memory consolidation into long-term memory.

Pages 511–513, Figure 23–2 •

Answer E

4. Procedural memory is

A. the explicit ability to report facts and events of everyday life
B. predicated on the integrity of the medial temporal regions
C. the implicit ability to perform motor, perceptual, and cognitive skills
D. prominently impaired in Korsakoff's syndrome
E. all of the above

Discussion: Procedural memories involve the implicit ability to learn cognitive or behavioral-motor skills that are not accessible as specific facts, are not stored with respect to specific time or place, and do not require the integrity of the medial temporal regions that explicit declarative memory requires.

Page 512 •

Answer C

5. Amnestic disorders due to temporal lobe damage have been associated with conditions such as

A. viral encephalitis
B. degenerative neurological disorders
C. traumatic brain injury
D. B and C only
E. A, B, and C

Discussion: The critical importance of the medial temporal lobe regions in memory functioning has been demonstrated historically from early surgical cases involving temporal lobe resection. Lesions of medial temporal structures that occur in a wide variety of neuropathological conditions, including viral encephalitis, degenerative neurological disorders, traumatic head injury, posterior artery occlusions, and stroke, are associated with memory impairment.

Page 513 •

Answer E

6. Disturbance of memory functioning is

A. consistently organic in origin due to lesions from head injury, stroke, and neoplasms
B. readily diagnosed with a Mini-Mental State Examination
C. rarely displayed by the patients presenting with psychiatric disturbances
D. sometimes transient because of lethargic conditions or confusional states
E. typically independent of attentional capacity

Discussion: Memory disturbances are often the primary initial complaint of the early organic brain disorder, but not all memory difficulties are organic in origin because psychiatric patients often display memory dysfunction. Differential diagnosis of memory disturbance is difficult in the early stages and often requires additional evaluation, such as neuropsychological examination as well as integration from other sources of information. Transient memory difficulties may arise from inattention and hypervigilant, agitated, lethargic, or confusional states.

Page 513 •

Answer D

7. The Wechsler Adult Intelligence Scale–Revised (WAIS-R)

A. is a standard instrument for a clinical assessment of intelligence for individuals between the ages of 21 and 55 years
B. is composed of verbal and nonverbal subtests that are robust and resistant to decline from medical and psychiatric disorders
C. has a mean of 100 and a standard deviation of 15, which would predict that two thirds of the population in the United States has a Full-Scale IQ between 85 and 115
D. consists of six verbal subtests, which primarily measure nondominant hemisphere functioning, and five visual-spatial subtests, which measure dominant hemisphere functioning
E. is an exact quantitative measure, which can precisely pinpoint the level of intelligence at which a patient is functioning

Discussion: The WAIS-R was normed with a clinical assessment of intelligence for patients between 16 and 74 years old. Verbal subtests of Digit Span and Arithmetic rely heavily on attention and concentration abilities, and they are typically considered sensitive to brain injury in either hemisphere as well as attentional disturbance from psychiatric disorder. Visual-spatial abilities are generally more susceptible to variability or decline in cases of medical or psychiatric disorders. Verbal subtests are typically considered to primarily measure dominant hemisphere functioning; visual-spatial subtests are associated more with nondominant hemisphere functioning. Because of the standard error of measurement of the WAIS-R, an IQ score should be considered an index of an approximate level of intelligence because many medical and psychiatric conditions may adversely affect measured levels of intelligence.

Pages 514–515, Table 23–3 •

Answer C

8. In clinical evaluations that attempt to distinguish primary neurological disorders from primary psychiatric disorders:

A. Identical symptoms between patients may be secondary to a variety of causes.
B. A longitudinal history of a symptom's manifestation is often the best way to differentiate the cause of the symptom.
C. A history of prior psychiatric disorders and the presence of a family history of mental illness should be considered.
D. Cognitive dysfunction originating from a psychological origin is often associated with a pattern of inconsistent performance, decreased social skills, and the patient's intense concern over cognitive decline.
E. All of the above

Discussion: Answers A, B, C, and D are all important considerations in making a differential diagnosis between neurological and primary psychiatric disorders.

Page 515 •

Answer E

9. In the clinical evaluation of intelligence and memory:

A. The determination of subtle cognitive deficits in intelligence or memory can be reliably determined by a bedside evaluation.
B. Adults can be expected to demonstrate a capacity to repeat six numbers forward and five numbers backward to demonstrate intact remote memory functions.
C. Deficits in visual-spatial functioning are frequently evident from a patient's reduced ability to provide a linear and sequential history.
D. Verbal functions are often better preserved than visual-spatial functions in cases of diffuse or generalized brain damage.
E. Fugue states and amnesia related to traumatic or psychosocial precipitants typically have a gradual onset and progressive course of increasing memory deficits.

Discussion: Reliable determination of subtle or specific deficits in intelligence and memory typically requires more detailed neuropsychological testing than can be conducted at the bedside. Repetition of digits forward and backward provides indication of recent memory (registration) capacity. Deficits in visual-spatial functioning may not be readily apparent, should be closely evaluated with additional measures, and do not necessarily show a relationship to the way in which a patient relates his or her history. Amnesia and fugue states related to emotional changes associated with traumatic or psychosocial precipitants usually have a clear onset, and the impairment may benefit the affected individual either consciously or unconsciously.

Pages 515–516 •

Answer D

CHAPTER

24 Alterations of Speech, Thought, Perception, and Self-experience

Ralph E. Hoffman • Thomas H. McGlashan

1. What differentiates derailment (or loose associations) from flight of ideas?

A. Shifts in frame of reference are more idiosyncratic and difficult to follow in instances of derailment.
B. Loose associations reflect a sustained inability to coherently elaborate on a theme or topic, a competence that is retained in patients exhibiting flight of ideas.
C. Flight of ideas tends to be accompanied by pressured speech.
D. All of the above
E. None of the above

Discussion: In flight of ideas, the speaker seems capable of fleshing out particular themes or topics in a given frame of reference. In loosening of associations, there is a loss of the ability to elaborate on any topic and an overlapping of frames of reference.

Pages 518–519 •

Answer D

2. Which group of speakers never produces formal thought disorder?

A. patients with personality disorder
B. patients with depression
C. patients with cyclothymia
D. normal speakers
E. none of the above

Discussion: Formal thought disorder is generally associated with the more severe psychiatric illnesses but does not inevitably occur in conditions such as schizophrenia, mania, or substance-induced disorders. Milder examples of formal thought disorder are observed in an even wider range of psychiatric illnesses.

Page 519 •

Answer E

3. What factor differentiates Wernicke's aphasic speech disorder from schizophrenic speech disorder?

A. loose associations
B. frequent production of neologisms-paraphasias and paragrammatisms
C. inability to notice and correct speech errors
D. none of the above

Discussion: There are similarities between the speech disorders of aphasic and schizophrenic individuals. Both can produce nonwords called neologisms in psychiatry and paraphasias in neurology. Also shared are word-finding difficulties, paragrammatisms (utterances in which word order or word combinations may deviate from syntactical norms), and word salad. Prolonged social isolation or sustained alienation coupled with bizarre ideation may lead severely psychotic schizophrenic patients to disregard linguistic conventions. Aphasic patients will persistently deviate from normal speech by producing nonwords and ungrammatical word combinations.

Page 519 •

Answer B

4. What finding is useful in differentiating a delusion from an obsession?

A. perseveration on the same theme, fear, or idea
B. reflects concerns, fears, or beliefs that are irrationally based
C. the patient knows that her or his concerns, fears, or beliefs are irrationally based
D. all of the above
E. none of the above

Discussion: Patients who are obsessed are intensely preoccupied, as are those with delusions; however, the former group are able to recognize, even if only for a moment, that concern is not rational. There is no such capacity for reality testing in a delusional individual.

Pages 520–521 •

Answer C

5. What finding is most useful in differentiating paranoia from a phobia?

A. danger is felt to be due primarily to human intentions rather than nonhuman environment
B. accompanied by fear or anxiety
C. may reach delusional proportions
D. none of the above

Discussion: Phobias reflect fearfulness about the nonhuman environment. Paranoia, which can become much more encompassing, involves a suspiciousness of the actions and motives of others.

Pages 522–523, Table 24–2 •

Answer A

6. A hypnotic state can be accompanied by

A. hallucination
B. disorders of will
C. amnesia
D. all of the above

Discussion: Hypnosis involves the induction of a trance state that is a mixture of intense absorption with one idea or activity, dissociation from other experiences and sensations, and heightened suggestibility to instruction. In such states, there is a liability to experience pseudohallucinations. The enhanced suggestibility mimics a disorder of will.

Page 525 •

Answer D

7. What finding is the least useful in differentiating patients with schizophrenia from those with dissociative identity disorder?

A. patient hears "voices"
B. disorganized speech
C. inappropriate affect
D. amnesia
E. catatonic symptoms

Discussion: Voices are described by patients who dissociate, and yet they differ from the hallucinations of schizophrenic patients. In dissociative states, these hallucinations are more conversational than idiosyncratic.

Page 524 •

Answer A

8. Recurrent or repetitive thought content is not characteristic of

A. delusions
B. flight of ideas
C. obsessions
D. depressive ruminations

Discussion: In flight of ideas, there is by definition a ceaseless change of content.

Pages 519, 521, Table 24–2 (p. 523) •

Answer B

9. Poverty of speech and poverty of content of speech are similar in that

A. both are negative symptoms
B. less meaning is expressed
C. both are consistent with the diagnosis of schizophrenia
D. mutism is the extreme case
E. all of the above

Discussion: Poverty of speech in which there is absence of spontaneous speech can be seen in schizophrenia, depression, and aphasia. Extreme poverty of speech is described as mutism. If there is perseveration and vagueness together, poverty of content of speech is also noted.

Pages 519–520 •

Answer E

10. Dissociation is a major aspect of

A. thought control
B. waxy flexibility
C. delusions of passivity
D. body dysmorphic disorder
E. all of the above
F. none of the above

Discussion: Dissociation is a complex phenomenon that involves the splitting off of thoughts, feelings, or behaviors from integrated awareness.

Page 525 •

Answer F

11. Autotopagnosia, astereognosis, and prosopagnosia all involve a loss of

A. sense of self
B. handedness
C. recognition
D. reactivity
E. awareness of illness

Discussion: Agnosias involve massive deficits in self-experience. In autotopagnosia, there is denial of hemiparesis or blindness secondary to right parietal lesions. In astereognosis, objects cannot be recognized by touch. In prosopagnosia, faces cannot be identified.

Page 526 •

Answer C

CHAPTER

25 Emotions

Robert Kohn • Martin B. Keller

For each numbered item, select the lettered heading most closely associated with it. Each letter may be selected once, more than once, or not at all.

1. Match the definition with the correct term.

____ 1. observable behavior of emotion	A. mood
____ 2. a pervasive and sustained emotion	B. affect
____ 3. inability to describe emotion	C. alexithymia
____ 4. mood within the normal range	D. apathy
	E. euthymia

Discussion: Mood is a pervasive and sustained emotional state and may not be readily discernible or observed but may need to be reported. Affect is the observable behavior of emotion and may fluctuate. Alexithymia is the inability of individuals to describe or be aware of their emotions or mood. Apathy is a dulled emotional tone associated with detachment or indifference. Euthymia is a mood that is considered to be within the normal range.

Pages 529–530, Table 25–2 •

Answers 1, B; 2, A; 3, C; 4, E

2. Match the diagnosis with the associated symptom:

____ 1. social phobia	A. situationally bound panic attacks
____ 2. acute stress disorder	B. unexpected panic attacks
____ 3. panic disorder	C. excessive worrying
____ 4. generalized anxiety disorder	D. compulsions to relieve anxiety
	E. reexperiencing

Discussion: Panic attacks as an expression of anxiety can be present in nearly all the anxiety disorders. There are three types of panic attacks: unexpected, situationally predisposed, and situationally bound. Panic disorder requires that unexpected panic attacks be present. Situationally bound panic attacks are characteristic of social phobia and specific phobia. The anxiety of generalized anxiety disorder is characterized as an excessive worrying often about routine life circumstances. Reexperiencing of a traumatic event, increased arousal and avoidance of the stimuli associated with the trauma, is characteristic of the anxiety symptoms seen in the acute stress disorder and posttraumatic stress disorder. The anxiety in obsessive-compulsive disorder is the obsession, and the compulsion is the behavior produced to relieve the anxiety.

Pages 531–533, Table 25–10 •

Answers 1, A; 2, E; 3, B; 4, C

3. Match the terms.

____ 1. anhedonia	A. psychological temperature
____ 2. demoralization	B. lack of interest
____ 3. learned helplessness	C. inability to initiate an adaptive response
____ 4. Cloninger's vulnerability model	D. inaccurate cognition
	E. heritable personality traits

Discussion: Demoralization is a term that describes what symptom checklists measure. This is a condition of low self-esteem, helplessness, hopelessness, sadness, and anxiety that is a continuum from normalcy to depression. It is at times described as the psychological temperature. Anhedonia is lack of interest or pleasure. This is a symptom of a major depressive episode and must be present in individuals who have major depressive disorder but do not express a depressed mood. Learned helplessness is one of the cognitive theories of depression developed from animal models. In the learned helplessness condition, the animal is unable to initiate an adaptive response. Another cognitive theory is that of Beck. Beck believed that the development of depression is due to the individual's having inaccurate cognitions. There are a number of models of personality that have attempted to explain the development of depressed mood. Cloninger used a vulnerability model that claimed that neurobiology interacts with heritable personality traits.

Pages 533–535, Table 25–11 •

Answers 1, B; 2, A; 3, C; 4, E

4. Match the definition with the term or syndrome.

____ 1. poverty of speech	A. abulia
____ 2. loss of will to act	B. alogia
____ 3. exaggerated emotional expression	C. dysprosody
____ 4. disorder of affective and inflectional speech	D. blunted affect
	E. pseudobulbar palsy

Discussion: Abulia is a severe state of apathy considered to be a loss of the will to act. Alogia is poverty of speech manifested by brief, laconic, and empty replies. Dysprosody is a disorder of prosody, the affective and inflectional coloring of speech. Individuals with dysprosody have difficulty in communicating their emotion. Pseudobulbar palsy is a neuropsychiatric disorder characterized by exaggerated emotional expression with unintended laughing or unmotivated crying. The emotion expressed is unrelated to the mood or in disproportionate intensity to the emotion experienced. This is mostly a result of cerebrovascular accidents involving the cortex or the internal capsule. The affect associated with significant reduction in the intensity of emotional expression is a blunted affect.

Pages 537–538, Table 25–14 •

Answers 1, B; 2, A; 3, E; 4, C

Choose the one best answer for the following questions.

5. The following is a true statement about the basic patterns of emotional expression:

A. Emotional expression varies across cultures.
B. Emotional expression varies with age.
C. Emotional expression is fully hard-wired.
D. Deep brain structures have a limited role in emotion.
E. Emotions can be combined.

Discussion: The basic patterns of emotional expression are present at birth and vary little with age or across cultures. This is most clearly seen in the facial expressions and emotions of infants. Facial expressions of infants and adults for certain emotions are similar. Emotional expression is hard-wired to an extent, but this is an incomplete view. The evidence for the lack of a fully hard-wired explanation of emotional expression is found in the behavioral, experiential, and somatic or physiological components of emotion often not being correlated. The areas of the brain mostly associated with emotion are the phylogenetically more ancient and primitive, the deep brain structures. The cortex is also involved in the expression of emotion. The 10 basic emotions that Izard identified can be combined to produce different behavioral reactions and can be modified through learning and maturation.

Pages 528–529, Table 25–1 •

Answer E

6. The following best describes a feature of the state-trait dichotomy of anxiety:

A. It is a stimulus-oriented theory.
B. Trait anxiety is stable over time.
C. State anxiety is a personality feature.
D. The stimulus must be an environmental source.
E. The state component has not been validated.

Discussion: The state-trait dichotomy of anxiety is an outgrowth of the response-oriented theories. The anxiety response is the same despite the stimulus. The stimulus-oriented theory states that stimulus events serve to initiate the emotional response. State anxiety is momentary, whereas trait anxiety is stable over time and impervious to stress. Trait anxiety may be a personality feature, whereby the individual is consistently anxious despite the situation. This dichotomy has been well validated and has been shown to be true for either intrapsychic or environmental stimulus.

Page 531, Figure 25–1 (p. 532) •

Answer B

7. The following condition is considered within the realm of normal experience in a pleasurable mood state and is not a symptom of a manic mood:

A. euphoria with sexual pleasure
B. affect with loud, difficult-to-interrupt speech
C. indiscriminate enthusiasm for occupational interactions
D. infectious mood
E. expansive mood

Discussion: The mood of a manic or hypomanic individual is characterized as euphoric, unusually good, cheerful, or high. It may be expansive, be excessive, and have an infectious quality. There is indiscriminate enthusiasm for interpersonal, sexual, and occupational interactions. The speech during a manic mood state is characterized as pressured, loud, rapid, and difficult to interrupt. Euphoria is part of normal experience as well. Feelings of euphoria can be achieved during sexual pleasure.

Pages 536–537 •

Answer A

8. In evaluating the affect of a psychiatric patient, the following is an important consideration:

A. The duration of the affect is of little importance.

B. The focus is mainly on facial expressions.
C. One observes that the underlying affect is being suppressed.
D. The reported emotional state is what really matters.
E. Behavioral gestures may mislead the interviewer.

Discussion: In evaluating affect, the quality, duration, appropriateness, intensity, range, and control over the affect should all be considered. Because adults frequently are capable of controlling facial expression in attempts to intentionally or unintentionally suppress their affect, other behavioral gestures and facial expressions should be monitored. Affect is the observed emotional state, not the reported emotional state. Mood, which is more stable than affect, is reported. The observed affect and the reported mood do not necessarily coincide.

Pages 529–530, Tables 25–3, 25–4 •

Answer C

CHAPTER

26 Physical Signs and Symptoms

Philip R. Muskin

1. A 43-year-old man presents with complaints of indigestion, fatigue, too little energy to engage in pleasurable activities, and drinking a beer nightly to aid in sleep. He believes his symptoms are secondary to lack of appetite and poor intake of food. He is requesting vitamin supplementation to return him to his former state of health. The diagnosis of a mood disorder would be compatible with which of the following information?

A. a recent immigrant from Beijing
B. someone from the Dominican Republic, living in New York City for 10 years, but who has never learned to speak English
C. a native Californian whose great-grandparents came to the United States in the 1800s
D. a businessman visiting from England
E. all of the above

Discussion: Patients with depression frequently present with physical symptoms including fatigue, insomnia, lack of energy, and poor appetite. Patients with insomnia will often attribute their symptoms to their lack of sleep. Such symptom sets are not culturally determined in their entirety.

Page 542 •

Answer E

2. A 61-year-old woman comes to a medical clinic after having fallen down and gives a history of 20 years of "palpitations." She claims to have briefly lost consciousness, but this cannot be confirmed. Her pulse is regular at 90, her blood pressure is 150/85. She takes no medication regularly except for 5 mg of diazepam, which she takes "as needed." The appropriate steps to take would include all of the following **except**

A. 24-hour Holter monitor
B. thyroid function test
C. referral to psychiatry clinic
D. urine toxicology screen
E. electrocardiogram

Discussion: Patients, such as the one described above, who have a variety of psychiatric and physical symptoms may be intoxicated or in withdrawal. Even though such a patient may appear typically anxious, the physician must have a strong suspicion that the individual might well have a medical condition. Such a diagnosis can be made or refuted only by careful medical and psychiatric evaluation and not just a psychiatric workup alone.

Pages 540–541, 544 •

Answer C

3. A patient complains of nervousness, some shaking of the hands, difficulty falling asleep, poor concentration, and irritability. These symptoms could be referable to which of the following medical conditions?

A. hyperthyroidism
B. multiple sclerosis
C. hypoparathyroidism
D. AIDS
E. all of the above

Discussion: Numerous medical disorders have behavioral components. There may be a direct effect of the disorder on the patient's brain by alterations of blood flow, infections, or parenchymal disease. Medical illness also has global effects on the body, such as fatigue. Endocrine and cardiovascular disorders are commonly the cause of psychiatric symptoms. In a review of 658 consecutive psychiatric outpatients, careful medical evaluation revealed that 9.1% of the psychiatric cases had a medical illness that produced the psychiatric symptoms.

Page 543 •

Answer E

4. A 25-year-old man presents to the clinic requesting surgery to correct a defect in his nose. He reports that his nose is unusually large and causes him considerable problems in relationships with other people who make fun of him. His activities are extremely curtailed by his concerns about his appearance; he thinks about his nose all day and frequently cannot fall asleep at night because of his ruminations about how this physical defect has ruined his life. He accepts that not all people find his nose unsightly but believes that most people think he is unattractive. The diagnosis that fits his symptom picture best is

A. obsessive-compulsive disorder
B. somatization disorder
C. Body dysmorphic disorder
D. delusional disorder, somatic type
E. hypochondriasis

Discussion: Body dysmorphic disorder is a preoccupation with a defect of physical appearance in an individual who has a consensually normal appearance. The distinction from delusional disorder, somatic type, and obsessive-compulsive disorder can be difficult in some patients.

Page 547 •

Answer C

5. A college student complains of anxiety, tremulousness, outbursts of crying, and fear of driving 3 weeks after an automobile accident in which she sustained no injuries of any type. The vehicle was destroyed but her air bag deployed, saving her life. Her thoughts are filled with what might have happened, and thoughts about the car that side-swiped her intrude into other activities. She has nightmares seeing her car smashing into the tree, from which she awakens in a sweat with palpitations and shortness of breath. At times, she sees the accident happening again, even when she is fully awake. Both her mother and her sister have been treated with desipramine for panic attacks. Her diagnosis is

A. panic disorder
B. posttraumatic stress disorder
C. generalized anxiety disorder
D. obsessive-compulsive disorder
E. brief psychotic disorder

Discussion: The classic symptoms of posttraumatic stress disorder are described above. This is one of the anxiety disorders and as such is associated with many of the physical symptoms of such disorders. It is important to distinguish signs from symptoms in the assessment of such a patient.

Pages 541–542, Table 26–1 •

Answer B

6. A confused, agitated patient cannot give a history that will aid in making a diagnosis. Vital signs are generally normal except for a heart rate of 100 and a blood pressure of 150/90. Which of the following findings is not valid to rule out withdrawal from a substance as the cause of the symptoms?

A. elevated white blood cell count
B. temperature of 39°C
C. negative urine toxicology screen
D. chest film with signs of consolidation in the right lower lobe
E. history that the patient is the head of a major corporation

Discussion: Patients who are withdrawing from a substance may well have a negative result of urine toxicological analysis as a matter of course. However, in cases of chronic substance abuse, particularly with alcohol, patients may have serum levels of alcohol that are, for them, too low to prevent withdrawal.

Page 544 •

Answer C

7. In the diagnostic decision regarding a patient who presents with a sudden inability to move the right hand, which of the following is **not** true as a component of the presentation of conversion disorders?

A. The person is distressed regarding the symptom.
B. There is no precipitant that can be found for the symptom.
C. The person seems unconcerned about the symptom.
D. The paralysis matches the known innervation of the hand.
E. There is a history of an injury during a sports activity during the same day.

Discussion: Patients with conversion disorder usually have symptoms in systems that are under voluntary control. They are not necessarily hysterical in their demeanor. Whereas some may seem unusually calm, others may be extremely distressed.

Pages 545–546 •

Answer B

8. A consultation is requested for an elderly patient who is alternatingly sedated and agitated, disoriented, hallucinating, and uncooperative. The patient is afebrile and has a normal electrocardiogram and a normal chest radiograph. The patient came from a nursing home before this admission. The papers from the nursing home have a diagnosis of "senile dementia." Which of the following needs to be evaluated as a possible cause of the patient's mental status?

A. infection

B. electrolyte abnormalities
C. medication effects
D. nutritional status
E. all of the above

Discussion: Elderly patients frequently manifest psychiatric symptoms as signs of an underlying medical condition. The recognition of delirium in such patients is essential.

Page 543 •

Answer E

CHAPTER

27 Behavior and Adaptive Functioning

Susan C. Vaughan • John M. Oldham

1. Which of the following is a precursor to personality?

A. temperament
B. capacity for adaptive functioning
C. defense mechanisms
D. adult development

Discussion: Temperament is the biological substrate that interacts with early development to shape personality. There is evidence of striking variation among neonates in their ability to tolerate frustration and in how susceptible to distress they are. Differences in temperament can make a baby "hard" or "easy" to his or her parents, thereby affecting the development of the relationships with caretakers.

Page 550 •

Answer A

2. All of the following influence the development of personality **except**

A. genetic factors
B. early life experiences
C. inborn temperament
D. adaptive functioning

Discussion: Adaptive functioning is a consequence of personality, not a factor that influences its development. Different personality styles give rise to different styles of coping and functioning in different people. In contrast, genetic factors, positive and negative early life experiences, and temperament affect the development of personality.

Page 550 •

Answer D

3. Categorical models of personality

A. are used in DSM-IV
B. evaluate the blend of traits that compose an individual's personality
C. do not involve diagnostic classification
D. are the same as dimensional models

Discussion: The DSM-IV diagnostic system for Axis II personality disorders is a categorical model in which a person is described as meeting or not meeting the criteria for a particular diagnosis. In contrast to dimensional models, categorical models do not attempt to capture the blend of traits a given individual possesses but rather decide whether a given disorder is present or absent. The five-factor model and Cloninger's seven-factor model are examples of dimensional classification systems for personality.

Pages 550–551, Tables 27–2, 27–3 •

Answer A

Directions for numbers 4 and 5: For each numbered item, select the lettered heading most closely associated with it. Each letter may be selected once, more than once, or not at all.

4. Match the trait with the appropriate model.

____ 1. novelty seeking, reward dependence, harm avoidance
____ 2. anxiety disorder, avoidant personality disorder
____ 3. neuroticism, extraversion, openness

A. five-factor model
B. Cloninger's seven-factor model
C. biogenic spectrum model

Discussion: Cloninger's seven-factor dimensional model of personality consists of four dimensions related to temperament (novelty seeking, reward dependence, harm avoidance, and persistence) and three related to character (self-directedness, cooperativeness, and self-transcendence). Siever and Davis' biogenic spectrum model of personality proposes that certain personality styles and disorders are associated with and are variants of various Axis I disorders. In this mode, Axis I anxiety disorders and Axis II avoidant personality disorders are seen as a spectrum. The five-factor model of personality is composed of the factors 1) neuroticism, 2) extraversion, 3) openness, 4) agreeableness, and 5) conscientiousness. Those with more obsessive personality styles typically score low on the factors of extraversion, openness, and agreeableness; those with more histrionic styles typically score low on conscientiousness and neuroticism.

Pages 551–552, Tables 27–2, 27–3, 27–4 •

Answers 1, B; 2, C; 3, A

5. Match the scale with its application.

____ 1. provides a means of assessing interpersonal behavior and functioning	A. Structural Analysis of Social Behavior (SASB)
____ 2. assesses domains of functioning: work; relationships with family, friends, and spouse or partner; and leisure.	B. Social Adjustment Scale (SAS)
	C. both
	D. neither

Discussion: Both measures assess interpersonal behavior. The SASB examines the typical focus of interpersonal contacts, the tone of a person's interactions with others, and whether the interaction is characterized by interdependence or independence. The SAS assesses the degree of overt fighting, friction, avoidance, and capacity for openness in a person's relationships with family, friends, and coworkers. The SAS is designed to provide an overview of the degree of impairment a person has in various domains of functioning, including 1) occupational functioning, 2) relationships with family and friends and spouse or romantic partner, and 3) how effectively a person uses and enjoys leisure time.

Pages 553–554, Table 27–5 •

Answers 1, C; 2, B

6. Those with impulsive behaviors

A. do not often have binge-like episodes of the behavior
B. tend to overestimate their chances of being caught
C. find the behaviors distinctly unpleasurable at the time
D. usually note a growing sense of tension that is relieved by the behavior
E. more frequently have high cerebrospinal fluid levels of serotonin metabolites

Discussion: Impulsive behaviors include pyromania, kleptomania, trichotillomania, pathological gambling, substance use, and paraphilias. These behaviors share common features, including that they often occur in binge-like episodes; that patients tend to underestimate the risk of being caught; and that the behaviors are initially pleasurable, although patients may later be troubled by the behaviors as they reflect on them. The behaviors are pleasurable in part because they relieve a growing sense of tension that is lessened by the behavior. Thus, the behavior often provides relief from this tension. The biochemical defect most commonly associated with impulse-control disorders is low, not high, levels of serotonin metabolites in the cerebrospinal fluid.

Pages 557–558 •

Answer D

7. Compulsive behaviors

A. almost never co-occur with impulse-control disorders in the same person
B. include food-restricting behavior in anorexics
C. seem purposeful to the individual at the time
D. rarely occur in response to aberrant patterns of thought
E. include pathological gambling

Discussion: Food-restricting behavior is an example of a compulsive behavior in patients who are struggling to control their eating. They tend to co-occur in patients who already have impulse-control disorders and may similarly involve a defect in serotoninergic pathways. Compulsive behaviors such as hand washing or compulsive masturbation often seem nonsensical to individuals who are nonetheless compelled to do them anyway and are often the result of obsession thoughts (e.g., compulsive hand washing in response to the obsession thought that one's hands are contaminated).

Pages 559–560 •

Answer B

8. Avoidant behaviors

A. are always positive responses to negative experiences
B. are rarely linked to a specific situation
C. involve attempts to avoid fear or panic
D. do not produce increased anticipatory anxiety
E. do not occur in children

Discussion: Avoidant behaviors such as school phobias in children and agoraphobia (fear of going outside alone) in adults are sometimes adaptive responses to negative experiences (i.e., avoiding an automated teller machine where one was robbed) but can also be negative or maladaptive responses (being unable to attend school because one fears having a panic attack while there). Most avoidant behaviors are initially linked to a specific experience or situation (i.e., having a panic attack in a tunnel), although they may generalize to other situations as the avoidance continues (i.e., beginning to fear crossing bridges as well). What is avoided in an avoidant behavior is the fear or panic a given situation causes, but a consequence of the avoidance is that the person begins to be more and more anxious, in effect teaching himself or herself to be afraid and to have a greater amount of anticipatory anxiety. School phobia is an example of an avoidant behavior that occurs during childhood.

Pages 560–561 •

Answer C

For each numbered item, select the lettered heading most closely associated with it. Each letter may be selected once, more than once, or not at all.

9. Match the following type of disorder to the behavior.

____ 1. suicide attempt by pill overdose
____ 2. agoraphobia
____ 3. trichotillomania (hair pulling)
____ 4. hand washing
____ 5. kleptomania
____ 6. excessive masturbation
____ 7. fear of spiders (arachnophobia)
____ 8. checking behaviors
____ 9. paraphilias

A. compulsive
B. impulsive
C. avoidant

Pages 557–561, Table 27-6 •

Answers 1, B; 2, C; 3, B; 4, A; 5, B; 6, A; 7, C; 8, A; 9, B

CHAPTER

28 Cultural Considerations in Psychopathology

David Taylor

1. The diagnosis and treatment of cognitive disorders

A. are not affected by cultural considerations
B. are influenced by socioeconomic, cultural, and ethnic variables
C. are remarkable for the finding of higher rates of Alzheimer's disease among the Chinese
D. are not affected by culture because the Mini-Mental State Examination is so objective

Discussion: Whereas cognitive disorders are not thought of as being culturally influenced syndromes because their biological basis is widely accepted, their presentation, epidemiology, evaluation, and management are shaped by socioeconomic, cultural, and ethnic variables. The prevalence rates of diseases of the brain are shaped by poverty, diet, and toxic exposures for which different nationalities are at risk. Culturally determined patterns of substance use and sexual behavior affect the rates of cognitive disorders caused by alcohol and human immunodeficiency virus. Chinese, Chinese-Americans, and African-Americans have been reported to have lower rates of Alzheimer's dementia.

Page 563 •

Answer B

2. Lifetime rates of alcoholism among Native Americans

A. are the same as those for other Americans
B. are less than those found in certain groups of Asians
C. are 23% in the Native American population
D. are spuriously elevated because of reporting biases

Discussion: Lifetime rates for alcoholism and substance abuse vary significantly across cultures. Rates vary from 23% among Native Americans to 0.45% among the population of Shanghai. Patterns of use, attitudes toward substance consumption, accessibility of the drug, physiological reactions to the same drug, and family norms and patterns all vary. Some factors, such as comorbidity patterns, nature of dependence syndromes, age at onset, and results of laboratory tests, are less affected by cultural factors.

Pages 563–564 •

Answer C

3. All of the following statements about schizophrenia are true **except**

A. catatonia is more common in India.
B. hebephrenia is more common in Japan.
C. the course of schizophrenia is markedly better in nonindustrialized countries.
D. perceptual alterations among distressed Puerto Ricans are rarely mistaken for schizophrenia.

Discussion: All of the above are true statements about the variation of schizophrenic phenomenology and course around the world. There is a higher rate of misdiagnosis of schizophrenia among patients from devalued and ethnic minority groups. Differences in cultural and gender-related conceptions regarding the expression of emotion complicate the assessment of flat affect; and culturally syntonic experiences may be mistaken for schizophrenic symptoms, such as hallucinations among bereaved Native Americans or perceptual alterations among Puerto Ricans.

Page 564 •

Answer D

4. The specific characteristics of the dysphoria of depressive illness vary cross-culturally, as which of the following examples illustrates?

A. Among the Hopi, irritability is frequently described.
B. Among Latinos, irritability, rage, and "nervousness" are prominent.
C. Among African-Americans, unique somatic complaints are common.
D. Studies of the Hopi show rates of somatic complaints equal to those of Cuban-Americans.

Discussion: The Hopi identify five indigenous syndromes related to depression. Feelings of guilt, shame, and sinfulness are separate experiences displaying distinct relationships to subtypes of depression. Unique somatic complaints such as "heat or water in the head" and "crawling sensation of worms and ants" are found in Nigerian cultures. A study comparing Puerto Ricans, Mexican-Americans, and Cuban-Americans on the Center for Epidemiologic Studies Depression (CES-D) Scale found that the women in all three groups tended to endorse depressive and somatic scale items together as a single factor significantly more often than men did.

Pages 564–565 •

Answer B

5. Examples of the cultural variation of anxiety disorders include all of the following **except:**

A. There is a higher rate of simple phobia, social phobia, and agoraphobia among African-Americans compared with whites.
B. Mexicans born in Mexico compared with those born in the United States show a markedly lower rate of anxiety disorders.
C. Japanese-Americans have a higher rate of panic disorder than do Americans of European descent.
D. Latinos experience a "culture-bound" type of anxiety disorder.

Discussion: The rate of anxiety disorders among African-Americans has been attributed to the effects of racial discrimination. Explanations for the differences in the rates of anxiety disorder between Mexicans and Mexican-Americans include selective migration and different thresholds for perceiving and reporting dysfunction. *Ataque de nervios* is an example of a syndrome with co-occurring anxiety, depression, and somatoform and dissociative symptoms among non-Western groups. The Japanese variant of this is known as *taijin kyofusho.*

Page 565 •

Answer C

6. Somatoform disorders are among the most problematical disorders from the perspective of international usage for all of the following reasons **except**

A. Many nosologies around the world do not distinguish between mood, anxiety, somatoform, and dissociative categories.
B. Idioms of distress in many societies rely on somatic complaints for the expression of nonpathological personal and social predicaments.
C. DSM-IV somatoform categories highlight symptoms relevant to all human organ systems, which is therefore an exhaustive list.
D. In most of the world, the degree to which symptoms are unexplained is difficult to ascertain because of the marked limitation of diagnostic tests and medical personnel.

Discussion: The symptoms listed in the DSM-IV system do not canvas the rich variety of somatic symptoms reported in other parts of the world, such as heat in the feet, chest, or head; "gas" that moves from the abdomen around the flank to the back; "brainache"; and feeling presences when alone.

Page 566 •

Answer C

7. Which of the following is **not** an example of a dissociative disorder?

A. *amok*
B. *ataque de nervios*
C. *indisposition*
D. *uu nung mo kiw ta*

Discussion: *Uu nung mo kiw ta* is an example of a Hopi depressive syndrome. Other dissociative conditions include Arctic *pibloktoq* and Bahamian "blacking out." Many indigenous illness syndromes around the world display salient features of pathological dissociation. Some of these syndromes are characterized by involuntary possession trance, which is distinguishable from dissociative identity disorder. Many of these disorders have been classified as culturally bound syndromes, and yet this is felt to be a limited and biased term given that Western psychiatry is itself culturally bound; therefore, the concept of "idiom of distress" has been put forth.

Pages 566–567, 568–569 •

Answer D

CHAPTER

29 Psychiatric Classification

Michael B. First • Allen Frances • Harold Alan Pincus

1. Which of the following is **not** a goal of the DSM-IV system of psychiatric classification?

A. to allow psychiatrists and researchers to communicate more effectively
B. to facilitate the management of psychiatric disorders
C. to educate patients and their families about the nature of their psychiatric conditions
D. to provide an all-encompassing list of those disorders that are worthy subjects of research

Discussion: Communication, management, and psychoeducation are all important goals of the DSM-IV classification system. DSM-IV represents a compendium of those psychiatric disorders for which the most solid data are available. Many disorders of potential research interest are not included as official categories because of lack of data. It is expected that additional research will ultimately determine whether including these disorders in future editions of the manual makes sense from the standpoint of clinical utility.

Page 572 •

Answer D

2. Which of the following is the main reason that DSM-IV did not adopt an etiological approach to classification?

A. lack of historical precedent
B. lack of precedent in other types of medical classifications
C. lack of firm understanding of the underlying etiology of mental disorders
D. lack of effective treatments for most mental disorders

Discussion: Given the lack of knowledge about the underlying etiology of mental disorders, an etiology-based system would have to be based on speculative theories linked to particular orientations, severely limiting their clinical utility and making them likely to become rapidly obsolete as we continue to gain more understanding about etiology.

Pages 572–573 •

Answer C

3. Which of the following is **not** an advantage of the descriptive syndromal approach to classification?

A. It is usable across theoretical orientations.
B. Syndromal definitions facilitate the understanding and treatment of mental disorders.
C. Syndromal definitions have a tendency to become reified.
D. Syndromal definitions provide a shorthand for clinical descriptions.

Discussion: One of the most unfortunate side effects of the DSM's descriptive system is the tendency for users to treat the syndromal definitions as if they truly represent disease entities. It is important for users of the manual to remember that the syndromal definitions represent only the state of the art as it existed during the time of the preparation of that version. It is expected that the syndromal definitions will continually evolve in accordance with our steadily increasing knowledge base about psychiatric disorders.

Page 573 •

Answer C

4. Which of the following statements about the early history of the DSM's classifications is true?

A. DSM-I was developed as an alternative to ICD-6, the first official international classification of mental disorders.
B. DSM-III was the first edition that contained diagnostic criteria.
C. The revision of DSM-III (which became DSM-III-R) was originally intended as a "fine-tuning" of DSM-III.
D. All of the above

Discussion: Each version of the *Diagnostic and Statistical Manual of Mental Disorders* (except DSM-III-R) was developed in response to (and in conjunction with) a new edition of the *International Statistical Classification of Diseases and Related Health Problems* (ICD): DSM-I with ICD-6, DSM-II with ICD-8, DSM-III with ICD-9, and DSM-IV with ICD-10. Diagnostic criteria were first introduced by DSM-III, and they greatly increased the reliability of DSM-III diagnoses compared with DSM-II diagnoses. DSM-III-R, although originally planned to be a minor updating of DSM-III, turned into a much more substantial revision.

Pages 573–574 •

Answer D

5. Which of the following statements is **not** true about the preparation of DSM-IV?

A. The goal of the DSM-IV revision process was modification and refinement rather than a reconceptualization.
B. The DSM-IV revision process was based on a systematic review of the empirical data.
C. Ten disorder-specific field trials were conducted as part of the empirical review process.
D. Expert opinion was given a higher priority than the review of empirical data.

Discussion: Expert consensus was the core of prior revision efforts because of the paucity of available empirical data at the time. The DSM-IV revision process had the advantage of the availability of a much larger knowledge base of empirical data. The cornerstone of the DSM-IV revision process was a comprehensive systematic review of this database so that all decisions would be maximally informed by the data.

Page 574 •

Answer D

6. Which of the five axes in the multiaxial system underwent the most significant change in DSM-IV?

A. Axis I
B. Axis III
C. Axis IV
D. Axis V

Discussion: In DSM-III-R, Axis IV was for rating the severity of psychosocial stressors. In DSM-IV, Axis IV is for listing clinically relevant psychosocial and environmental problems.

Page 574 •

Answer C

7. Which of the following statements are true regarding the elimination of the term "organic" from DSM-IV?

A. The term was eliminated because it reflected a reductionistic mind-body dualism.
B. The organic-nonorganic distinction is meaningless because all disorders have both biological and psychological components.
C. The DSM-III-R "organic mental disorders" have each been split into two disorders: substance-induced and due to a general medical condition.
D. All of the above

Discussion: This is perhaps the most significant change in DSM-IV. In addition to eliminating the term, the former organic mental disorders are distributed throughout the classification, each included in that section with those other disorders with which it shares phenomenology. For example, mood disorder due to a general medical condition and substance-induced mood disorder are in the mood disorders section in DSM-IV.

Pages 577–578 •

Answer D

8. Which of the following statements are true about the appendix of research categories in DSM-IV?

A. Of all the proposals for new disorders, only a handful were added to DSM-IV.
B. The categories were included in the appendix to provide a common language for researchers and psychiatrists.
C. Text and criteria have been provided for each appendix category.
D. All of the above

Discussion: Because of the high threshold for data required for inclusion of a category in DSM-IV, many proposed categories of potential research and clinical interest were not added to DSM-IV. This appendix afforded an opportunity to present these categories with suggested research criteria sets. Whether any of these categories are ultimately added to DSM-V will depend on the quantity and quality of data collected about them in the next 10 years.

Page 583, Table 29–3 (p. 582) •

Answer D

CHAPTER 30

Diagnostic Classification in Infancy and Early Childhood

Megan Hester • David Taylor

1. Which of the following are factors to take into account in doing a full diagnostic work-up and planning intervention for children younger than 4 years?

A. presenting symptoms and behaviors
B. parents as individuals
C. caregiver-infant interactive patterns
D. affective, language, cognitive, motor, and sensory patterns
E. all of the above

Discussion: All of the above factors are important in developing an understanding of why an infant or toddler is having problems. A full evaluation includes all of these factors and other additional factors, such as developmental history; family functioning and cultural and community patterns; the infant's maturational characteristics; the family's psychosocial, medical, and pregnancy-delivery history; and current environmental conditions and stressors.

Page 585 •

Answer E

2. The result of a comprehensive evaluation of children younger than 4 years should lead to preliminary notions about

A. a plan for pharmacological therapy
B. the nature of the infant's or child's difficulties
C. the relative contribution of the areas assessed (i.e., family relationships) to the child's difficulties
D. answers B and C
E. answers A and B

Discussion: A comprehensive evaluation should lead to preliminary notions about the nature of the infant's or child's difficulties as well as strengths. The evaluation should show the level of the child's overall adaptive capacity and functioning in the major areas of development in comparison to age-expected developmental patterns. The evaluation should also show the relative contribution of the different areas assessed by the evaluation and how they relate to the child's difficulties. Comprehensive treatment or preventive intervention planning should flow from a careful evaluation. Pharmacological treatment, if ever indicated, would only be a component of a broader plan.

Page 585 •

Answer D

3. The types of relationship problems in infancy and childhood disorders are

A. overinvolved relationship
B. angry-hostile relationship
C. abusive relationship
D. anxious-tense relationship
E. all of the above

Discussion: Axis II in the Diagnostic Classification 0–3 is reserved not for personality disorders, which the infant by definition cannot manifest, but rather for a relationship classification. All of the above are types of relationship problems listed in the Diagnostic Classification 0–3. Additional relationship problems also include underinvolved relationship and a mixture of all these relationships.

Pages 588–589 •

Answer E

4. Axis IV in the proposed diagnostic classification for infants and children refers to

A. physical, neurological, developmental, and mental health disorders
B. psychosocial stress
C. functional emotional development level
D. relationships classification
E. none of the above

Discussion: Axis IV in this system is identical to that in DSM-IV for adults and older children.

Page 589 •

Answer B

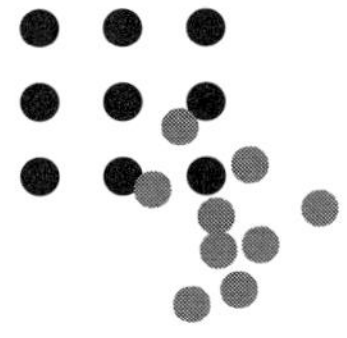

SECTION **V**

Section Editor: Harold Alan Pincus

Associate Section Editors

Harold S. Koplewicz • *Chapters 32–40, Childhood Disorders*

Thomas R. Kosten • *Chapters 41–50, Substance Use Disorders*

Disorders

CHAPTER 31 Introduction

Harold Alan Pincus

There are no questions for this chapter.

CHAPTER

32 Childhood and Adolescent Manifestations of Adult Disorders

Harold S. Koplewicz • Richard F. Morrissey • Stanley Kutcher

1. Which of the following statements is true regarding the prevalence of major depressive disorder (MDD) among prepubertal children?

A. Sex ratios in prepubertal children are roughly equal.
B. Sex rates in prepubertal children roughly parallel adult rates, with female rates exceeding male rates.
C. Sex ratios in prepubertal children roughly reverse those found in adult populations, with rates among prepubertal boys exceeding those found in girls.
D. Not enough empirical research has been conducted to determine prevalence rates in prepubertal children.

Discussion: In prepubertal children, prevalence rates for MDD in boys and girls are roughly equal. By adolescence, the sex ratio approximates that of adults, with female rates about twice the male rates, although this differential may not be true for early adolescence.

Page 595 •

Answer A

2. Early onset of MDD has **not** been associated with which of the following variables?

A. female gender
B. suicidal ideation
C. a chronic course
D. comorbid attention-deficit/hyperactivity disorder (ADHD) diagnosis

Discussion: MDD with onset in childhood or adolescence is often the first episode of a chronic mood disorder characterized by relapse and functional impairments. The most common age at onset is estimated to be midadolescence, with early onset of MDD.

Page 595 •

Answer D

3. Recent epidemiological investigations of MDD among the young have suggested

A. a later age at onset and decreased prevalence
B. an earlier age at onset and decreased prevalence
C. a later age at onset and increased prevalence
D. an earlier age at onset and increased prevalence

Discussion: Recent investigations suggest a cohort effect. Younger cohorts show both an earlier age at onset and an increased prevalence of the disorder.

Page 595 •

Answer D

4. Which of the following has **not** been identified as a specific risk factor in the onset of MDD?

A. substance abuse
B. female gender
C. parental history of MDD
D. dysthymia

Discussion: Predictive risk factors for MDD in this population have not been well characterized, and those factors that have been correlated with depressive *symptoms* may not be associated with the syndrome of MDD. Relatively specific risk factors include all of the above with the exception of substance abuse. Persistent subsyndromal depressive symptoms can be understood in and of themselves to be a risk factor for MDD.

Page 595 •

Answer A

5. Neuroendocrine investigations of MDD in young people have established that:

A. Abnormalities of the hypothalamic-pituitary-adrenal (HPA) axis are found relatively frequently in children and adolescents.
B. Hypothalamic-pituitary-thyroid (HPT) abnormalities are found frequently in children and adolescents.
C. HPA and HPT dysregulations, when they occur, do so in a fashion different from that found in the older population.
D. Dysregulated hypothalamic–pituitary growth hormone functioning has been demonstrated in children and adolescents, with the occurrence of abnormal basal stimulation secretion.

Discussion: Neurobiological studies show some differences yet some similarities among child, adolescent, and adult MDDs. HPA and HPT abnormalities are rare in children and adolescents as opposed to dysregulation of growth hormone production. Studies of sleep physiology have been contradictory.

Page 596 •

Answer D

6. Which of the following statements correctly characterizes MDD in younger populations?

A. There is little evidence of comorbidity.
B. MDD among the young is not generally predictive of a persistent and chronic disorder.
C. Dysthymia and separation anxiety disorder are common comorbid diagnoses.
D. Psychopharmacological treatments have been conclusively demonstrated to be useful.

Discussion: Comorbidity with MDD is significant and is related to more severe functional impairment. Dysthymia and separation anxiety disorder are most commonly comorbid. Other studies have shown associations with eating, substance use, and anxiety disorders.

Page 596 •

Answer C

7. Which of the following statements is correct regarding the presence of dysthymia in young people?

A. Prevalence rates are roughly comparable to those found in adults.
B. Prevalence rates are generally accepted to be about 1% to 2%.
C. It is not especially associated with significant morbidity.
D. Psychosocial treatments have been demonstrated to have significant utility.

Discussion: The prevalence rates for dysthymia are comparable to those in adults, that is, they range from 4% to 8%. As in MDD, dysthymia in children and adolescents is associated with significant morbidity and often signals the onset of a chronic mood disorder.

Pages 596–597 •

Answer A

8. In diagnosing bipolar disorder in young people, special care should be taken to differentiate the disorder from

A. separation anxiety disorder
B. schizophrenia
C. phobic avoidance
D. anorexia nervosa

Discussion: The diagnosis of bipolar disorder in young people is often confused with schizophrenia, which has somewhat different precursors and outcome, or with personality disorders, especially borderline personality disorder. Other complicating factors in a differential are nonaffective psychoses, unipolar depression, organic syndromes, and ADHD.

Pages 597–598 •

Answer B

9. One recognized early marker of bipolar disorder is

A. early-onset schizophrenia
B. substance abuse
C. prepubertal MDD
D. the presence of a learning disorder

Discussion: More than 30% of youngsters with prepubertal MDD have bipolarity on 2- to 5-year follow-up.

Pages 597–598 •

Answer C

10. Two major sources of concern in prescribing lithium in the treatment of bipolar disorder in adolescents are side effects of

A. weight gain and acne
B. weight loss and acne
C. weight gain and height attenuation
D. weight loss and height attenuation

Discussion: Lithium is the treatment of choice in this population. Weight gain and acne are of particular concern to adolescents.

Page 598 •

Answer A

11. Premature termination of prophylactic lithium maintenance for bipolar adolescents has been found to be associated with

A. sudden weight gain
B. relatively high relapse rates
C. relatively low relapse rates
D. headache and nausea

Discussion: Strober and coworkers found that the relapse rate of bipolar illness in 13 bipolar I adolescents who discontinued prophylactic lithium therapy shortly after hospital discharge was nearly three times higher than the rate in patients who continued lithium without interruption.

Page 598 •

Answer B

12. Which of the following statements is true regarding the occurrence of anxiety disorders in children and adolescents?

A. They are relatively uncommon, affecting no more than 5% of the population.
B. They often occur comorbidly with other psychiatric diagnoses.
C. They are more likely to be present in behaviorally disinhibited children.
D. Familial heritability has not been well established.

Discussion: These disorders are often comorbid with MDD, dysthymia, ADHD, and Tourette's disorder. High rates of familial prevalence have been reported. The hallmark of these disorders is behavioral inhibition.

Page 598 •

Answer B

13. One of the most common signs of an underlying anxiety disorder in children is

A. oppositional behavior
B. conduct disorder
C. fire setting
D. school refusal

Discussion: Among the above, only school refusal is a sign of behavioral inhibition and a precursor of anxiety disorder.

Page 598 •

Answer D

14. "Behavioral inhibition" among normal children is considered a common precursor to the development of

A. MDD
B. dysthymia
C. anxiety disorders
D. ADHD

Discussion: As originally conceptualized by Kagan and colleagues, behavioral inhibition refers to characteristics of a subgroup of normal children who are irritable as infants, fearful as toddlers, and cautious and introverted as school-age children. In one study, rates of anxiety and psychiatric disorders in general were markedly higher among inhibited children.

Page 598 •

Answer C

15. Childhood fears can be considered to be indicative of specific phobias when

A. they include objects other than common fears of the dark, thunderstorms, or strangers
B. there is significant functional interference
C. typical parental limit setting is ineffective
D. normal parental reassurance is ineffective

Discussion: Childhood fears are among the most common psychological characteristics of youth. Objects of fear may be developmentally idiosyncratic or fairly universal, such as fears of the dark, strangers, dogs, or thunderstorms. These fears warrant little more than reassurance and patience. When there is impairment, such as an unwillingness to play outdoors or attend school because of a particular fear, the diagnosis of specific phobia is suggested.

Pages 598–599 •

Answer B

16. The treatment of choice for specific phobias of childhood and adolescence is

A. family therapy
B. psychodynamically oriented play therapy
C. behavioral therapy
D. pharmacotherapy

Discussion: Behavioral interventions, such as systematic desensitization and progressive relaxation, are the treatment of choice for these problems.

Page 599 •

Answer C

17. One of the major changes in DSM-IV's listing of childhood and adolescent anxiety disorders is the omission of

A. separation anxiety disorder
B. avoidant disorder
C. social phobia
D. specific phobia

Discussion: The omission of avoidant disorder was based on the finding that there was insufficient evidence to distinguish it from social phobia.

Page 599 •

Answer B

18. Which of the following is **not** recommended treatment for social phobia in children?

A. monoamine oxidase inhibitors
B. fluoxetine
C. buspirone
D. cognitive-behavioral treatment

Discussion: Whereas monoamine oxidase inhibitors such as phenelzine are useful in treating adults with social phobia, they are not recommended for use in children and adolescents.

Pages 599–600 •

Answer A

19. Which of the following could best be considered to be a relatively unusual obsession in childhood obsessive-compulsive disorder?

A. fears of contamination
B. fears of homicidal impulses
C. fears of harm to self
D. fears of harm to parents

Discussion: Whereas children with this condition may commonly be afraid that they might harm their parents, a generalized fear of homicidality is unusual.

Pages 600–601 •

Answer B

20. Which of the following has **not** been associated with the occurrence of early-onset schizophrenia?

A. male gender
B. premorbid schizotypal personality
C. neurodevelopmental abnormalities
D. ADHD

Discussion: Presentation of schizophrenia in children, although rare, is similar to that in adults, including negative and positive signs. The most commonly reported symptoms are auditory hallucinations, affective disturbance, thought disorder, and delusions. ADHD is not part of a prodrome to schizophrenia.

Pages 601–602 •

Answer D

CHAPTER

33 Mental Retardation

Ludwik S. Szymanski • Maija L. Wilska

Select the one best answer or completion.

1. The following are sufficient for the diagnosis of mental retardation:

A. external phenotype of a known syndrome associated with mental retardation
B. mental age of 6 years or younger
C. IQ of 75 or below, if onset is before 21 years of age
D. IQ of 70 or below in the presence of impaired adaptive skills and onset before 18 years of age
E. IQ one standard deviation below normal, in the presence of impaired adaptive skills and onset before 18 years of age

Discussion: There are several modern and many older definitions of mental retardation. Mental retardation is not a specific disease but rather a behavioral syndrome of multiple causes and presentations. Psychiatrists use the DSM-IV criteria, which are summarized in answer D. Another definition, which is similar, is that of the American Association on Mental Retardation: "Mental Retardation refers to substantial limitations in present functioning. It is characterized by significantly subaverage functioning, existing concurrently with related limitations in two or more of the following applicable adaptive skill areas: communication, self-care, home living, social skills, community use, self-direction, health and safety, functional academics, leisure and work. Mental retardation manifests before age 18."

Pages 605–606 •

Answer D

Instructions for questions 2 to 5: For each numbered item, select the lettered heading most closely associated with it. Each letter may be selected once, more than once, or not at all.

2. Match the characteristic feature with the syndrome:

____ 1. tendency to hyperactivity and social withdrawal, especially in boys
____ 2. increased risk for thyroid dysfunction
____ 3. 14:21 chromosomal translocation
____ 4. described only in girls
____ 5. obesity

A. Down's syndrome
B. fragile X syndrome
C. Rett's syndrome
D. Prader-Willi syndrome
E. fetal alcohol syndrome

Discussion: Many of the classification systems for mental retardation have been based on the timing of the insult to the central nervous system. Thus, there are prenatal causes, such as the genetic disorders of a chromosomal basis (Down's syndrome), gene mutations (fragile X syndrome, Rett's syndrome), and malformation syndromes due to DNA microdeletions (Prader-Willi syndrome) or unknown causes. There are also external prenatal causes such as maternal infection or intoxication (fetal alcohol syndrome), perinatal causes, and postnatal causes.

Pages 608–615, Tables 33–2 to 33–5 •

Answers 1, B; 2, A; 3, A; 4, C; 5, D

3. Match the clinical problem with the description:

____ 1. major depression
____ 2. bipolar I disorder
____ 3. aggression
____ 4. personality change due to medical condition (organic personality disorder)
____ 5. anxiety disorders

A. cannot be diagnosed in persons with mental retardation
B. never occurs in persons with mental retardation
C. is the most common personality feature of persons with mental retardation
D. occurs in persons with mental retardation
E. is seen in virtually all persons with mental retardation

Discussion: All major psychiatric diagnoses occur in persons with mental retardation. Depression in particular has been underdiagnosed in this population. This was because of several assumptions and assessment difficulties. It was thought that they could not be depressed because of insufficient intelligence. Poor language skills made the diagnosis difficult, and depressed patients may not have disturbed others and thus may have gone unnoticed.

Pages 627–630 •

Answers 1, D; 2, D; 3, D; 4, D; 5, D

4. Match the treatment with the indication:

____ 1. is the specific treatment for aggression in persons with mental retardation
____ 2. is indicated primarily for treatment of psychotic disorders
____ 3. requires higher dosage in persons with mental retardation
____ 4. might be helpful for rage episodes associated with brain disorder symptoms
____ 5. has same indications whether mental retardation is present or not

A. antipsychotics, especially thioridazine
B. carbamazepine
C. β-blockers
D. lithium
E. none of the above

Discussion: Psychotropic medications have a sad history of indiscriminate use and abuse in this population. Antipsychotics, which accounted for half of all such prescribed medications, were used primarily for their side effect of sedation. At the height of the institutional era, more than half of mentally retarded individuals living in institutions were receiving medication. As a result, there was backlash in which medication use was discouraged and came to be seen, in the aggregate, as an indication of an inferior program or hospital. There is not good research on the use of drugs in this population, and the general principles of use are the same as for persons without mental retardation.

Pages 631–632 •

Answers 1, E; 2, A; 3, E; 4, C; 5, A, B, C, D

5. Match the treatment issue with the setting:

____ 1. can be effective with persons with mental retardation, if sufficient communication skills are present
____ 2. may interfere with making a diagnosis of a mental disorder in persons with mental retardation
____ 3. should be obtained before use of medications with persons with mental retardation
____ 4. is a common treatment for self-injurious behavior

A. legally valid informed consent
B. behavioral treatment
C. individual and group psychotherapy
D. "diagnostic overshadowing"

Discussion: Psychotherapy with this population is not different in nature from treating persons with average intelligence and resembles work with children. The prerequisites are some communication skills and the ability to maintain a relationship. Group therapy is useful in social skills development. Behavioral treatment, particularly for self-injurious behavior, should focus on replacing maladaptive behaviors with newer ones, not just elimination of behavior. "Diagnostic overshadowing" refers to the psychiatrist's tendency to overlook comorbid mental disorders in patients with a diagnosis of mental retardation.

Pages 632–633 •

Answers 1, C; 2, D; 3, A; 4, B

Instructions for questions 6 to 9: Select the one best answer or completion for the following.

6. Adults with mental retardation do best if they

A. live in institutions
B. work in sheltered workshops
C. stay with their families all their lives
D. live in community-based residences or apartments, with supports as needed
E. are sterilized before achieving puberty

Discussion: The principles of treatment of mental retardation involve the normalization principle and the right to community living. These ideas include the right to live with a family, no institutionalization of children, deinstitutionalization of adults, education and training for all children (mainstreaming), employment of adults in the community, training, advocacy, and movement toward full inclusion. The treatment of persons with mental retardation involves multiple caregivers and providers because they have multiple disabilities and needs.

Page 623 •

Answer D

7. Aggression in persons with mental retardation

A. is aimed at obtaining attention
B. usually is a symptom of psychosis
C. is best handled by behavior modification
D. requires diagnostic assessment just as in patients without mental retardation
E. is due to organic brain damage

Discussion: Aggression is one of the most frequent reasons for referral in this population. It can range from swearing to violence. The assessment of aggression involves considering whether there is a defined mental disorder, whether it is a learned behavior, or whether it is due to a particular brain lesion or seizure disorder. Often there are multiple causes.

Page 630 •

Answer D

8. Psychiatric diagnosis of persons with mental retardation

A. is established with the help of behavior rating scales
B. cannot be done, unless the person has good verbal language
C. requires diagnostic assessment as in persons without mental retardation
D. can be based on caregiver's theory
E. can be done by psychometric testing

Discussion: Assessment of a mentally retarded patient should involve history from all involved caregivers and should focus on the reasons, both overt and covert, for the current referral, behavioral symptoms, and medication history. Interviewing patients themselves requires special techniques such as assessment of communication skills. Directiveness and structure are important, although, paradoxically, open-ended questions are often useful to avoid repetition. Patients may often answer repetitively to avoid appearing to misunderstand a particular question.

Pages 625–627 •

Answer C

9. Personality of persons with mental retardation

A. commonly is characterized by aggression
B. commonly is characterized by passivity
C. commonly is characterized by lack of sexual interest
D. commonly is characterized by hypersexuality
E. is not unique

Discussion: Myths about the personality patterns of mentally retarded individuals include that they have uniform personality characteristics owing to organic brain damage and are more commonly passive, aggressive, or dependent. These patients are shaped in their behavior by cognitive deficits, neurological dysfunction, and environmental experiences. The last in particular can lead to unusual personality development especially in those institutionalized since childhood.

Pages 629–630 •

Answer E

CHAPTER

34 Learning and Motor Skills Disorders

Larry B. Silver

1. In DSM-IV, learning disorders are listed

A. under mental retardation
B. as a disorder first diagnosed in infancy, childhood, or adolescence
C. on Axis II
D. as a form of pervasive developmental disorder
E. as synonymous with a learning disability

Discussion: In DSM-IV, the learning disorders are listed under the category identified earlier. Learning disorders were first delineated in DSM-III as the academic skills disorders; the changed nomenclature reflects the underlying learning disability rather than simply the general area of difficulty. Learning disability is a term in educational law.

Pages 637–638 •

Answer B

2. Within the public school system, children and adolescents can be identified as having a learning disability if

A. they have a learning disorder
B. they are failing in all skill areas
C. they are of above-average intelligence
D. they have a motor skills disorder
E. they meet the educational guidelines for a learning disability

Discussion: Criteria for learning disabilities as defined in recent federal guidelines are as follows: 1) documented evidence that general education has been ineffective, 2) evidence of a disorder in the basic psychological process of learning, 3) evidence of academic achievement below the student's level of intellectual function, and 4) evidence that the difficulty is not due to another particular problem (e.g., visual or hearing difficulties).

Page 638 •

Answer E

3. For a public school system to identify a student as having a learning disability, it is essential that the individual have

A. above-average intelligence
B. failing grades in the majority of subjects
C. a central processing deficit
D. hyperactivity or distractability
E. a reading problem

Discussion: A central processing deficit in the functions required for learning is essential for the diagnosis of a learning disability in the context of a public school system. In other words, this deficit must be present in isolation, or if other handicapping conditions are present, it must be evident in addition.

Pages 638–639 •

Answer C

4. When a child or adolescent presents to a psychiatrist as having academic difficulties and behavior problems, which of the following possibilities is **not** relevant to the differential thinking?

A. if there is a learning disorder
B. if there is family dysfunction
C. the age of the student
D. if the behavior problems are secondary to academic difficulties
E. if the student has mental retardation

Discussion: Because many children, regardless of age, may be referred to mental health professionals rather than special education professionals, it is critical that mental health workers recognize potential referral bias. Clarification of the relative contributions of emotional, social, or family problems is essential.

Pages 638–640, Figure 34–1 (p. 641) •

Answer C

5. Learning disorders and motor skills disorder are caused by

A. bad parenting
B. bad schools
C. bad communities
D. mental retardation
E. neurological dysfunction

Discussion: These disorders are thought to have a neurological basis. Neuropathological studies have shown a pattern of cortical cells that maintained an earlier stage of migration and development. Possible causes are genetic, prenatal, perinatal, and postnatal.

Page 644 •

Answer E

6. Reading disorders are caused by

A. difficulty with decoding of words
B. poor teaching
C. a lack of interest by the student
D. anxiety
E. depression

Discussion: The process of reading involves both decoding or word recognition and reading comprehension. Decoding is the transcribing of a printed word into speech, and comprehension is its interpretation. Decoding is unique to reading as opposed to comprehension, which is a more universal linguistic skill. If the ability to decode is impaired but comprehension is intact, the problem is one of dyslexia. Rarely the difficulties are reversed, and the disorder is termed hyperlexia. If both decoding and comprehension are impaired, then a diagnosis of reading backwardness is made.

Page 644 •

Answer A

7. Some children and adolescents identified by a teacher as having a mathematics disorder in reality do not. The cause is probably

A. parents' lack of interest in math
B. poor instruction by the teacher
C. the student is a girl
D. peer pressure
E. student's lack of interest in math

Discussion: Because math achievement is highly dependent on the quality of instruction offered students, it may be that a significant number of those students who are coded as having a learning disability by the school system do not have intrinsic math disorders but have not had appropriate instruction.

Pages 644–645 •

Answer B

CHAPTER

35 Autistic Disorder and Other Pervasive Developmental Disorders

Megan Hester • David Taylor

1. Pervasive developmental disorders (PDDs) possess which characteristic(s) that differentiate them from other specific developmental disorders?

A. early age at onset
B. developmental delays
C. developmental deviations
D. answers A and C
E. answers B and C

Discussion: The presence of deviations differentiates PDDs from other specific developmental disorders such as mental retardation. The prototypical PDD is autism; however, other PDDs include Rett's disorder, childhood disintegrative disorder, Asperger's disorder, and PDD not otherwise specified.

Page 650 •

Answer C

2. Studies of autistic disorder have shown that:

A. It is more prevalent in boys than in girls.
B. It is associated strictly with lower socioeconomic status.
C. The majority of people afflicted have IQs of below 50.
D. The majority of people afflicted have phenomenal abilities.
E. It is extremely common.

Discussion: Autism is four times more prevalent in boys than in girls. According to Kanner (1943), there is an association between *high* socioeconomic status and autism. More recent studies have indicated that autistic disorder is seen at all socioeconomic levels. Approximately 25% to 30% of children with autism have IQs below 50; 20% to 30% have IQs of 70 or greater. A small number of people with autistic disorder display "savant" or phenomenal abilities. Autistic disorder itself is rare.

Pages 651–652 •

Answer A

3. All but one of the following etiological theories about PDD is still thought to be plausible:

A. PDD is a genetic disorder.
B. PDD is related to developmental neuropathological processes.
C. PDD shares a common etiology with syndromes causing mental retardation.
D. PDD is caused by environmental factors (nurture).

Discussion: The most recent theories about PDD suggest that either genetic factors or early developmental disruptions in brain functioning contribute to the onset of the disorder. PDD is often associated with mental retardation (e.g., fragile X syndrome) and other nonspecific neurological abnormalities. Genetic disorders such as phenylketonuria and tuberous sclerosis have been linked to autism. However, although some theorists still argue for environmental factors, "nurture," as a cause, PDD are influenced more by medical factors, or "nature."

Pages 652–655 •

Answer D

4. The central feature associated with PDD is

A. low IQ
B. hyperactivity
C. disturbance of social development
D. obsessive movements
E. adaptability to change

Discussion: The central feature associated with PDD is disturbance of social development. A child with autistic disorder has trouble functioning socially. Typically, abnormal patterns of eye contact and facial expression, lack of empathy for others' feelings, difficulty with use of language, resistance to change, incapability of shifting attention, and trouble picking up on social cues are all characteristic of autism and other PDDs.

Pages 655–657, Table 35–1 (p. 654) •

Answer C

5. Rett's disorder

A. preferentially strikes girls
B. with onset of the disorder, there is deceleration of head growth
C. may show improved social capabilities with time, despite cognitive and motor deterioration
D. has some of the same manifestations as autistic disorder in toddlerhood
E. all of the above

Discussion: Rett's disorder is a disorder that manifests itself similarly to autistic disorder in toddlerhood, although manifestations after toddlerhood are substantially different. There is loss of acquired language; restricted interest in social contact or interactions; and the start of handwringing, hand clapping, or tapping in the midline of the body. This motor activity is seen together with lubrication of the hands with saliva.

Page 656 •

Answer E

6. Means of evaluating a child for autism include

A. the Draw-A-Person Test
B. observation
C. neurological examination
D. answers B and C
E. answers A and B

Discussion: The Draw-A-Person Test is not a recommended means of evaluation for autistic disorder. However, observation in a variety of settings is an essential part of evaluating a child for autism. Several structured observations may be used, such as the Autism Diagnostic Observation Schedule, the Prelinguistic Autism Diagnostic Observation Scale, and the Childhood Autism Rating Scale. A complete physical examination including a neurological examination should be performed. The examination should also include audiological tests and vision testing.

Pages 657–658, Table 35–4 •

Answer D

7. The goals of treatment defined by Rutter include **all but one** of the following:

A. the advancement of normal development, particularly regarding cognition, language, and socialization
B. the cure for autism through pharmacological treatment
C. the promotion of learning and problem solving
D. the reduction of behaviors that impede the learning process
E. the assistance of families coping with autism

Discussion: Rutter includes all of these as goals of treatment except answer B. There is no "cure" for autism. There is no specific pharmacological treatment that substitutes for appropriate educational, behavioral, psychotherapeutic, vocational, and recreational programming. Pharmacological treatment should be used in conjunction with other treatment, and it should be understood by parents, teachers, and others that medication will not provide a cure for the disorder.

Pages 659–660, Table 35–6 •

Answer B

8. Psychosocial interventions include

A. behavioral techniques
B. social skills therapy
C. psychotherapy
D. all of the above

Discussion: A variety of psychosocial interventions are helpful in autistic disorder. Most fundamental is tending to the unique educational needs of this population. Behavioral techniques and social skills therapy are beneficial. Brief individual psychotherapy for those individuals with sufficient verbal skills and comorbid anxiety or depression can be helpful but is not a mainstay of psychosocial treatment.

Pages 660–661 •

Answer D

CHAPTER

36 Attention-Deficit and Disruptive Behavior Disorders

Vanshdeep Sharma • Jeffrey H. Newcorn • Kristin Matier-Sharma • Jeffrey M. Halperin

1. All of the following statements about the attention-deficit and disruptive behavior disorders (AD-DBDs) in DSM-IV are true **except**

A. The attention-deficit/hyperactivity disorder (ADHD) has been broadened to include individuals with primarily inattentive or primarily hyperactive symptoms.
B. A diagnosis of conduct disorder (CD) preempts oppositional defiant disorder (ODD).
C. In prepubertal children, boys predominate over girls in each diagnostic category.
D. The subtyping of CD is determined according to age at onset of symptoms.
E. All of the above

Discussion: Answers A, B, C, and D are each taken directly from the DSM-IV definitions. There is a strong gender bias in favor of boys for ADHD and CD, although the gender bias for ADHD may become much smaller with age. However, the male/female predominance for ODD is mainly confined to prepubertal years, after which the ratio is about equal.

Pages 667–670 •

Answer E

2. The developmental trajectory of symptoms in the AD-DBDs is characterized by which of the following?

A. ADHD symptoms always have their onset by the beginning of school.
B. Inattention symptoms usually decrease substantially with age in individuals with ADHD.
C. ODD is usually a precursor to CD.
D. Late-onset CD generally predicts more favorable outcome.
E. None of the above

Discussion: By definition, at least some symptoms of ADHD must be present by age 7 years. Whereas these are often observed by the beginning of school, this is not necessarily the case—particularly for inattention symptoms. Decline in symptoms is most dramatic for hyperactivity rather than inattention, although some decrease in severity of inattention may also be seen. ODD is a precursor to CD for most individuals who have CD; however, the majority of children with ODD do not progress to CD.

Pages 671–672 •

Answer D

3. It is of considerable clinical importance to recognize the presence of aggression in children with ADHD because:

A. ADHD children with comorbid aggression are at increased risk for the development of CD, antisocial personality, and substance abuse.
B. The comorbid group is more likely to require hospital admission.
C. It is likely that children with both conditions will require multiple medication treatments.
D. All of the above
E. None of the above

Discussion: Children with ADHD who are aggressive have been shown to have a more malignant course than children with either condition alone. Multiple interventions are likely in the case of comorbidity, which increases the likelihood that polypharmacy would be required. However, this is by no means the rule. Also, whereas the comorbid group is probably at increased risk for requiring inpatient treatment, the majority can be treated as outpatients.

Page 674 •

Answer A

4. Which of the following neurochemical findings have been reported in children with AD-DBDs?

A. The prolactin response to fenfluramine challenge differs in younger aggressive and nonaggressive ADHD children.
B. Cerebrospinal fluid 5-hydroxyindoleacetic acid (5-HIAA) level is low in children with aggressive behavior disorders and predicts the subsequent development of CD.
C. Plasma dopamine β-hydroxylase is low in children with aggressive behavior disorders.
D. There is decreased uptake on positron emission tomography (PET) scan in the frontal lobes of adult ADHD patients.
E. All of the above

Discussion: Halperin and coworkers (1994) reported increased prolactin in response to acute challenge with the serotoninergic releaser–reuptake blocker fenfluramine in prepubertal ADHD boys, although there may be age effects. [Note: Other studies have indicated a blunted response in older aggressive (non-ADHD) individuals.] Kruesi and associates (1990, 1992) found low cerebrospinal fluid 5-HIAA levels in aggressive children and adolescents, about two thirds of whom also had ADHD. Rogeness and colleagues have reported that plasma dopamine β-hydroxylase is low in aggressive children, including those with comorbid ADHD. Zametkin and colleagues found reduced uptake in the frontal lobes of adults with ADHD on PET scan.

Pages 670–671, Table 36–1 •

Answer E

5. The hypothesis that ADHD and CD have distinct genetic substrates is best supported by which of the following findings?

A. increased rate of antisocial personality in parents of children with ADHD and CD
B. an increase in CD among siblings of ADHD children
C. cosegregation of ADHD and CD in the pedigrees of children with comorbid ADHD and CD
D. the results of PET scan studies, which indicate frontal lobe abnormalities in adults with ADHD but not antisocial personality
E. All of the above

Discussion: The increased rate of antisocial personality in the parents of children with ADHD and CD may be consistent with the interpretation that there is likely to be a familial pattern of these disorders, but it does not necessarily argue that there are distinct genetic mechanisms for the two disorders. Similarly, an increased frequency of CD in the siblings of ADHD children would not argue for a distinction between these disorders, although it might be consistent with genetic as well as other hypotheses. However, the finding that ADHD and CD cosegregate in first-degree relatives of ADHD probands is more consistent with a genetic basis for the two conditions. PET scan studies, which indicate pathology in adults with ADHD, might ultimately be helpful in elucidating the genetics of the disorder but are not sufficient to invoke a genetic basis alone. Also, this same study was not conducted in adults with antisocial personality disorder.

Page 671 •

Answer C

6. The longitudinal course of ADHD is best described by which of the following statements?

A. The majority of children with ADHD will continue to have the full disorder as adolescents and adults.
B. Development of antisocial personality at follow-up may be predicted by the early onset of aggression or the maintenance of ADHD symptoms.
C. Data indicate that psychostimulant treatment increases the risk of substance abuse in the adult outcome of ADHD children.
D. Data indicate that the psychostimulant treatment improves the long-term outcome of ADHD children.
E. All of the above

Discussion: Whereas many ADHD children will continue to have some symptoms of the disorder causing impairment, the majority do not have the full disorder. There are no data to indicate that psychostimulant treatment increases the risk of substance abuse. However, the studies have also failed to indicate that long-term outcome is improved by this treatment. The risk of antisocial personality disorder (which is itself a risk factor for substance abuse) is increased in individuals who have an early onset of aggression or who maintain their ADHD symptoms at impairing levels.

Pages 671–672 •

Answer B

7. Which of the following techniques is most useful in the assessment of children with ADHD?

A. structured interview with the teacher rating the presence of ADHD symptoms at school
B. clinical interview with the child
C. comprehensive psychometric testing battery
D. data from parent and teacher rating scales
E. all of the above

Discussion: Obtaining information from the teacher regarding ADHD symptoms is essential, but this need not come in the form of a structured interview. The clinical interview with the child is usually less helpful. Comprehensive psychometric testing may be necessary in some cases (usually those with comorbid learning disorder), but it is not required for diagnosis of ADHD. In contrast, parent and teacher rating scales are inexpensive, easy to integrate into clinical practice, and sensitive to treatment effects.

Pages 672–674 •

Answer D

8. Which of the following statements regarding treatment of children with AD-DBDs is most accurate?

A. Psychostimulant treatment has been demonstrated to be the most successful intervention in children with CD.
B. Pharmacological treatment has been conclusively shown to be superior to psychosocial treatment in the long term in children with ADHD.
C. The most effective psychosocial treatment techniques in ADHD children involve behavioral interventions with the child.
D. School-based psychosocial interventions are superior in children with ADHD because the symptoms are often most evident at school.
E. Cognitive-behavioral therapy has been found to be effective in children with CD but not so clearly with ADHD children.

Discussion: There have been no studies to assess the utility of psychostimulant treatment in aggression independent of ADHD. Also, whereas pharmacological treatments using psychostimulant and other agents have been clearly shown to be effective in children with ADHD, and studies of multimodal treatments have yielded conflicting results, no studies have directly compared pharmacological and psychosocial treatments. Effective psychosocial treatments in ADHD children may involve training of parents and consultation with teachers as well as behavioral work with the child. These interventions may be applied in a range of settings. Cognitive-behavioral therapy has been demonstrated to be effective in children with CD but not so clearly with ADHD, but it may well be suited for use in the comorbid group.

Pages 674–678 •

Answer E

9. Which of the following statements best describes the clinical use of psychostimulants in the treatment of the AD-DBDs?

A. Methylphenidate, dextroamphetamine, and pemoline have been shown to be essentially equal in terms of group response to treatment, but some children may respond better to one of these medications than to another.
B. Sustained-release preparations are more effective than short-acting preparations.
C. Short-acting methylphenidate and dextroamphetamine are roughly equal in potency and half-life and can be used interchangeably.
D. Appetite suppression and insomnia are frequently occurring adverse effects of all psychostimulants and often limit the utility of these medications.
E. All of the above

Discussion: Although all of the psychostimulants are roughly effective in terms of treatment response on group data, there is evidence that some children may respond better to one medication than to another. Sustained-release preparations are extremely useful for many children but are not more effective than short-acting preparations. Short-acting dextroamphetamine is actually more potent than methylphenidate and should be used in lower dose. Also, the half-life is slightly longer, even though both are usually given on a 4-hour schedule. Appetite suppression and insomnia are frequently occurring but do not usually limit treatment. This applies even to three-times-a-day dosing schedules.

Pages 674–675 •

Answer A

10. Treatment studies using psychostimulant medication in children with ADHD who are aggressive suggest that

A. Children with comorbid ADHD and CD may have a greater response to stimulant treatment in terms of reduction of ADHD symptoms.
B. Stimulant treatment produces a decrease in aggressive behavior in ADHD children.
C. Clonidine may have a role in the treatment of children with ADHD, aggressive children, or children with ADHD who are aggressive.
D. All of the above
E. None of the above

Discussion: Several studies examining the magnitude of stimulant response in ADHD children have indicated that those with comorbid CD, who may have the most severe ADHD symptoms, appear to demonstrate the most robust reduction in symptoms. These children seem to show a decrease in aggressive as well as ADHD symptoms. Clonidine has also been shown to be effective in these conditions in several studies.

Pages 677–678 •

Answer D

CHAPTER

37 Feeding and Other Disorders of Infancy or Early Childhood

Irene Chatoor

1. Failure to thrive is frequently **not** associated with which one of the following feeding disorders?

A. feeding disorder of homeostasis
B. feeding disorder of attachment
C. infantile anorexia
D. pica
E. rumination disorder

Discussion: Failure to thrive is a commonly used term in pediatric practice. The DSM-IV category of feeding disorders encompasses a wider group of abnormal feeding behaviors. Pica is not associated in particular with demonstrable failure in physical growth or with delay of social or motor development, all of which are components of failure to thrive syndromes.

Pages 683, 697–698 •

Answer D

2. Food refusal is diagnostic of which one of the following disorders?

A. feeding disorder of attachment
B. rumination disorder
C. infantile anorexia
D. pica
E. feeding disorder of homeostasis

Discussion: Infantile anorexia is characterized by food refusal during the infant's transition to self-feeding. There is failure to thrive despite the mother's intense efforts to get the child to eat.

Pages 690–693 •

Answer C

3. Anticipatory anxiety about eating is seen primarily in which one of the following disorders?

A. pica
B. rumination disorder
C. infantile anorexia
D. feeding disorder of attachment
E. posttraumatic feeding disorder

Discussion: Infants with posttraumatic feeding disorder have intense anxiety when they are exposed to food. This usually follows an episode of choking, vomiting, or gagging, and the stimulus may be limited to a particular feared food. Infants with complex medical problems may be at greater risk for this disorder.

Pages 693–696 •

Answer E

4. The onset of which feeding disorder is characteristically between 9 and 18 months of age, during the transition to self-feeding?

A. rumination disorder
B. infantile anorexia
C. posttraumatic feeding disorder
D. pica
E. feeding disorder of attachment

Discussion: Infantile anorexia is initially noted at this particular developmental stage. This distinguishes it from other types of feeding disorders that are manifested either later, such as pica, or earlier, such as feeding disorder of attachment.

Pages 690–693 •

Answer B

5. Removal from the home and foster placement may be indicated in

A. feeding disorder of homeostasis
B. feeding disorder of attachment
C. infantile anorexia
D. posttraumatic feeding disorder
E. rumination disorder

Discussion: Feeding disorder of attachment, which has been described as psychosocial dwarfism, is a syndrome of developmental delay and growth failure that is a part of a continuum of neglect and maltreatment of the child leading to insecure attachment of the infant. Mothers, who frequently suffer from character pathology, affective illness, or substance abuse, often have themselves had traumatic childhoods. Because of the psychological problems of the parent and the risk of other forms of child neglect or abuse, infants with this type of disorder may need to be removed from the home. Treatment ranges from home-based interventions to hospitalization, and decisions must be made on a case by case basis. There is not an indication for this type of intervention in the other disorders listed.

Pages 686–690 •

Answer B

6. Internal regulation of eating in infantile anorectics can be facilitated by the parents by which one of the following?

A. establishing a regular meal pattern
B. allowing the child to eat whenever he or she wants
C. treating the child with sweets
D. praising the child for eating
E. distracting the child with television

Discussion: Treatment of infantile anorexia has the primary goal of facilitating internal regulation of eating by the infant. This involves an assessment of the infant's temperamental characteristics and exploration of the mother's psychology and upbringing. In addition, the development of rules to govern eating, such as scheduled mealtimes and snacks, is essential to the infant's development of an internal regulation mechanism.

Pages 691–692 •

Answer A

7. Treatment through desensitization has been effective in which one of the following disorders?

A. pica
B. posttraumatic feeding disorder
C. feeding disorder of homeostasis
D. feeding disorder of attachment
E. infantile anorexia

Discussion: Desensitization treatment for posttraumatic feeding disorder involves helping the parents understand the dynamics of the anticipatory anxiety, identifying triggers of anxiety, obtaining a professional assessment of the infant's oral motor coordination, and behavioral manipulation of the infant's feeding through the use of reinforcers

Pages 694–695 •

Answer B

8. Pica should be considered in the differential diagnosis if the child presents with which of the following symptoms?

A. overweight
B. intellectual precocity
C. lead intoxication
D. foul oral odor
E. nightmares

Discussion: The diagnosis of pica should be considered only if the behavior is persistent and inappropriate for the child's developmental level. Pica should be considered in cases of accidental poisoning, lead intoxication, and worm infestation. Any children with signs of malnutrition or iron deficiency should also be considered for the diagnosis of pica.

Pages 697–698 •

Answer C

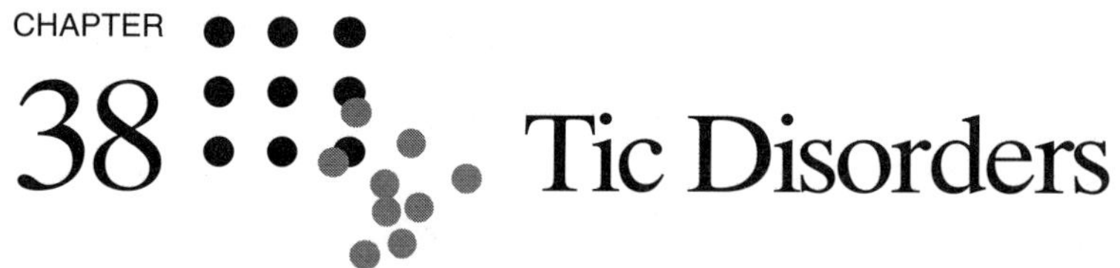

CHAPTER 38 Tic Disorders

John T. Walkup • Mark A. Riddle

1. Tic severity tends to increase

A. when patients are stressed
B. when patients are anxious
C. when patients are excited
D. all of the above

Discussion: Tics wax and wane in severity and change in character and quality over time. They can be exacerbated by both excitement and tension.

Page 702 •

Answer D

2. Tic severity tends to decrease

A. during the lifetime of the patient
B. when the patient is involved in focused productive activity
C. when the patient is asleep
D. all of the above

Discussion: Tics decrease in severity during periods of focused productive activity and during sleep. Tics are involuntary, yet because they are briefly suppressible or can be triggered by an environmental stimulus, they may appear as volitional acts.

Page 702 •

Answer D

3. Coprolalia is

A. uncommon in Tourette's disorder patients
B. essential for the diagnosis of Tourette's disorder
C. difficult to distinguish from normal swearing
D. all of the above

Discussion: Coprolalia, although often incorrectly considered essential for the diagnosis of Tourette's disorder, is infrequent; only 2% to 6% of cases are affected.

Page 702 •

Answer A

4. Differences in the diagnostic criteria for Tourette's disorder between DSM-III-R and DSM-IV include

A. a decrease in the age at onset criterion to before 15 years in DSM-IV
B. the inclusion of an impairment criterion in DSM-IV
C. the need for two vocal tics in DSM-IV
D. a duration greater than 6 months in DSM-IV

Discussion: There are four diagnostic categories in the tic disorders section of DSM-IV. These include Tourette's disorder, chronic motor or vocal tic disorder, transient tic disorder, and tic disorder not otherwise specified. The impairment criterion was added in DSM-IV.

Pages 702–703 •

Answer B

5. The most common co-occurring disorder in Tourette's disorder is

A. attention-deficit/hyperactivity disorder
B. obsessive-compulsive disorder (OCD)
C. learning disabilities
D. oppositional defiant disorder

Discussion: All of these other disorders may be comorbid with Tourette's disorder. The most common disorder is attention-deficit/hyperactivity disorder (50% to 60%). OCD co-occurs in 30% to 70% of cases.

Pages 704–705 •

Answer A

6. Which of the following best characterizes the differences in obsessive-compulsive symptoms observed in patients with OCD compared with those with Tourette's disorder and OCD?

A. In Tourette's disorder with OCD, there is usually greater concern with dirt, germs, and contamination.
B. In OCD, there is greater concern with physical symmetry.
C. Symptoms are more sensorimotor in Tourette's disorder with OCD.
D. Symptoms are more sensorimotor in OCD.

Discussion: Patients with Tourette's disorder frequently have concerns regarding physical symmetry, evenness, exactness, and impulse control. Patients with OCD are usually more preoccupied with contamination than Tourette's disorder patients are. The number of independent concerns in Tourette's disorder is greater than in OCD, in which there is often a single major concern. Some investigators have argued that the obsessions and compulsions in Tourette's disorder are more sensorimotor in character and in OCD are more cognitive and autonomic.

Pages 704–705, Table 38–1 •

Answer C

7. Evidence that Tourette's disorder is a genetic condition is best supported by which of the following studies?

A. linkage studies, which have identified the genes involved in the transmission of Tourette's disorder
B. the family studies that have conclusively identified the specific model of inheritance of Tourette's disorder
C. twin studies, which have identified that the concordance rate for any tic disorder is greater than 90% in monozygotic twins
D. twin studies, which have identified the concordance rate for Tourette's disorder to be significantly higher in monozygotic twins than in dizygotic twins

Discussion: Comparison of concordance rates for Tourette's disorder in monozygotic and dizygotic twins identifies Tourette's disorder as an inherited condition. In two large studies, the concordance rate for Tourette's disorder in monozygotic twins was more than 50%, and the rate for the presence of any tic disorder approached 100%. The twin studies are unable to identify a particular mode of transmission or to identify the breadth of the clinical phenotype.

Pages 705–707, Tables 38–2, 38–3 •

Answer D

8. The best scientific evidence supports which one of the following neuroanatomical sites for the pathological change of Tourette's disorder?

A. temporal lobes
B. frontal lobes
C. parietal lobes
D. basal ganglia

Discussion: Neuroanatomical studies have focused on the basal ganglia and their interconnections with the frontal cortex and limbic system. Volumetric magnetic resonance studies have identified the absence of the usual left-right asymmetry in the basal ganglia compared with control subjects and suggest hypoplasia or atrophy of the left basal ganglia. Single-photon emission computed tomography scans have found decreased blood flow to the left lenticular region.

Pages 707–708 •

Answer D

9. Which of the following is most true about neurotransmitter abnormalities in Tourette's disorder?

A. The dopamine system has been implicated.
B. The serotonin system has been implicated.
C. The noradrenergic system has been implicated.
D. All of the above

Discussion: All of these neurochemical systems have been implicated in Tourette's disorder. Much of this is speculation based on medication responsiveness of tics to dopamine blockers, α-adrenergic agonists, and the use of serotonin reuptake inhibitors in OCD. In addition, the opioid system has been implicated.

Page 708 •

Answer D

10. The mean age at onset for Tourette's disorder is

A. 6 years old
B. 7 years old
C. 8 years old
D. 9 years old

Discussion: In Tourette's disorder, tic symptoms usually begin in childhood with a mean age at onset of 7 years. Although the first tic may develop during adolescence, this is unusual.

Pages 709–711 •

Answer B

11. All of the following statements are true about the clinical course of Tourette's disorder **except:**

A. Tics most often begin in the face.
B. Eye-blinking tics are often the first tic and are the most common tic.
C. Motor tics most often precede the development of phonic tics.
D. Obsessive-compulsive symptoms usually follow the development of tics.
E. Tics tend to increase in severity over time.

Discussion: Longitudinal studies suggest that tic severity is greatest in most patients during the latency and early teenage years. Most patients experience a decline in tic severity as they get older; only a small percentage of patients (10%) experience a stable or deteriorating course.

Pages 709–711 •

Answer E

12. Neuroleptic medication for tic suppression

A. is part of the treatment plan for the majority of patients with Tourette's disorder
B. is usually side effect free
C. can be associated with unusual side effects in children, such as separation anxiety, depression, and school avoidance
D. is associated with a higher than normal frequency of tardive dyskinesia

Discussion: Neuroleptics are often effective at low doses, and low doses minimize side effects. Side effects include not just those seen traditionally with this class of medications but also more unusual and subtle side effects such as those listed above. Dosage reductions can lead to withdrawal dyskinesias with tic worsening above pretreatment baseline levels. Tardive dyskinesia has been rarely reported.

Pages 712–713 •

Answer C

13. All of the following statements are true about impairment in Tourette's disorder **except:**

A. Large muscle movements that call attention to oneself are relatively more impairing than tics of small muscle groups.
B. Tics with an associated premonitory urge are relatively more impairing than tics without a premonitory sensation.
C. Vocal tics that disrupt the flow of speech or call attention to oneself are relatively more impairing than simple sniffing, grunting, and throat-clearing tics.
D. Impairment is essential for diagnosis in DSM-IV.
E. Impairment due to tics is uniformly present in people with motor and phonic tics.

Discussion: Impairment in Tourette's disorder is not always correlated with severity. All of the above concerns with one exception are associated with impairment, including large, disruptive, and painful motor movements and socially unacceptable tics.

Page 710 •

Answer E

CHAPTER

39 Communication Disorders

William M. Klykylo

1. Disorders of communication in DSM-IV include all but

A. expressive language disorder
B. receptive language disorder
C. mixed receptive-expressive language disorder
D. stuttering
E. phonation disorder

Discussion: Receptive language disorders in children generally do not exist without accompanying expressive language disorders.

Pages 720–721 •

Answer B

2. The diagnosis of a language disorder is not made in the presence of

A. attention-deficit/hyperactivity disorder
B. mental retardation
C. sensory deficits
D. pervasive developmental disorder
E. environmental deprivation

Discussion: The language disorders of pervasive developmental disorder transcend this category; language disorder may be diagnosed in the presence of the other conditions if the deficits are sufficiently severe.

Page 720 •

Answer D

3. Communication disorders occur

A. in less than 1% of the pediatric population
B. in girls more often than in boys
C. in older more frequently than in younger children
D. almost always singly in individual children
E. in the company of other Axis I disorders in about half the cases reported

Discussion: These are common conditions with high comorbidity. Numbers from 1% to 13% have been posited for the prevalence of language disorders and as high as 32% for speech disorders. Acquired disorders are less common than developmental ones.

Pages 722–723 •

Answer C

4. The most common additional communication disorder associated with the language disorders is

A. phonological disorder
B. stuttering
C. stammering
D. cluttering
E. voice disorder

Discussion: Children with phonological disorder have a higher prevalence of language disorders.

Page 723 •

Answer A

5. Causal influences cited for communication disorders include all **except**

A. genetic predisposition
B. sensory deficits
C. environmental deprivation
D. internal conflict
E. prenatal factors

Discussion: Psychodynamic factors have not been shown to have a clear relationship with the development of these disorders.

Pages 723–724 •

Answer D

6. A pathognomonic finding in children with mixed receptive-expressive language disorder is

A. patterns of laterality on positron emission tomography scan
B. stuttering
C. difficulty with phonation
D. difficulty understanding certain categories of language
E. difficulty in patterns of inflection

Discussion: All other findings are associated with but not essential for the diagnosis.

Pages 724–725 •

Answer D

7. Assessment of communication disorders in children should make note of **all but**

A. comprehension
B. pragmatics
C. production
D. accent

Discussion: Accent may vary in populations and is not inherently pathological.
Pages 725–726 •

Answer D

8. Interventions necessary in the management of patients with communication disorders include **all but**

A. medications such as selective serotonin reuptake inhibitors to reduce the intensity of stuttering
B. special education consultation
C. multidisciplinary diagnostic evaluation
D. referral to a speech and language pathologist
E. parent counseling

Discussion: No indication or evidence of efficacy for the use of medication presently exists. The use of medications is limited to the treatment of comorbid psychiatric problems.

Pages 728–730 •

Answer A

CHAPTER

40 Elimination Disorders

Christopher P. Lucas • David Shaffer

1. Nocturnal enuresis

A. is pathological at age 4 years
B. is three times as common in boys as in girls at the age of 11 years
C. is associated with urinary tract infection in 25% of cases
D. will also affect a first-degree relative in 70% of enuretics
E. is more common in epileptic children

Discussion: The evidence for some genetic predisposition is strong. Approximately 70% of children with nocturnal enuresis will have a first-degree relative who also wets or has wet the bed in the past. Twin studies have shown greater monozygotic (68%) than dizygotic (36%) concordance.

Page 732 •

Answer D

2. Imipramine

A. is effective in diurnal enuresis
B. is more effective in enuretics who are depressed
C. can cause cardiac arrhythmia
D. has relapse rates similar to the "night alarm"
E. should be administered at a dose of 3.5 mg/kg

Discussion: Imipramine is one of several pharmacological treatments for nocturnal enuresis. Other options include intranasal synthetic antidiuretic hormone (DDAVP) and stimulants. Imipramine has been shown to be effective in many randomized placebo-controlled double-blind trials. Toxic effects can include the possibility of sudden death, presumably due to cardiac arrhythmia.

Pages 733–735, Table 40–1 •

Answer C

3. In nocturnal enuresis, the night alarm

A. acts much more quickly than drug treatment
B. works more quickly if it is used together with methylamphetamine
C. requires little or no explanation to subjects
D. works less well in secondary enuresis
E. cures almost 90% of all cases

Discussion: The use of a night alarm, which is triggered by the presence of wet urine, has led to high rates of cure. However, cure is usually achieved only after 2 months. Adjuvant use of stimulants may speed the treatment, as might a louder alarm. A common problem is the failure of families to persist with treatment long enough.

Page 735 •

Answer B

4. Encopresis

A. is associated with constipation in more than 90% of cases
B. is often indicative of severe psychiatric illness
C. is equally common in boys and girls at the age of 8 years
D. can be caused by hypercalcemia
E. frequently is associated with "pot phobia"

Discussion: Although the majority of patients with encopresis are medically normal, a small proportion will have disease of etiological significance. Physical causes of encopresis without retention include inflammatory bowel disease, central nervous system disorders, and sensory disorders of the anorectal region. Encopresis with retention can be caused by Hirschsprung's disease, neurogenic megacolon, hypothyroidism, hypercalcemia, chronic codeine or laxative use, and anal-rectal stenosis or fissure.

Page 737 •

Answer D

5. Retentive encopresis

A. can be caused by Crohn's disease
B. is usually associated with smearing of feces
C. should usually be treated by oral laxatives alone
D. is associated with abnormal external anal sphincter functioning
E. is usually associated with coercive toilet training

Discussion: Encopretics with constipation or overflow are found to have rectal and colonic distention, massive impaction with hard feces, and a number of specific abnormalities of anorectal physiology. These abnormalities include elevated anal resting tone, decreased anorectal motility and weakenss of the internal anal sphincter, and dysfunction of the external anal sphincter (e.g., contraction during defecation).

Page 737 •

Answer D

CHAPTER

41 Generic Substance and Hallucinogen Use Disorders

Thomas R. Kosten

1. The dependence syndrome involves the following criteria:

A. tolerance, withdrawal, intoxication
B. intoxication, withdrawal, compulsive use
C. intoxication, compulsive use, tolerance
D. tolerance, withdrawal, compulsive use

Discussion: The dependence syndrome, defined by Edwards in 1976, had 10 criteria. The DSM-IV definition has seven criteria, of which tolerance and withdrawal are the first two. A pattern of compulsive use and its severity are delineated by the additional criteria. Tolerance and withdrawal are related to a higher risk of medical problems. Intoxication is a separate phenomenon.

Page 743 •

Answer D

2. Treatment-seeking substance abusers who are *most* likely to meet *all* seven of the DSM-IV criteria for dependence are dependent on

A. heroin
B. LSD
C. alcohol
D. cannabis
E. toluene

Discussion: Opioid abusers who seek treatment are more likely to meet all criteria for substance dependence. Hallucinogen abusers are less likely to have as severe a dependence by DSM-IV criteria. Alcoholic individuals and cocaine abusers have a more variable presentation.

Page 743 •

Answer A

3. Physical dependence on drugs such as heroin or alcohol is most likely to develop for the first time between ages

A. 15 and 20 years
B. 20 and 30 years
C. 30 and 40 years
D. 40 and 50 years

Discussion: There is a high prevalence for substance abuse between ages 18 and 24 years. The initial problem is one of intoxication. Tolerance and withdrawal phenomena take longer to develop and, if they develop, are evident in the third decade of life.

Page 744 •

Answer B

4. Rates of substance abuse in monozygotic twins compared with dizygotic twins are

A. three times higher in monozygotic twins
B. equal
C. two times higher in dizygotic twins
D. six times higher in monozygotic twins

Discussion: Family genetic studies have found rates of substance abuse three to four times higher in monozygotic than in dizygotic twins. No single marker has been confirmed. There is an association with alleles for dopamine receptors.

Pages 744–745 •

Answer A

5. The most common comorbid psychiatric disorder in substance abusers is

A. schizophrenia
B. antisocial personality
C. borderline personality
D. depression
E. obsessive-compulsive disorder

Discussion: In both the Epidemiological Catchment Area study and the National Comorbidity Survey, substance abuse and dependence were the most common comorbid disorders, usually in combination with affective and anxiety disorder. Antisocial personality disorder is also frequent, but major depression is most common.

Page 744, Table 41–1 (page 746) •

Answer D

6. "Gateway drugs" that in adolescents later lead to drug dependence, as first suggested by Kandel, include

A. alcohol, cocaine, heroin
B. alcohol, marijuana, cocaine
C. tobacco, alcohol, marijuana
D. tobacco, diazepam, marijuana
E. cocaine, diazepam, heroin

Discussion: Longitudinal studies by Kandel suggest that tobacco, alcohol, and marijuana are gateway drugs if they are used in the early teens. Adolescents who use these substances early are more likely to have substance dependence than are those who use them later in life. Postponement leads to decreased risk. There is an association between use of gateway drugs and conduct disorder.

Pages 746–747 •

Answer C

7. A biological test that can help determine the physiological manifestations of substance dependence is

A. breath alcohol analysis
B. urine toxicology screen
C. naloxone injection
D. serum liver enzyme activity
E. serum drug level measurement

Discussion: Naloxone injection precipitates withdrawal and is thus a challenge test for opioid dependence. Another test of dependence is a barbiturate tolerance test. Urine toxicological analysis, serum drug level measurements, and breath alcohol analysis can detect use within specific time frames, but positive results do not indicate dependence.

Page 748 •

Answer C

8. The most critical component in the following list for treating recently detoxified substance abusers as outpatients is

A. meeting with family "enablers"
B. getting vocational rehabilitation
C. regular urine or breath monitoring for substance abuse
D. avoiding psychotropic medications
E. insisting on Alcoholics Anonymous attendance

Discussion: Meeting with enablers, attending Alcoholics Anonymous, and vocational rehabilitation can and should all be part of the treatment of a newly abstinent substance abuser. The relative necessity and timing of these interventions will vary. Psychotropic medication is often essential in patients with comorbid disorders. Regular urine or breath monitoring is a requisite for an outpatient treatment.

Pages 750–752, Table 41–2 •

Answer C

9. After oral ingestion, LSD typically has its onset of psychoactive effects at

A. 10 minutes
B. 30 minutes
C. 60 minutes
D. 3 hours
E. 6 hours

Discussion: Whereas there are physiological sympathomimetic effects of LSD within 20 minutes, the psychoactive effects usually begin by 2 to 4 hours after the dose. There is no known physiologically lethal dose.

Answer D

10. Hallucinogens such as LSD are most likely to be associated with the following clinical symptoms:

A. auditory hallucinations
B. visual distortions
C. depersonalization
D. retarded depression
E. disorientation

Discussion: Hallucinogen intoxication is characteristic but can be of variable duration. A special issue is "flashbacks" to the drug-induced state, which are usually visual in nature. They can also be somatic or emotional and involve depersonalization.

Answer B

11. From the early 1970s to 1988, the lifetime prevalence of hallucinogen abuse among high-school seniors had changed by

A. increasing threefold
B. increasing twofold
C. decreasing fourfold
D. no significant amount
E. decreasing twofold

Discussion: In the late 1960s and early 1970s, at least one third of college students were estimated to have tried hallucinogens. The 1988 high-school senior survey estimated that 8% had ever tried LSD, 5% had used it in the last year, and 2% had used it in the previous month. Thus, a fourfold decrease has occurred. Polydrug abusers may commonly use hallucinogens.

Answer C

12. The "designer drug" MDMA most likely leads to damage to neurons associated with which neurotransmitter?

A. dopamine
B. norepinephrine
C. acetylcholine
D. serotonin

Discussion: MDMA is a ring-substituted amphetamine. Designer drugs of this class are associated with damage to serotonergic neurons. Another class of designer drugs that are opioid-like is toxic to dopamine neurons and can cause parkinsonian symptoms.

Pages 746, 750 •

Answer D

CHAPTER

42 Alcohol Use Disorders

Henry R. Kranzler • Thomas F. Babor • Pamela Moore

1. In the United States, the prevalence of abstention from alcohol

A. increases with increasing educational level
B. is higher in young men than in young women
C. exceeds 50% in women
D. is higher in whites than in blacks
E. decreases with increasing age

Discussion: The data from the 1988 U.S. National Health Interview Survey suggest that more than half of women do not drink alcohol. Increased age and lower level of education are associated with higher rates of abstention. Blacks and Hispanics also abstain more than whites do.

Page 756, Tables 42–1 and 42–2 (page 757) •

Answer C

2. In studies of psychiatric comorbidity:

A. Antisocial personality disorder is relatively uncommon in the community but is commonly found in association with alcoholism.
B. There is a relatively low prevalence of mood disorders among alcoholic individuals.
C. The high prevalence of anxiety disorders in community samples of alcoholic individuals reflects the inordinately increased risk of these disorders in alcoholic individuals.
D. Men are about twice as likely as women to have a diagnosis of major depression in clinical samples of alcoholic patients.
E. It has been clearly demonstrated that treatment of comorbid psychiatric disorders in alcoholic patients translates into improved drinking outcomes.

Discussion: The most common comorbid diagnoses with alcohol use disorders are major depression, antisocial personality disorder, drug dependence, and anxiety disorders. Indeed, the overlap between diagnoses of antisocial personality disorder and alcohol dependence suggests a commonality of etiology (73.6% of the Epidemiological Catchment Area study respondents with antisocial personality disorder met criteria for alcohol abuse or dependence).

Pages 757–759 •

Answer A

3. In DSM-IV, a diagnosis of alcohol dependence is given

A. only if tolerance or withdrawal is present
B. only if efforts to cut down or stop drinking (i.e., impaired control) are evident
C. only if a patient manifests three or more of the criteria for the diagnosis during a 12-month period
D. if a patient who previously met criteria for alcohol dependence has six or more drinks on an occasion
E. in any patient with characteristic signs and symptoms of alcohol withdrawal

Discussion: The DSM-IV diagnosis of dependence is made when three or more criteria are met. These include tolerance, withdrawal, and loss of control. Symptoms of alcohol withdrawal, a separate disorder, are also considered in a diagnosis of alcohol dependence.

Pages 760–761, Table 42–3 •

Answer C

4. For the assessment of heavy alcohol consumption during the preceding 8 hours, the most sensitive, widely available test is

A. the ratio of aspartate transaminase to alanine transaminase
B. γ-glutamyl transpeptidase
C. mean corpuscular volume of erythrocytes
D. alkaline phosphatase
E. breath alcohol level

Discussion: γ-Glutamyl transpeptidase elevations occur in three fourths of alcoholic patients before evidence of clinical liver disease. Elevated mean corpuscular volume of erythrocytes also indicates heavy drinking but can return to normal in 2 to 4 months of abstinence. Transaminase ratios are less sensitive than γ-glutamyl transpeptidase. Breath alcohol level is the best, most readily available measure of alcohol intoxication. This measures acute intoxication, not the sequelae of chronic intoxication. A level greater than 150 mg/dL in a patient who is not intoxicated is a sign of tolerance.

Pages 762–763 •

Answer E

5. Potentially life-threatening conditions that may be associated with alcohol use disorders

A. are rare
B. do not occur when only a diagnosis of alcohol abuse is present
C. can usually be adequately treated without medication
D. include acute withdrawal, serious medical complications (e.g., pancreatitis or bleeding esophageal varices), and acute psychiatric syndromes (e.g., psychosis or suicidal intent)

Discussion: There are several life-threatening conditions for which those who use alcohol are at increased risk. Age, gender, and specific alcohol-related diagnosis do not limit the risk. Appropriate emergency treatment is essential.

Page 766 •

Answer D

For each numbered item, select the lettered heading most closely associated with it. Each letter may be selected once, more than once, or not at all.

6. A. in a controlled environment
B. early full remission
C. early partial remission
D. sustained full remission

____ 1. Patient X has maintained sobriety, living at home with his wife during the 14 months after completion of alcoholism rehabilitation.
____ 2. Patient Y has been in prison for the past 6 months.
____ 3. In a 2-month period, Patient W has reduced his drinking and now meets only two criteria for alcohol dependence, after having met five criteria.
____ 4. Patient Z reports 4 months of continuous sobriety, during which time she has attended at least one AA meeting daily.

Discussion: In DSM-IV, course specifiers should be made with a diagnosis of alcohol dependence in remission. Early remission is used if either no criteria (full remission) or less than three criteria (partial remission) are noted in a period between 1 and 12 months. Sustained remission is greater than 12 months. A controlled environment is reserved for those with no access to alcohol.

Page 761 •

Answers 1, D; 2, A; 3, C; 4, B

7. A. buspirone
B. disulfiram
C. bupropion
D. naltrexone
E. fluoxetine

The following is true concerning the pharmacotherapy of alcoholism:

____ 1. This medication reduced the frequency of drinking and resulted in fewer drinks per drinking day than placebo in alcoholic individuals after withdrawal.
____ 2. Independent of whether a specific anxiety disorder was present, this medication has been shown to reduce drinking among anxious alcoholic individuals.
____ 3. This medication has a mechanism of action that involves binding to aldehyde dehydrogenase.
____ 4. This selective antidepressant may be useful for treating depression in alcoholic patients.

Discussion: Medications are used to treat alcohol withdrawal, maintain abstinence, or treat comorbid psychiatric disorders. Benzodiazepines are useful for withdrawal. An aversive drug such as disulfiram in conjunction with a psychosocial program of rehabilitation may prevent relapse. Naltrexone, an opioid antagonist, can also adjunctively be helpful in preventing relapse. Fluoxetine and buspirone have been studied for treatment of depression and anxiety, respectively, in alcoholic patients. Buspirone has also been shown to improve retention in treatment.

Pages 769–771 •

Answers 1, D; 2, A; 3, B; 4, E

8. A. zimeldine
B. desipramine
C. lithium carbonate
D. fluoxetine
E. diazepam

Concerning the treatment of comorbid depression in alcoholics:

____ 1. A higher oral dosage of this tricyclic antidepressant may be needed to compensate for the increased clearance of the drug that results from heavy drinking.

____ 2. This central nervous system depressant can be used to treat insomnia in alcoholic patients after detoxification, but it can also produce dependence.

____ 3. A large, multicenter study showed this medication to be no more effective than placebo in the prevention of relapse in either depressed or nondepressed drinkers.

____ 4. Although studies with this selective serotonin reuptake inhibitor have shown it to reduce drinking in heavy drinkers, it was withdrawn from commercial development because of adverse events.

Discussion: Treatment of comorbid depression in alcoholic patients is complicated by the challenge of making a correct diagnosis. Depressive symptoms are common in withdrawal but may remit spontaneously. If symptoms persist, use of a medication is warranted. Studies of tricyclic antidepressants have used more sophisticated dosing strategies to compensate for the fact that cigarette smoking and heavy drinking can stimulate hepatic enzymes. In a large Veterans Administration study, lithium was found to be no better than placebo. Zimeldine, a serotonin reuptake inhibitor, does reduce alcohol consumption. Studies of other selective serotonin reuptake inhibitors such as citalopram, fluoxetine, fluvoxamine, and viqualine have shown mixed results in terms of reduction of alcohol consumption.

Page 770 •

Answers 1, B; 2, E; 3, C; 4, A

CHAPTER

43 Caffeine Use Disorders

Eric C. Strain • Roland R. Griffiths

1. High levels of caffeine consumption in smokers may be partially due to

A. decreased absorption of caffeine
B. decreased metabolism of caffeine
C. increased absorption of caffeine
D. increased metabolism of caffeine
E. the synergistic subjective effects produced by the combination of caffeine and nicotine

Discussion: Excessive caffeine consumption has repeatedly been observed to be associated with smoking tobacco (nicotine dependence), and this higher consumption of caffeine in smokers may be partly due to the increased metabolism of caffeine in smokers. Significantly higher levels of caffeine consumption have also been noted in abstinent alcoholic versus nonalcoholic individuals, and usage levels of coffee, cigarettes, and alcohol have been shown to be positively related.

Page 780 •

Answer D

2. Typical features of caffeine intoxication can include all of the following **except**

A. gastrointestinal disturbance and diarrhea
B. muscle twitching and diuresis
C. pupillary constriction and drowsiness
D. restlessness and nervousness
E. tachycardia and flushed face

Discussion: Caffeine intoxication can produce restlessness, nervousness, excitement, insomnia, flushed face, diuresis, gastrointestinal disturbance, muscle twitching, rambling flow of thought and speech, tachycardia or cardiac arrhythmias, periods of inexhaustibility, and psychomotor agitation. It does not produce pupillary constriction and drowsiness.

Pages 779–782 •

Answer C

3. The most common feature of caffeine withdrawal is

A. depression
B. influenza-like symptoms
C. headache
D. impaired concentration
E. sleepiness-drowsiness

Discussion: Whereas each of these answers can be associated with caffeine withdrawal, the most common feature is headache. Studies suggest that up to 50% of people can experience headache if they abruptly stop moderate caffeine use, that is, 200 to 300 mg/d.

Pages 782–786 •

Answer C

4. Caffeine can be in all of the following **except**

A. analgesics
B. chocolate
C. cold remedies
D. fruit juices
E. weight loss aids

Discussion: Coffee, tea, and certain sodas (including some noncola sodas) can contain caffeine. In addition, chocolate and several over-the-counter medications, such as certain analgesics, cold remedies, and weight loss aids, can contain caffeine. However, fruit juices do not contain caffeine.

Page 782 •

Answer D

5. The average daily consumption of caffeine in the United States is

A. less than 100 mg
B. 101–200 mg
C. 201–300 mg
D. 301–400 mg
E. greater than 400 mg

Discussion: In the United States, it is estimated that more than 80% of adults consume caffeine on a daily basis, and the average daily consumption among adults is approximately 280 mg. The average daily consumption in other countries can be considerably higher. For example, in Sweden, it is 425 mg/d; in the United Kingdom, it is 444 mg/d.

Pages 786–787, Table 43–6 •

Answer C

For each numbered item, select the lettered heading most closely associated with it. Each letter may be selected once, more than once, or not at all.

6. Match the beverage with caffeine concentration:

____ 1. the amount of caffeine in brewed coffee

____ 2. the amount of caffeine in instant coffee

____ 3. the amount of caffeine in tea

A. 100 mg/6 oz
B. 70 mg/6 oz
C. 40 mg/6 oz
D. 20 mg/6 oz
E. 4–5 mg/6 oz

Discussion: Brewed coffee contains the highest concentration of caffeine for a beverage (100 mg/6 oz), followed by instant coffee (70 mg/6 oz). Caffeinated soda and tea contain approximately equal concentrations of caffeine (45 mg/6 oz and 40 mg/6 oz, respectively). Cocoa beverage (5 mg/6 oz), chocolate milk (4 mg/6 oz), and milk chocolate (6 mg/1 oz) each contain relatively low amounts of caffeine, but dark chocolate contains 20 mg/1 oz.

Page 781, Table 43–1 •

Answers 1, A; 2, B; 3, C

CHAPTER

44 Cannabis-Related Disorders

Amanda J. Gruber • Harrison G. Pope, Jr.

1. Individuals with cannabis dependence

A. frequently use other drugs of abuse
B. display a high prevalence of Axis II disorders
C. frequently exhibit cannabis-induced anxiety or psychotic disorders
D. often do not exhibit cannabis in their urine samples
E. usually have a preexisting Axis I disorder

Discussion: Cannabis use disorders are frequently comorbid with other substance abuse disorders. Surveys of psychiatric populations with mixed Axis I diagnoses, but not panic disorder, have found a high prevalence of cannabis use. There is also an association with conduct disorder in youth and antisocial personality disorder in adulthood.

Page 796 •

Answer A

2. Cannabis use in the United States

A. is more common in the lower socioeconomic classes
B. frequently progresses from initial experimentation to frank dependence
C. is responsible for a substantial portion of psychiatric admissions in college health centers
D. frequently begins in the early teens
E. usually does not escalate from experimentation to dependence for many years

Discussion: Cannabis is among the first drugs of experimentation (often in the teenage years) for all cultural groups in the United States. As with most other illicit drugs, cannabis use disorders appear more often in men, and these disorders are most common in persons between the ages of 18 and 30 years.

Pages 796, 800 •

Answer D

3. Negative effects of cannabis use do **not** include

A. bronchitis
B. residual impairment of neuropsychological function
C. cerebellar degeneration
D. "morning-after" impairment documented on flight simulators or driving simulators
E. possible exacerbation of preexisting Axis I disorders

Discussion: Residual effects of cannabis use have been observed 24 to 48 hours after acute intoxication. These include impairment on neuropsychological testing and in tests on driving and flight simulators. Individuals with preexisting Axis I disorders such as psychotic or anxiety disorders may be at risk for exacerbation of symptoms.

Pages 798–800 •

Answer C

4. In a longitudinal study of cannabis use at one American college, the percentage of students who reported weekly use of cannabis in 1978 was 26%. What was the prevalence of weekly use at the same college in 1989?

A. 51%
B. 36%
C. 22%
D. 12%
E. 6%

Discussion: Cannabis use seems to have increased in younger age groups, as the Monitoring the Future Study (1992–1993) of high-school students suggests. However, a survey of college students done at the same American college in 1969, 1978, and 1989 found that the prevalence of weekly cannabis use was 16%, 26%, and 6%, respectively. These findings suggest that only a small percentage of individuals who have tried cannabis are currently exhibiting frank cannabis abuse or dependence.

Page 796 •

Answer E

5. The treatment of cannabis dependence may require all **except**

A. treatment of an underlying Axis I disorder
B. group therapy

C. treatment of other associated drug abuse
D. a brief detoxification period with benzodiazepines
E. a brief detoxification period with methadone

Discussion: Some heavy users of cannabis may experience a withdrawal state during detoxification. Usually this is mild and requires no treatment. Symptoms may include restlessness, irritability, insomnia, decreased appetite, nausea, diarrhea, fever, yawning, depression, and others. One author has suggested long-acting benzodiazepines as a treatment if there is great discomfort or abnormal vital signs. There are frequently other drugs of abuse, and this complicates withdrawal and treatment. Patients with comorbid Axis I disorders or other substance dependence may need inpatient hospitalization.

Pages 801–803 •

Answer E

6. Cannabis-induced psychotic disorder

A. may linger for weeks, even after cannabis is withdrawn
B. occurs commonly but is almost invariably self-limited
C. in the United States, is apparently more common in women
D. may frequently represent an exacerbation of a preexisting psychotic disorder
E. occurs more frequently when cannabis is smoked in conjunction with opium

Discussion: Cannabis-induced psychotic disorder rarely persists beyond the period of acute intoxication. A review of the literature was unable to exhibit a series of unequivocal cases in which such symptoms persisted in the absence of an underlying Axis I disorder. For this reason, the presence of such symptoms should prompt a further work-up.

Pages 799–800 •

Answer D

7. Urine testing for cannabinoids

A. is currently still unreliable
B. may be compromised in accuracy by the presence of other drugs, especially phenyclidine
C. shows a good correlation between THC levels and the user's psychiatric illness
D. may show positive results for weeks after a cannabis-dependent individual has ceased smoking
E. can detect even picogram quantities of cannabinoids

Discussion: Tetrahydrocannabinol (THC) is highly lipophilic and is widely distributed throughout the body. It is metabolized by hydroxylation to other active metabolites with half-lives exceeding 50 hours. It is also conjugated to water-soluble metabolites that are slowly excreted in the bile, urine, hair, and feces. Because it is stored in adipose tissue, THC can be detected for up to 30 days after the individual's last exposure to cannabis.

Page 796 •

Answer D

8. Individuals with cannabis dependence

A. usually voluntarily seek treatment eventually
B. usually do not come for treatment until the disorder has been in progress for a decade or more
C. frequently enter treatment in the wake of an episode of cannabis-induced psychosis or anxiety
D. rarely seek treatment at all
E. respond quickly to treatment with a low probability of relapse, provided the treatment is begun early in the course of the disorder

Discussion: Individuals with cannabis dependence rarely seek treatment independently. They may, however, respond positively to an offer of treatment. In one investigation, a public service announcement directed at chronic marijuana users resulted in interviews of 225 people who responded. It was found that 74% reported negative consequences of their marijuana use, and 92% wanted to be treated.

Page 801 •

Answer D

CHAPTER

45 Cocaine Use Disorders

Elinore F. McCance

1. Risk factors for cocaine use disorders include

A. poverty
B. age
C. psychiatric illness
D. use of other street drugs
E. gender

Discussion: Epidemiological studies have not identified demographical characteristics that predict cocaine abuse. The only well documented predisposing condition related to cocaine abuse is psychiatric illness.

Page 808 •

Answer C

2. Tachyphylaxis refers to

A. increased heart rate during cocaine abuse
B. rapidly diminishing effects of cocaine despite continued presence of cocaine in plasma
C. a severe medical complication related to binge use of cocaine
D. a condition unique to cocaine use in which there is an increase in heart rate followed by cardiovascular collapse
E. physiological changes observed after a dose of cocaine

Discussion: The elimination half-life of cocaine is approximately 90 minutes, but cocaine-associated euphoria is of significantly shorter duration (depending on route of administration). This accounts for both the binge pattern of abuse and medical complications because plasma levels increase as multiple doses are consumed.

Pages 808–809 •

Answer B

3. Among the following conditions, the least likely medical complication of cocaine abuse is

A. myocardial infarct
B. seizures
C. hyperpyrexia
D. cardiac arrhythmia
E. vasculitis

Discussion: The major medical complications of cocaine abuse are cardiac or central nervous system related. Myocardial infarct and arrhythmia probably result from peripheral catecholaminergic effects of cocaine. Cocaine produces hyperpyrexia. Seizures may result from cocaine's ability to lower seizure threshold or from cardiac events related to cocaine use.

Pages 811, 813–814 •

Answer E

4. Acute abstinence after binge cocaine use

A. often precipitates an episode of major depression
B. is the time in which patients are at highest risk for cardiac events related to cocaine toxicity
C. often is associated with agitation, depression, and paranoia, which may result in emergent medical evaluation
D. is not associated with significant morbidity because cocaine is not physiologically addicting
E. is the period during which the cocaine abuser is most likely to decide to seek treatment for cocaine addiction

Discussion: The "crash" that follows a cocaine binge can be characterized by extreme agitation, depression, and paranoia. Suicidal ideation or attempts are not uncommon and may result in emergent medical and psychiatric treatment.

Pages 812–813 •

Answer C

5. The neurotransmitter most important to cocaine-induced euphoria is

A. norepinephrine
B. serotonin

C. dopamine
D. γ-aminobutyric acid (GABA)
E. glycine

Discussion: Cocaine inhibits dopamine reuptake and increases extracellular dopamine concentration. These effects in reward pathways (nucleus accumbens) are considered the best explanation of cocaine-induced euphoria at this time.

Page 809 •

Answer C

6. Dysphoria after cocaine use has been hypothesized to occur as a result of

A. inhibition of excitatory amino acids
B. noradrenergic postsynaptic receptor supersensitivity
C. chronic serotonin depletion
D. dopaminergic autoreceptor supersensitivity
E. GABAergic hyperfunction

Discussion: Chronic high-dose binge cocaine use has been associated with depression, irritability, and anhedonia during periods of abstinence in humans. Animal studies have shown chronic cocaine administration to decrease intracranial electrical self-stimulation (ICSS) of dopaminergic reward areas, and increased voltage is required to induce ICSS. Animal studies have also confirmed decreased dopaminergic neurotransmission after chronic cocaine exposure. This implies that brain reward regions may be down-regulated or less sensitive to neurotransmitters after chronic cocaine exposure. Alteration of receptor sensitivity including autoreceptor supersensitivity could decrease dopaminergic neurotransmission, which may be important to the development of dysphoria often seen after cocaine abuse.

Pages 809–810 •

Answer D

For each numbered item, select the lettered heading most closely associated with it. Each letter may be selected once, more than once, or not at all.

A. amantadine
B. bromocriptine
C. desipramine
D. fluoxetine
E. disulfiram

____ 7. a dopamine agonist with high affinity for the D_2 receptor

Discussion: Bromocriptine, which has D_2 agonist effects, has been put forward as a potential pharmacotherapy to be used in early abstinence. Its proposed efficacy is based on animal studies showing that long-term cocaine use may result in dopaminergic autoreceptor supersensitivity, which would effectively reduce dopaminergic neurotransmission. Bromocriptine may reverse this deficit, but its usefulness has yet to be shown in clinical trials.

Pages 817–818 •

Answer B

____ 8. some studies have shown reduced cocaine craving during early treatment at dosages of 200 to 300 mg daily

Discussion: Amantadine is a dopamine agonist that has been shown to have short-term beneficial effects on cocaine craving and use at 200 to 300 mg daily. As with bromocriptine, the ability of amantadine to enhance dopaminergic neurotransmission is thought to underlie any therapeutic effect. Amantadine's clinical benefit has yet to be shown in controlled clinical trials.

Pages 817–818 •

Answer A

____ 9. may be useful for those in whom alcohol use is a trigger for cocaine use

Discussion: Comorbid cocaine-alcohol abuse is common. For many addicts, alcohol use is a trigger for cocaine use. Because disulfiram (Antabuse) prevents alcohol use, it may reduce cocaine use in such individuals. This was demonstrated in a pilot study but has yet to be shown in controlled clinical trials.

Page 819 •

Answer 3

____ 10. reduction in cocaine use, but not abstinence

Discussion: Fluoxetine has been shown to reduce cocaine use as shown by urine benzoylecgonine quantitation. Fluoxetine has not been shown to be effective in producing abstinence.

Pages 818–819 •

Answer D

____ 11. serum concentration should be observed to maximize therapeutic benefit

Discussion: Desipramine administered at dosages of 200 to 250 mg daily for 4 to 6 weeks has been shown in some studies to be effective in decreasing cocaine craving and maintaining abstinence. Serum desipramine level should be monitored because levels of 220 ng/mL and greater have been associated with side effects, including anxiety and agitation, which may contribute to relapse.

Page 818 •

Answer C

CHAPTER

46 Phencyclidine Use Disorders

Ilana Zylberman • Joyce H. Lowinson • Stephen R. Zukin

1. Acute psychotomimetic effects of phencyclidine (PCP) result from

A. inhibition of dopamine reuptake
B. disruption of glutamatergic neurotransmission
C. anticholinergic effects
D. occupation of sigma receptors
E. inhibition of serotonin reuptake

Discussion: PCP binds to a high-affinity PCP receptor that is located within the *N*-methyl-D-aspartate (NMDA) receptor complex. Binding of PCP uncompetitively inhibits NMDA receptor activation by L-glutamate. This disrupts NMDA receptor–mediated glutamatergic neurotransmission. Higher or repeated doses of PCP result in activity at other sites, such as catecholamine and indolamine receptors, leading to other effects such as coma, seizures, and respiratory arrest.

Pages 828–829, Figs. 46–1 and 46–2 •

Answer B

2. Choose the correct answer:

A. PCP is difficult to synthesize.
B. Hemodialysis is an effective therapeutic measure for PCP overdose.
C. PCP is highly hydrophilic.
D. In the stomach, PCP is largely nonionized.
E. PCP may undergo enterohepatic recirculation.

Discussion: PCP, which is easy to synthesize, is extremely lipid soluble. In the stomach and urinary tract, it is ionized owing to a pK_a of 8.5. In the nonacidic environment of the small bowel, it is nonionized, readily diffuses into the portal circulation, and is subject to enterohepatic recirculation. This last phenomenon may account for the fluctuating clinical course. Hemodialysis is ineffective because of PCP's large volume of distribution.

Pages 827, 829 •

Answer E

3. The peak of PCP popularity occurred in the

A. early 1970s
B. late 1970s
C. early 1980s
D. late 1980s
E. early 1990s

Discussion: Illicit PCP use was first reported in 1965. By 1979, 13% of high-school seniors had tried it. Emergency department visits and deaths also peaked in 1978 to 1979. There have been episodic, geographically localized increases in PCP abuse since that time.

Pages 827–828 •

Answer B

4. Proper assessment and treatment measures should **not** include

A. minimization of sensory stimulation
B. serum creatine kinase levels
C. benzodiazepines
D. haloperidol
E. "talking the patient down"

Discussion: PCP users must be placed in an environment with minimal sensory stimuli in an acute evaluation. Talking the patient down, as may be done with those using LSD, is not safe. Serum creatine kinase levels, along with uric acid and aspartate and alanine transaminase elevations, were found to be associated with rhabdomyolysis. There is no pharmacological antagonist for PCP. Benzodiazepines can reduce agitation. Neuroleptics can lower the seizure threshold.

Pages 831–832 •

Answer E

5. Which of the following drugs has the same mechanism of action as PCP?

A. LSD
B. amphetamine
C. cocaine
D. ketamine
E. marijuana

Discussion: PCP was developed as a general anesthetic in the 1950s under the brand name Sernyl. PCP and ketamine are both considered "dissociative anesthetics" because they induce semiconsciousness with sharp dissociation from the environment. Ketamine tolerance has been studied and is postulated to be similar to that which develops for PCP.

Pages 827, 829 •

Answer D

6. Features of PCP intoxication do **not** include

A. waxing and waning of symptoms
B. coma
C. psychosis
D. violent behavior
E. synesthesia

Discussion: PCP abusers may present in a variety of ways, either medically or psychiatrically. There is usually an acute psychosis, which can occur at low serum levels of drug. Users do not have subjective feelings of drunkenness and can be impulsively violent. Schizophrenia-like symptoms may persist for days to weeks. Patients are at high risk for coma, seizures, hypertension, and rhabdomyolysis. Nystagmus is found in 57% of patients.

Pages 829–831 •

Answer E

7. PCP-related deaths result more frequently from

A. acute renal failure
B. hyperthermia
C. seizures
D. homicides and accidents
E. hypertensive crisis

Discussion: Whereas there are several potentially life-threatening reactions to PCP, such as acute renal failure, hyperthermia, seizures, and hypertensive crisis, many PCP-related deaths involve external events, such as homicides or accidents. In 1983, 66% of PCP-related deaths reported involved at least one other drug.

Pages 828, 830–831 •

Answer D

8. Which of the following statements is **incorrect?**

A. PCP stimulates activation of the ion channel gated by the NMDA receptor in the presence of glycine.
B. The usual precursor for PCP synthesis is piperidine.
C. Negative results of urine toxicology screen do not rule out PCP intoxication.
D. Physical injury is frequently found in PCP-intoxicated patients because of anesthesia and violence.
E. The clinical picture of PCP intoxication can be indistinguishable from schizophrenia.

Discussion: PCP inhibits NMDA receptor activation in the presence of glutamate. Glycine is a coagonist.

Page 828, Fig. 46–1 •

Answer A

CHAPTER

47 Inhalant Disorders

Charles W. Sharp • Neil Rosenberg

1. Inhalant intoxication is least likely to include the following symptom:

A. incoordination
B. blurred vision
C. dysarthria
D. lethargy
E. hyperreflexia

Discussion: Signs and symptoms of inhalant intoxication include visual disturbances, incoordination, dysarthria, and depressed reflexes.

Page 837 •

Answer E

2. Solvent abusers are most likely to be

A. white teenage boys
B. minority preteenagers
C. minority college-age women
D. white adult men
E. preteenagers of different ethnic groups

Discussion: The highest rates of inhalant abuse are among eighth-graders. In this age group, the rate compares with that for marijuana use and is higher than for cocaine use.

Pages 837–838, Table 47–3 •

Answer E

3. The comorbid psychiatric disorder most likely to be associated with inhalant abuse is

A. depression
B. panic
C. schizophrenia
D. antisocial personality
E. organic brain syndrome

Discussion: Comorbidity in this population has not been well studied. Antisocial personality disorder is common. Inhalant abusers have been found to be more self-destructive than other drug abusers in a study of psychiatric emergency department patients. Psychotic disorders are commonly reported, but no systematic study has been done.

Pages 838–839 •

Answer D

4. Ototoxicity is most likely associated with the following abused substance:

A. nitrous oxide
B. toluene
C. butane
D. fluorocarbons
E. leaded gasoline

Discussion: Clinically, toluene abusers have midhigh-frequency loss and abnormal brain stem auditory evoked responses. In animal models, there is destruction of cochlear cells caused by toluene and trichloroethylene, but benzene and trichloroethane do not produce these changes. Structure-activity relationships have been studied, and interactions with other compounds such as *n*-hexane have been examined. Lead causes a characteristic syndrome that can be treated. Nitrous oxide produces a sensorimotor polyneuropathy.

Pages 842–843, Tables 47–7 and 47–8 •

Answer B

5. Toluene inhalation is most likely to lead to the following abnormality on brain imaging:

A. increased fluorodeoxyglucose uptake in frontal lobes on positron emission tomography
B. multifocal loss of white matter on MRI
C. increased fluorodeoxyglucose uptake in occipital cortex on positron emission tomography
D. increased lateral ventricular size on MRI
E. reduced lateral ventricular size on MRI

Discussion: Clinically, toluene abusers frequently suffer from cognitive dysfunction and even dementia. Magnetic resonance imaging (MRI) findings show diffuse cerebral, cerebellar, and brain stem atrophy; loss of differentiation of gray and white matter; and increased periventricular white matter signal intensity on T2-weighted images. On pathological examination, there is leukoencephalopathy with changes similar to adrenoleukodystrophy.

Pages 840–842, Figs. 47–1 and 47–2 •

Answer B

6. Urine toxicological analysis in toluene abusers is most likely to show high levels of

A. homovanillic acid
B. hippuric acid
C. benzene
D. benzoylecgonine
E. ketones

Discussion: High levels of hippuric acid or cresols in the urine indicate toluene exposure. Urine trichloroacetate is useful in diagnosing trichlorinated hydrocarbon exposure. Ketones and homovanillic acid are natural metabolites, and benzoylecgonine is a metabolite of cocaine. Screens for hippuric acid can be an adjunct in treatment.

Pages 842, 847 •

Answer B

7. The target organ that is least likely to be adversely affected by inhalant abuse is the

A. cerebellum
B. liver
C. otic nerve
D. kidney
E. none of the above; each solvent affects any one organ differently

Discussion: Toxic effects are manifold and overlapping. Effects on the kidney can precipitate acidosis, which may be the basis for neurological disease. Solvents also affect the liver, lungs, heart, and hematopoietic system.

Pages 839–846 •

Answer E

8. Most abused inhalants affect the brain directly, but the inhalant most likely to act primarily through cardiovascular smooth muscle is

A. butane
B. chloroform
C. toluene
D. nitrites
E. leaded gasoline

Discussion: Aliphatic nitrites act on cardiovascular smooth muscle as vasodilators and have been reported to cause bradycardia. In the 19th century, amyl nitrite was used to treat angina pectoris. Although the primary site of action of other inhalants is not the heart, arrhythmia is one of the most common causes of death among inhalant abusers.

Pages 835, 845 Table 47–1 (page 836) •

Answer D

9. Abused products containing solvents are most likely to

A. contain a variety of substances
B. have solvents clearly labeled
C. be one type of substance
D. be swallowed
E. be illegal

Discussion: Most solvents that are abused are not illegal substances and are widely available. There are many different chemicals in products such as aerosols, degreasers, and glue. They are not specifically labeled.

Pages 835–836 •

Answer A

CHAPTER

48 Nicotine Use Disorders

Susan J. Fiester

1. Nicotine withdrawal syndrome includes all of the following symptoms **except**

A. depressed mood
B. insomnia
C. nausea
D. irritability or frustration
E. restlessness

Discussion: Nicotine withdrawal is accompanied by four of eight symptoms that include, in addition to the above, anxiety, difficulty concentrating, decreased heart rate, and increased appetite or weight gain.

Pages 853, 855 •

Answer C

2. Which of the following is true regarding the epidemiology of cigarette smoking and tobacco dependence?

A. The lifetime prevalence of nicotine dependence in the United States is 20%.
B. More women than men have successfully stopped smoking in recent years.
C. The current prevalence of smoking is 14%.
D. Most women stop smoking during pregnancy and do not start smoking again after delivery.
E. The prevalence of smoking has been increasing in industrialized countries.

Discussion: The prevalence of smoking is increasing in most developing countries while it is decreasing in most industrialized countries. In the United States, there has been increasing societal pressure for individuals to stop smoking. However, despite an increase in the proportion of smokers who are quitting, 25% of the U.S. population continues to smoke, with a lifetime prevalence of nicotine dependence of 20%. Only 45% of the population has never smoked. Slightly more men than women smoke, although a greater proportion of men successfully stop smoking.

Page 853 •

Answer A

3. Nicotine effects include all of the following **except**

A. decreased anxiety
B. decreased heart rate and blood pressure
C. increased concentration and vigilance
D. increased metabolic rate
E. increased appetite

Discussion: Nicotine is a powerful psychoactive substance with a host of actions. It improves mood, decreases anxiety, decreases distress in response to stressful stimuli, and decreases aggression; improves overall cognitive function and performance; decreases appetite for simple carbohydrates, decreases stress-induced eating, and increases resting metabolic rate.

Pages 854–855 •

Answer E

4. All of the following are true of the natural history and course of nicotine addiction **except:**

A. History of depressive disorder or substance use disorder predicts a proven outcome in smoking cessation.
B. Relapse rates are much lower than those for alcohol and other substances of abuse.
C. Repeated attempts at cessation are often necessary before abstinence can be achieved.
D. Withdrawal symptoms can continue for 3 to 4 weeks or longer.
E. Significant health benefits can result after cessation even in long-term smokers.

Discussion: Cessation attempts result in high relapse rates. The relapse curve for smoking cessation parallels that for opiates: 65% of those who stop smoking relapse in 3 months, and another 10% relapse in 3 to 6 months. The relapse rate is 80% by 1 year. Less than a quarter of people who have quit smoking are successful on their first attempt. The average smoker attempts cessation two or three times before success.

Page 855, Table 48–1 •

Answer B

5. Which of the following is true of the treatment of nicotine addiction?

A. Behavioral therapy should always be provided.
B. Nicotine replacement provides the best outcome.
C. Replacement by the transdermal nicotine patch combined with behavioral therapy produces the best cessation rates.
D. Antidepressant therapy provides no benefit.
E. Nicotine nasal spray is the most effective and safest form of nicotine replacement.

Discussion: A summary of overall quit rates demonstrates that quit rates are the highest for combined psychosocial and psychopharmacological interventions, although transdermal nicotine alone and behavioral therapy alone result in substantial success in smoking cessation. Essentially, nicotine replacement therapy, particularly transdermal nicotine, doubles the long-term abstinence rate; behavioral therapy doubles the effectiveness of transdermal nicotine.

Pages 861–862, Table 48–4 •

Answer C

6. Which of the following medications has been shown in controlled trials to be beneficial in treating nicotine addiction?

A. fluoxetine
B. buspirone
C. alprazolam
D. amphetamines
E. benzodiazepines

Discussion: Buspirone has been shown to decrease craving, anxiety, and fatigue during withdrawal from nicotine. Although it failed to reduce withdrawal symptoms in some studies, it significantly increased the cessation rate in other studies. Equivocal results have been found for anxiolytics such as alprazolam. Selective serotonin reuptake inhibitors such as fluoxetine have not been found to be effective; tricyclics such as doxepin decrease craving and cigarette use.

Page 859 •

Answer B

CHAPTER

49 Opioid-Related Disorders

George E. Woody • Laura F. McNicholas

1. Recent estimates put the number of opioid addicts in the United States at

A. 500,000 persons
B. 1,000,000 persons
C. 2,000,000 persons
D. 4,000,000 persons
E. 5,000,000 persons

Discussion: Exact figures are difficult to obtain, but recent estimates indicate that there may be as many as 2 million opioid addicts in the United States. The Epidemiological Catchment Area study found that 0.7% of those surveyed ever met criteria for opioid dependence or abuse.

Pages 867–868 •

Answer C

2. The most common route of administration for heroin is

A. inhaled
B. intravenous injection
C. oral
D. smoked
E. subcutaneous injection

Discussion: Heroin is usually injected intravenously. When very pure heroin is available, smoking and inhalation (snorting) can become common as well.

Page 869 •

Answer B

3. Which of the following signs or symptoms of withdrawal is specific to opioid withdrawal or abstinence?

A. agitation
B. drug craving
C. increased systolic blood pressure
D. lacrimation
E. restlessness

Discussion: Lacrimation and rhinorrhea are characteristic of opioid withdrawal only. Drug craving, agitation, and restlessness are evident in other withdrawal states also. Blood pressure changes are not a criterion of opioid withdrawal.

Pages 869–870 •

Answer D

4. Severe opioid intoxication is most effectively treated by

A. administration of a respiratory stimulant
B. gastric lavage
C. intravenous hydration for hypotension
D. naloxone injected intravenously
E. supportive care, including respiratory support

Discussion: Naloxone, an opioid antagonist, reverses acute and severe intoxication. It can be administered as an intravenous infusion if necessary. Other supportive measures may be necessary, but naloxone should, for instance, reverse respiratory depression.

Pages 869, 874 •

Answer D

5. The initial dose of methadone necessary to treat opioid withdrawal is most likely to be

A. 10 mg
B. 30 mg
C. 45 mg
D. 60 mg
E. 100 mg

Discussion: An initial dose of 20 to 30 mg of methadone should stop signs and symptoms of withdrawal. This may not last 24 hours, and a second dose may be necessary 2 to 16 hours after the first. The Food and Drug Administration does not permit administering more than 30 mg in a single dose or more than 40 mg in divided doses on the first day of methadone treatment.

Pages 875–876 •

Answer B

6. The most common appropriately used medication for opioid detoxification, other than methadone, is

A. clonidine
B. clonazepam
C. clozapine
D. diazepam
E. lorazepam

Discussion: Clonidine, an α-adrenergic agonist with inhibitory action at the locus coeruleus, has been used to suppress sympathetic overactivity in patients withdrawing from opioids. It was found to be 80% to 90% effective in inpatient populations in decreasing signs and symptoms of withdrawal. Problems with this medication include hypotension, lethargy, insomnia, dizziness, and oversedation.

Page 875 •

Answer A

7. The euphorigenic, analgesic, and respiratory depressant effects of opioid agonists are thought to be mediated by which opioid receptor?

A. δ (delta)
B. ε (epsilon)
C. κ (kappa)
D. μ (mu)
E. σ (sigma)

Discussion: The μ receptor, for which morphine is a prototypical agonist, appears most closely related to opioid analgesic euphoriant and respiratory depressant effects.

Page 867 •

Answer D

8. Of the drugs listed, the substance of abuse least likely to be concomitantly abused by opioid addicts is

A. alcohol
B. alprazolam
C. cocaine
D. lysergic acid diethylamide
E. marijuana

Discussion: Alcohol, cocaine, and benzodiazepines are a significant problem among opioid addicts. Polysubstance abuse complicates acute management of withdrawal states as well as long-term rehabilitation.

Pages 869, 872 •

Answer D

CHAPTER

50 Sedative, Hypnotic, or Anxiolytic Use Disorders

Donald R. Wesson • Walter Ling • David E. Smith

1. Which of the following medications is usually considered a sedative-hypnotic?

A. phenobarbital
B. amitriptyline
C. zolpidem
D. chlorpromazine
E. buspirone

Discussion: Although many antidepressants produce sedation and are often prescribed as alternatives to sedative-hypnotics, they are not usually classified as sedative-hypnotics. Like the antidepressants, neuroleptics may produce significant sedation; however, they are not usually classified as sedative-hypnotics. Phenobarbital is not considered a barbiturate hypnotic, but amobarbital, pentobarbital, and secobarbital among others are classified as such. Although buspirone is used for treatment of anxiety, its pharmacological profile is not the same as that of classic sedative-hypnotics, and it is not typically classified with them.

Pages 881–882, Table 50–1 •

Answer C

2. Which of the following signs or symptoms is **not** common in sedative-hypnotic withdrawal?

A. vivid nightmares
B. slurred speech
C. anxiety
D. tachycardia
E. grand mal seizures

Discussion: Slurred speech is usually a sign of sedative-hypnotic intoxication but not of withdrawal. Other symptoms of withdrawal include tremor, insomnia, nausea, postural hypotension, seizures, delirium, and hyperpyrexia.

Pages 883–884 •

Answer B

3. Which of the following is a DSM-IV criterion for sedative-hypnotic abuse?

A. loss of control (i.e., the drug is often taken in larger amounts or for a longer period than was intended)
B. intense craving for sedative-hypnotics
C. continued use despite having persistent or recurrent social or interpersonal problems caused or exacerbated by the effects of the substance
D. frequent or daily use of a sedative-hypnotic without a prescription
E. using sedative-hypnotics to come down from cocaine

Discussion: Loss of control is a criterion for substance dependence but not abuse. Craving is not a criterion for abuse or dependence. Continued use despite persistent problems is a criterion of abuse. The clinical difficulty may be determining whether the recurrent social problems or interpersonal problems are caused or exacerbated by the effects of the substance rather than the underlying disorder for which the medication is being prescribed. The source of the medication is not a criterion for abuse or dependence, nor is use of the medication for nonmedical purposes.

Page 885 •

Answer C

4. In a patient who has been taking sedative-hypnotics daily at doses beyond the usual therapeutic range, which of the following approaches is **not** acceptable medical practice?

A. Immediately stop all sedative-hypnotics and substitute a sedating neuroleptic, such as chlorpromazine.
B. Substitute adequate doses of phenobarbital and gradually reduce the phenobarbital.
C. Gradually reduce the daily dose of the sedative-hypnotic.

D. Immediately stop all sedative-hypnotics and lecture on sleep hygiene.
E. Use carbamazepine to prevent withdrawal seizures.

Discussion: Abruptly stopping sedative-hypnotics in a patient who may be physically dependent is medically contraindicated. Neuroleptics may reduce seizure threshold and should be avoided during withdrawal, if possible. If an antipsychotic is necessary for control of acute psychosis, haloperidol, in conjunction with adequate doses of sedatives or anticonvulsants, is the preferred regimen. Gradually reducing the daily dose of the sedative hypnotic is a reasonable approach for long-acting sedative-hypnotics if the patient's access to medications can be controlled. Phenobarbital or other long-acting medication substitution is preferable for short-acting sedative-hypnotics. Antidepressants may lower seizure threshold and should not be started until detoxification is complete.

Pages 886–887 •

Answer A

CHAPTER

51 Dementia, Delirium, and Other Cognitive Disorders

Robert L. Frierson

1. False-positive VDRL results can be caused by all of the following **except**

A. autoimmune disorders
B. AIDS
C. old age
D. drug abuse

Discussion: False-positive VDRL test results are encountered among the elderly, drug abusers, and patients with autoimmune disorders. In addition, because the VDRL response may revert to negative in time, 20% to 30% of patients in later stages of syphilis will have a false-negative result.

Page 912, Table 51–4 (page 901) •

Answer B

2. Myoclonus can result from all of the following **except**

A. Alzheimer's disease
B. attempted hanging
C. carbon monoxide poisoning
D. AIDS
E. meperidine

Discussion: Myoclonus can be seen in all of these conditions except carbon monoxide poisoning. Other movement disorders are common in dementia, including tremor, chorea, and asterixis. Carbon monoxide poisoning can cause chorea.

Pages 900–901, Tables 51–3 and 51–8 •

Answer C

3. Blackouts

A. represent structural brain damage
B. occur only in chronic drinkers
C. never result from sedative-hypnotic use
D. correlate with amount of alcohol consumed per episode

Discussion: Blackouts are periods of amnesia for events that occur during heavy drinking. They are not related to chronicity of alcohol abuse but frequently occur in binge drinkers. They can occur with use of benzodiazepines.

Pages 912, 923 •

Answer D

4. Wernicke-Korsakoff syndrome is associated with

A. gastric carcinoma
B. peripheral neuropathy
C. amnestic disorder
D. all of the above

Discussion: Wernicke-Korsakoff syndrome, an amnestic disorder, is associated with alcoholism as well as other malnourished states, such as marasmus, gastric carcinoma, and human immunodeficiency virus (HIV) spectrum disease. Peripheral neuropathy is commonly associated. These patients only rarely recover.

Page 923 •

Answer D

5. With which parameter is the severity of dementia in Alzheimer's disease most closely correlated?

A. increased ventricular size
B. increase in concentration of neurofibrillary tangles
C. increase in concentration of senile (neuritic) plaques
D. degree of cortical atrophy
E. decrease in cerebral somatostatin concentration

Discussion: The concentration of neuritic plaques is directly associated with the severity of Alzheimer's disease. Neurofibrillary tangles are not so connected.

Pages 902–904 •

Answer C

6. The inheritance pattern in Wilson's disease is

A. sex-linked recessive
B. autosomal recessive
C. autosomal dominant
D. unknown

Discussion: Wilson's disease is inherited in an autosomal recessive manner. Features of Wilson's disease include dementia, movement disorder, and hepatic dysfunction.

Page 914 •

Answer B

7. Pseudodementia is characterized by which of the following?

A. remote memory preservation
B. guesswork on mental status examination
C. slow progression
D. good insight into cognitive deficits
E. consistently poor performance on testing

Discussion: Differentiation between dementia and the pseudodementia seen in depressive states can be challenging. Patients with pseudodementia, in addition to signs and symptoms of depression, may also have a rapid course of decline, seek treatment early, and have insight into their condition. Some authors have criticized this term because many patients have both dementia and depression.

Pages 899–900, Fig. 51–2 •

Answer D

Questions 8 to 10: For each numbered item, select the lettered heading most closely associated with it. Each letter may be selected once, more than once, or not at all.

8. Match the characteristic with a form of dementia.

____ 1. more common in men
____ 2. prominent physical impairments
____ 3. multiple lucencies on magnetic resonance imaging
____ 4. homonymous hemianopia
____ 5. reduced central nervous system acetylcholine levels

A. vascular dementia
B. Alzheimer's dementia
C. both

Discussion: Vascular dementia, which is usually the result of advanced cerebrovascular disease, is the second most common cause of dementia. There is usually an early appearance of lateralizing neurological signs. Radiographical evidence and cerebral ischemia are also common. Change in central nervous system acetylcholine levels is characteristic of Alzheimer's disease.

Pages 907–908 •

Answers 1, A; 2, A; 3, A; 4, A; 5, B

9. Match the infectious agent with the condition.

____ 1. prion
____ 2. slow virus
____ 3. RNA-associated retrovirus
____ 4. mutant measles virus

A. Creutzfeldt-Jakob disease
B. Pick's disease
C. kuru
D. AIDS
E. subacute sclerosing panencephalitis

Discussion: Infectious causes of dementia are less frequent but some are increasingly seen, such as AIDS dementia and neurosyphilis. The latter may also overlap with HIV disease. Pick's disease is not of infectious etiology.

Pages 908–912 •

Answers 1, A; 2, C; 3, D; 4, E

10. Match the finding with the appropriate condition.

____ 1. progressive dementia
____ 2. neuron loss in nucleus basalis of Meynert
____ 3. parietal lobe spared
____ 4. argentophilic inclusion bodies
____ 5. Down's syndrome

A. Pick's disease
B. Alzheimer's disease
C. both

Discussion: Pick's disease is a rare form of progressive dementia that is also characterized by reduced acetylcholine levels. On pathological examination, there is atrophy and sclerosis of the frontal and temporal lobes with notable argentophilic inclusion bodies. The relative sparing of the parietal and occipital lobes accounts for the different clinical presentation from Alzheimer's disease.

Pages 906–907 •

Answers 1, C; 2, C; 3, A; 4, A; 5, B

CHAPTER

52 Schizophrenia

Debra A. Pinals • Alan Breier

1. Schizophrenia, paranoid type, is distinguished from other subtypes by

A. bizarre mannerisms and posturing
B. disorganized speech or behavior
C. flat or inappropriate affect
D. good prognosis and earlier age at onset
E. prominent hallucinations or delusions

Discussion: The subtypes of schizophrenia listed in DSM-IV are based on most prominent symptoms observed and may not be stable over time. There is also a dimensional descriptor to characterize the presence or absence of psychotic, disorganized, or negative symptom dimensions during the entire course of the illness. Paranoid type is marked by hallucinations and delusions in the face of a clear sensorium and unchanged cognition. Disorganization of speech or behavior and negative symptoms are not usually present to a significant degree. Delusions (usually persecutory or grandiose) may be organized around a theme. There is usually later age at onset and better prognosis.

Pages 930–932 •

Answer E

2. Suicide accounts for what percentage of the mortality rate of schizophrenia?

A. 1%
B. 5%
C. 10%
D. 15%
E. 20%

Discussion: The mortality rate of schizophrenia is estimated to be twice that of the general population. Approximately 10% of the mortality is secondary to suicide. Young schizophrenic men are most likely to complete suicide. Degree of social isolation, agitation, depression, sense of hopelessness, history of prior suicide attempts, and recent loss may be associated with an increased risk of suicide among schizophrenic individuals.

Page 936 •

Answer C

For each numbered item, select the lettered heading most closely associated with it. Each letter may be selected once, more than once, or not at all.

3. Match the term with the correct definition:

____ 1. repetition of words spoken by others	A. tangentiality
____ 2. repetition of actions of others	B. echolalia
____ 3. linking sounds in speech pattern	C. echopraxia
____ 4. repetition of words or phrases	D. perseveration
____ 5. weak connections of ideas	E. clang association

Discussion: Because there is no specific laboratory test that will yield a diagnosis of schizophrenia, the mental status examination is crucial in making a correct diagnosis. Thought processes, which cannot be measured, are assessed by extrapolation from the organization of speech. Subtleties of thought disorder may not be obvious, and careful listening by trained psychiatrists is often required. In addition to the disturbances mentioned above, there are thought process abnormalities characteristic of negative symptoms. These include thought blocking, paucity of thought content, and increased latency of response time.

Pages 946–948 •

Answers 1, B; 2, C; 3, E; 4, D; 5, A

4. The concordance rate of schizophrenia among monozygotic twins is approximately

A. 20%
B. 30%
C. 40%
D. 50%
E. 60%

Discussion: Twin studies are an approach to understanding the relative genetic contribution to schizophrenia. The concordance rate among dizygotic twins is 8% to 12%, which is much greater than the 1% prevalence in the general population and is similar to the rate observed for first-degree siblings. The concordance rate for monozygotic twins is approximately 50%. Even though this high rate is compelling evidence for genetic contributions, that it is not higher is evidence of additional nongenetic factors in the etiology of schizophrenia.

Pages 936–937 •

Answer D

5. Working memory and emotional expression are functions of the

A. anterior cingulate
B. entorhinal cortex
C. inferior parietal cortex
D. prefrontal cortex
E. superior temporal gyrus

Discussion: All of the above areas, with the exception of the inferior parietal cortex, have been implicated in studies of the pathophysiology of schizophrenia. In addition, the amygdala, hippocampus, thalamus, and striatum have been studied. The prefrontal cortex, one of the largest regions of the human brain, is responsible for sophisticated functions including temporary storage of information, attention, suppression of interference from internal and external sources, and emotional expression. Computed tomography studies have demonstrated prefrontal atrophy; positron emission tomography studies have shown decreased frontal glucose use and blood flow, which is known as hypofrontality. It is not clear whether impaired activation of the frontal lobes during cognitive tasks is a primary frontal deficit or is secondary to other difficulties with cognitive task performance.

Pages 938–940 •

Answer D

6. Clozapine is considered an atypical antipsychotic agent because

A. it is associated with antipsychotic efficacy and no extrapyramidal symptoms
B. it is more effective in the treatment of negative symptoms than typical neuroleptics
C. it exerts its effects through multiple neurotransmitter symptoms
D. it is a weaker D_2 antagonist than typical antipsychotic agents
E. it is a dibenzodiazepine

Discussion: Clozapine, which had been used in Europe in the 1970s, was approved by the Food and Drug Administration in 1989. It is considered atypical because it is an effective antipsychotic that is not associated with a risk of extrapyramidal symptoms. All the other statements are true with the exception that its effect on negative symptoms is controversial. Clozapine does have an antagonistic effect on the 5-HT_2 receptor, but it primarily acts as a D_4 receptor blocker.

Pages 956–958 •

Answer A

CHAPTER

53 Bipolar Disorders

Mark S. Bauer

1. The following is true of the occurrence of bipolar disorder:

A. It is more prevalent in women than in men.
B. Its peak onset is in the early 20s.
C. Bipolar disorder remits by the early 60s.
D. Episodes tend to come in couplets or cycles.
E. Bipolar disorder is easily differentiated from unipolar depression because the initial episode is by definition manic or hypomanic.

Discussion: Bipolar disorder, which has peak onset between the ages of 15 and 30 years, has an approximately equal gender distribution. The natural history of the non–rapid-cycling type of bipolar disorder is one of multiple episodes, but in no particular sequence in a patient's lifetime. The illness does not remit by the early 60s. This disorder is differentiated from unipolar depression by longitudinal course; cross-sectional symptom profile during depression also does not differentiate between unipolar and bipolar disorder.

Pages 968, 973–975, 976–978 •

Answer B

Questions 2 to 5: For each numbered item, select the lettered heading most closely associated with it. Each letter may be selected once, more than once, or not at all.

Match the syndrome with the treatment result:

____ 2. rapid cycling	A. refractory to anticonvulsants
____ 3. hypomanic episodes	B. refractory to lithium
____ 4. bipolar depressive episodes	C. responsive to lithium
____ 5. manic episodes	D. no data on treatment outcome

2. Discussion: Approximately 20% to 40% of patients with bipolar disorder do not respond well to lithium, and that proportion may increase to as much as 80% for certain subgroups, such as patients who experience a rapid-cycling pattern (four or more affective episodes per year) or mixed manic and depressive episodes.

Pages 977, 980, Table 53–9 •

Answer 2, B

3. Discussion: The treatment of hypomania is not as well studied as that for mania or bipolar depression. In particular, issues such as maintenance treatment are complicated by the recognition of hypomanic states.

Pages 978–981 •

Answer 3, D

4. Discussion: Although the evidence is scarce regarding efficacy of specific agents in bipolar depression, lithium appears to be an effective antidepressant in bipolar depression. This is not the case in unipolar depression. Lithium is also the only antidepressant treatment that is not promanic. Lithium should be the first-line treatment for unmedicated bipolar patients in the depressed phase.

Page 980 •

Answer 4, C

5. Discussion: Lithium has been shown to be effective in the treatment of acute mania. The anticonvulsants carbamazepine and sodium valproate have also been found to be effective antimanic agents in placebo-controlled trials. This property is not shared by all anticonvulsants.

Page 980 •

Answer 5, A

6. All of the following are true about the course of bipolar disorder **except**

A. Resolution of comorbid substance dependence usually leads to resolution of mood symptoms.
B. Rapid cycling can occur and remit at any time during the disorder.
C. Social and occupational deficits may far outlast individual episodes.
D. Rapid cycling is not truly cyclic.
E. In women, depressive episodes predominate over manic episodes.

Discussion: Rapid cycling may occur at any time during the disorder and is not an "end stage" of the illness. It is based not on any inherent cyclicity but rather on increased number of episodes per year. Risk factors for this subtype include female gender, hypothyroidism, and antidepressant use. Social and occupational impairment is high in bipolar disorder type I, and the functional deficits may endure well beyond the resolution of manic or depressive symptoms. In the course of a lifetime, men have an approximately equal number of manic and depressive episodes; in women, depressive episodes outnumber manic episodes. Substance abuse may worsen the course of bipolar disorder. However, true bipolar disorder symptoms continue despite the resolution of substance dependence.

Pages 970, 973–975, 976–978 •

Answer A

7. The following is true about complications of treatment of bipolar disorder:

A. Adolescents are particularly susceptible to antidepressant-induced mania.
B. Lithium-induced hypothyroidism necessitates discontinuation of lithium as the first line of treatment.
C. Anticonvulsants are the treatment of choice for bipolar disorder during pregnancy because lithium is clearly teratogenic whereas the anticonvulsants are not.
D. Medications often contribute to functional impairment despite their efficacy in treatment of mood episodes.
E. Psychotherapy, beyond medical model counseling, is not indicated in bipolar disorder.

Discussion: Unwanted side effects of certain medications, such as sedation and impaired concentration or memory, may become burdensome to patients and contribute to functional impairment. In addition, medication side effects may lead to noncompliance, which in turn leads to worsening of symptoms and greater functional impairment.

Page 984 •

Answer D

8. All of the following are true about the pathophysiological process of bipolar disorder **except**

A. Several organic illnesses may produce a manic-like episode.
B. The amine hypothesis is supported by the tendency of antidepressants to precipitate manic episodes.
C. The probable gene for bipolar disorder lies on chromosome 11, at or near the locus for tyrosine hydroxylase.
D. Family studies cannot separate genetic from congenital risk factors for bipolar disorder.
E. Rapid cycling is associated with several physiological risk factors, which include female gender, hypothyroidism, and antidepressant use.

Discussion: Whereas single genes on several chromosomes have been studied in some large family groups with bipolar disorder, these findings have typically not been replicated across families or studies. Thus, different genes may be responsible in different families. It may also be that the expression of a psychiatric illness like bipolar disorder may be due to modifying pieces of DNA, such as trinucleotide repeats.

Pages 970–973, Tables 53–2 and 53–3 •

Answer C

For each numbered item, select the lettered heading most closely associated with it. Each letter may be selected once, more than once, or not at all.

9. Match the adverse effect with the medication.

____ 1. lithium
____ 2. carbamazepine
____ 3. sodium valproate
____ 4. antidepressants

A. can impair bone marrow function
B. can impair renal function
C. can cause hair loss
D. can induce mania

Discussion: Lithium can impair renal function, but the frequency of serious renal disease is small. Carbamazepine can cause both dose-dependent, reversible decreases in white blood cell count that are not clinically meaningful and irreversible, life-threatening agranulocytosis. Valproate can cause hair loss, which is usually reversible. All antidepressant treatments, including light and electroconvulsive therapy, may be promanic.

Pages 976, 981–983, Tables 53–10 and 53–15; see also Chapter 83 •

Answers 1, B; 2, A; 3, C; 4, D

CHAPTER

54 Depressive Disorders

Alan M. Gruenberg • Reed D. Goldstein

1. Which of the following symptoms is **not** a criterion symptom for major depressive disorder in DSM-IV?

A. diminished interest or pleasure in activities
B. insomnia or hypersomnia
C. tearfulness
D. psychomotor agitation or retardation
E. diminished ability to think or concentrate

Discussion: Tearfulness is not part of the DSM-IV criteria for major depressive disorder. Tearfulness is an affect commonly associated with a sad or depressed mood.

Page 991 •

Answer C

2. Individuals with major mood disorders are typically vulnerable to all of the following **except**

A. episodes
B. psychosis
C. neurovegetative signs
D. sociopathy
E. cognitive distortions

Discussion: Individuals with a major mood disorder such as depression suffer from a syndrome that is episodic in nature. There is usually an alteration in mood complicated in some instances by neurovegetative signs, psychosis, and cognitive distortions but not by sociopathy.

Page 990 •

Answer D

3. What is the estimate of suicide risk for individuals hospitalized with major depressive disorder?

A. 5%
B. 10%
C. 15%
D. 20%
E. 25%

Discussion: The definition of major depressive disorder includes suicidal ideation and recurrent thoughts of death. In fact, suicidality is the major cause of mortality due to this condition and the reason for immediate treatment or hospitalization. The risk for subsequent suicide for an individual hospitalized for an episode of severe major depression is estimated to be 15%.

Page 991 •

Answer C

4. According to the National Comorbidity Survey, which of the following is **not** associated with comorbid major depressive disorder as opposed to major depressive disorder in the absence of other conditions?

A. younger age at onset
B. lower intelligence
C. lower level of education
D. lower income
E. treatment in mental health settings

Discussion: The National Comorbidity Survey identified risk factors for comorbid depression as opposed to pure major depressive disorder. These included younger age, lower level of education, and lower income. Lower intelligence is not a risk factor. Data from the Epidemiological Catchment Area study indicated that the lowest income group manifested twice the risk of major depressive disorder than the highest income group.

Page 992 •

Answer B

5. The estimated overall lifetime prevalence for major depressive disorder in adults is

A. 0% to 9%
B. 10% to 19%
C. 20% to 29%
D. 30% to 39%
E. 40% to 49%

Discussion: Lifetime prevalence refers to those individuals who, up to the time of assessment, have met diagnostic criteria at some point in their lives. The National Comorbidity Survey estimated overall lifetime prevalence of major depression as 17.1%. The prevalence for women is twice as high as that for men.

Page 992 •

Answer B

6. Risk factors for major depressive disorder include all of the following **except**

A. male gender
B. female gender
C. prior history of depression
D. family history of depression
E. active alcohol or substance abuse

Discussion: The Depression Guideline Panel has listed 10 primary risk factors for depression. Female but not male gender is a risk. Additional factors include a history of suicide attempts, onset before age 40 years, postpartum period, comorbid medical illness, absence of social support, negative stressful life events.

Page 993 •

Answer A

7. Which of the following medical illnesses is **not** associated with excess risk for major depressive disorder?

A. cerebrovascular disease
B. dementia
C. diabetes mellitus
D. cancer
E. pneumonia

Discussion: Whereas a 4% to 5% current prevalence rate of major depressive disorder exists in community samples, symptoms of depression are found in 12% to 36% of patients with general medical conditions. The conditions typically associated with depression include stroke, dementia, Parkinson's disease, diabetes mellitus, coronary artery disease, and cancer.

Pages 993–994 •

Answer E

8. In the sleep laboratory, abnormalities in sleep of depressed patients are characterized by all of the following **except**

A. increased REM density
B. reduced REM latency
C. increased awakening during sleep
D. reduced sleep time
E. increased arousal threshold

Discussion: In polysomnography studies of patients with major depressive disorder, the electroencephalographical recordings demonstrate a shorter than normal onset of rapid eye movement (REM) sleep termed reduced REM latency. There is also a greater frequency of eye movements during REM sleep, which is termed increased REM density. Because of frequent awakenings, there is overall less sleep time recorded. The arousal threshold is decreased, not increased.

Page 998 •

Answer E

9. Among the biological findings associated with major depressive disorder, which of the following is **not** reported?

A. hypercortisolism
B. increased corticotropin-releasing factor (CRF) secretion
C. decreased adrenocorticotropic hormone secretion (ACTH)
D. thyroid-stimulating hormone (TSH) abnormalities
E. decreased cerebrospinal fluid 5-hydroxyindoleacetic acid (5-HIAA) concentration

Discussion: All of the above biological abnormalities are seen in major depression except decreased ACTH secretion. In melancholic depression, there is adrenocortical hyperactivity with increased CRF and hence ACTH secretion. This phenomenon is the basis of the use of the dexamethasone suppression test in the study of depression.

Page 998 •

Answer C

10. Which of the following is consistent with psychological theories of depression?

A. introjection of ambivalently held object
B. aggression toward others
C. generally positive thoughts about self, world, and future
D. limited interpersonal deficits
E. consistent social support

Discussion: Freud and Abraham emphasized the connection between mourning and melancholia through the introjection of an ambivalently held lost object. The depressive experience occurs because anger and aggression associated with the ambivalence are turned inward, not against others. Cognitive theory emphasizes the role of pervasive negative thoughts about one's self, the world, and the future. Behavioral theory focuses on lack of sufficient social supports.

Pages 999–1000 •

Answer A

11. The specifier with melancholic features suggests the presence of all of the following **except**

A. loss of interest or pleasure in activities
B. worsening of the syndrome in the morning
C. profound guilt
D. reactivity to external events or usual pleasurable stimuli

Discussion: Melancholia is a subtype of depression characterized by a lack of reactivity to external events and usual pleasurable stimuli. In addition, there is diurnal variation, early morning awakening, marked psychomotor change, prominent weight loss, and profound guilt. Recognition of this subtype is important given the usual good response to somatic treatments. Hypercortisolism and reduced REM latency are both found in melancholic depression.

Pages 1000–1001 •

Answer D

12. Which of the following is **not** part of the DSM-IV definition of dysthymic disorder?

A. depressed mood most of the day
B. symptoms present for at least 2 years
C. person has not been without symptoms for more than 2 months at a time
D. vulnerability to psychosis
E. no major depressive episode has been present during the first 2 years of the disturbance

Discussion: Psychosis is not a criterion of dysthymic disorder. If patients with dysthymic disorder have psychosis, it is not a result of that particular syndrome.

Pages 1012–1014 •

Answer D

CHAPTER

55 Panic Disorder With and Without Agoraphobia

M. Katherine Shear

1. Which of the following was **not** an earlier precursor of panic disorder?

A. agoraphobia
B. effort syndrome
C. neurasthenia
D. anxiety neurosis
E. soldier's heart

Discussion: Freud distinguished neurasthenia, a syndrome characterized by weakness and lethargy, from anxiety neurosis, described as similar to panic disorder.

Page 1020 •

Answer C

2. Which of the following is true of epidemiological studies of panic disorder?

A. The most common age at onset for panic disorder is the late 20s or early 30s.
B. Panic disorder patients are afraid of dying and are not suicidal.
C. Rates of panic disorder are about the same across the life span.
D. A majority of the population has at least a limited symptom panic attack at some point in their lives.
E. Panic occurs on a continuum of severity and frequency with a higher community prevalence of less frequent and less severe episodes.

Discussion: Most common age at onset is in the late teens and early 20s. Panic disorder is associated with an increased risk of suicidality. Rates of panic are lower in the elderly. Only a minority of the population ever experience any kind of panic symptom.

Pages 1022–1024 •

Answer E

3. Which of the following is true of comorbidity in panic disorder?

A. Although important, comorbidity is found only in slightly more than half of panic disorder patients.
B. Comorbid panic with major depression represents a manifestation of the major depression.
C. In family studies, family members of probands with panic disorder have a higher prevalence of both major depression and panic disorder than control subjects do.
D. Personality disorder comorbidity is seen in the majority of panic disorder patients.
E. Comorbidity of panic disorder with other anxiety disorders is rare.

Discussion: Comorbidity is found in 80% to 90% of panic disorder patients. Comorbid panic disorder and major depression are a heterogeneous group, with some having depression secondary to panic. Family members of panic disorder probands have a heightened prevalence of panic but not major depression. Comorbidity of panic disorder with other anxiety disorders is common.

Pages 1023–1024 •

Answer D

4. Which of the following premises of the neurobiological theory best differentiates it from the cognitive-behavioral theory?

A. Panic is distinct from other forms of anxiety.
B. A panic attack occurs because of a seizure-like neurophysiological discharge and has no identifiable trigger.
C. Phobic avoidance, fear of panic, and panic-related body sensations occur only as a consequence of panic.
D. Onset of illness occurs with the first panic—there are no earlier antecedents.

Discussion: According to cognitive-behavioral theory, panic attacks are triggered by frightening but innocuous body sensations, such as a racing heart, which occurs on running up the stairs.

Pages 1024–1025, Table 55–3 •

Answer B

5. Which of the following statements about nocturnal panic attacks is true?

A. They are exceedingly rare.
B. They are found only during rapid eye movement sleep.
C. They occur among patients with more severe panic attacks.
D. Nocturnal panic attacks are definitely associated with poor prognosis.

Discussion: Nocturnal panic attacks, which are poorly understood, have been reported by up to 25% of patients in one study. These episodes generally occur during deep sleep and are not associated with dreams. They are found in patients with more severe panic attacks and in patients with childhood onset as well as high degrees of comorbidity.

Page 1026 •

Answer C

6. The long-term outcome of panic disorder is characterized by

A. complete remission in more than 80% of cases
B. some improvement in 80% of cases
C. progression to other psychiatric disorders of greater severity
D. persistent, disabling panic disorder in more than 25% of patients

Discussion: The natural history of panic disorder is variable. One study summarized available studies of long-term outcome and concluded that whereas 80% of patients have at least some improvement, only half of those showed marked improvement or recovery. Almost 20% remained severely debilitated.

Page 1030 •

Answer B

7. Tricyclic antidepressants are considered the pharmacological treatment of choice for panic disorder. Which of the following is **not** seen in tricyclic antidepressant therapy?

A. frequent development of jitteriness syndrome
B. immediate symptom relief at low doses
C. good response to careful and gradual titration of medication
D. benefits of combination with benzodiazepines

Discussion: Imipramine has proven antipanic effects. Patients with panic disorder usually require gradual dose titration and low starting doses, such as 10 to 25 mg/d of imipramine. This is required because these patients are frequently sensitive to medication side effects and there is a 20% to 40% incidence of a syndrome of jitteriness, tachycardia, insomnia, irritability, and increased energy. Combination with a benzodiazepine, often sequentially or overlapping, can ameliorate the jitteriness syndrome and is helpful in the management of complicated patients. Panic patients usually require moderate to high doses of tricyclic antidepressants with a high rate of response (70% to 90%).

Pages 1031–1032 •

Answer B

8. Cognitive-behavioral treatments for panic disorder focus on all of the following issues **except**

A. presentation of the fear of sensation model
B. instruction in slow abdominal breathing
C. correction of cognitive misinterpretations of body sensations
D. an explanation of the "cognitive triad"
E. exposure to interoceptive cues

Discussion: The advent of cognitive-behavioral treatment has transformed the psychotherapeutic treatment of this illness. The cognitive triad is part of the cognitive therapy of depression. In cognitive-behavioral treatment of panic, patients learn to avoid hyperventilation by the use of abdominal breathing, decatastrophize the meaning of body sensations, and decondition automatic reactions by the use of exposure techniques.

Pages 1032–1033 •

Answer D

CHAPTER

56 Social and Specific Phobias

Martin M. Antony • David H. Barlow

1. Which of the following is **not** relevant to differentiating between specific phobia and panic disorder with agoraphobia?

A. the focus of apprehension (symptom focused versus situation focused)
B. the number of situations that are feared or avoided
C. the intensity of fear experienced in the feared situation
D. the presence of panic attacks outside the phobic situation
E. the types of situation avoided

Discussion: Differentiating between panic disorder with agoraphobia and situational or social phobia is often difficult because patients may have similar patterns of avoidant behavior. Four variables should be considered 1) type and number of panic attacks, 2) focus of apprehension, 3) number of situations avoided, and 4) level of intercurrent anxiety. Patients with panic disorder experience unexpected panic attacks and heightened anxiety outside of phobic situations, whereas those with specific or social phobias typically do not.

Pages 1044–1045 •

Answer C

2. Which of the following statements about comorbidity and phobic disorders is **least** true?

A. Specific phobias are more likely to co-occur with other specific phobias from the same DSM-IV type than from different DSM-IV types.
B. Individuals with principal diagnoses of specific phobia often have additional anxiety disorder diagnoses of lesser severity.
C. Individuals with principal anxiety disorder diagnoses often have additional specific phobia diagnoses of lesser severity.
D. Individuals with principal diagnoses of social phobia often have additional anxiety disorder diagnoses of lesser severity.
E. Individuals with principal anxiety disorder diagnoses often have additional social phobia diagnoses of lesser severity.

Discussion: Specific phobias tend to cluster by type of phobia. In addition, specific phobias often co-occur with other DSM-IV diagnoses. However, relative to other anxiety disorders, individuals with a primary diagnosis of specific phobia are less likely to have an additional diagnosis. Unlike specific phobias, social phobia is frequently associated with additional disorders of lesser severity.

Pages 1040–1041 •

Answer B

3. Which of the following is **least** likely to be considered a pathway to fear development?

A. misinformation about the feared stimulus
B. experiencing a trauma in the feared situation
C. witnessing a trauma in the feared situation
D. observing someone behave fearfully in the feared situation
E. lack of experience with the feared situation

Discussion: Rachman proposed three pathways to the development of fear. The first is *direct conditioning,* which involves an actual personal experience. Second is *vicarious acquisition,* and the third is through *informational and instructional pathways.* This model, developed in response to problems with classical and operant conditioning as explanations for phobia development and maintenance, seeks to account for the development of phobias in the absence of direct experiences.

Pages 1041–1043 •

Answer E

Question 4: For each numbered item, select the lettered heading most closely associated with it. Each letter may be selected once, more than once, or not at all.

4. Match the phobia with the statement:

A. is often associated with fainting in the phobic situation

B. a phobia from the situational type
C. is often treated with phenelzine
D. a phobia from the natural environment type
E. associated with recurrent unexpected or uncued panic attacks

____ 1. water phobia
____ 2. injection phobia
____ 3. social phobia
____ 4. claustrophobia

Discussion: DSM-IV criteria for specific phobia include the type of phobia. Natural environment type includes heights, storms, and water phobias. Situational phobias include airplanes, elevators, and enclosed places. In addition, there is an animal type and a blood-injection-injury type. One of the most consistent findings in the study of specific phobia is the tendency of patients with blood-injection-injury type of phobia to faint in the phobic situation. This is distinct from other phobic reactions that commonly resemble panic attacks and is perhaps unique.

Pages 1039, 1044–1045, 1051–1053, Table 56–5 •

Answers 1, D; 2, A; 3, C; 4, B

5. Behavioral approach tests

A. are conducted to help decrease a patient's fear
B. are useful for identifying specific fear triggers in a phobic patient
C. should not be conducted when a patient is feeling anxious
D. should be conducted in conjunction with pharmacotherapy
E. are among the most useful questionnaire measures for specific phobias

Discussion: Behavioral testing is an important part of any comprehensive evaluation of phobia. Because of a history of avoidance and distortions about the amount of fear experienced, a behavioral approach test can be useful in identifying specific triggers as well as assessing the intensity of the patient's fear in the actual situation. Such testing usually takes place at the onset of behavioral therapy. During the behavioral approach test, patients are asked to approach the feared object or situation and describe their response (e.g., intensity of anxiety, specific sensations, negative thoughts).

Page 1046 •

Answer B

6. The treatment of choice for animal phobias is

A. social skills training
B. propranolol
C. alprazolam
D. phenelzine
E. none of the above

Discussion: The treatment of choice for a variety of specific phobias is an exposure-based treatment. These treatments work best if the sessions are spaced closely together. Prolonged exposure is more effective. During exposure sessions, patients should be discouraged from avoidance strategies such as distraction. Real-life exposure works better than imagination, and the therapist's involvement is important. These treatments can be done gradually or quickly.

Page 1053 •

Answer E

7. Which of the following is **not** generally considered to be an effective treatment for generalized social phobia?

A. phenelzine
B. cognitive-behavioral therapy
C. clonazepam
D. moclobemide
E. atenolol

Discussion: In contrast to specific phobia, social phobia has been treated effectively with medications as well as with cognitive-behavioral psychotherapy. The monoamine oxidase inhibitors phenelzine and moclobemide both are effective, although phenelzine is more effective. Clonazepam and perhaps alprazolam are useful. Buspirone and β-blockers such as atenolol are not helpful. β-Blockers have a role in discrete social phobia, such as heightened performance anxiety.

Pages 1051–1053 •

Answer E

8. Which of the following statements about the treatment of phobic disorders is **least** true?

A. Phenelzine and cognitive-behavioral therapy are both effective treatments for social phobia.
B. Applied relaxation training is effective for some patients with social phobia.
C. Buspirone is effective for patients with generalized social phobia but not for those with only performance-related phobias.
D. The majority of patients with animal phobias can overcome their phobia in as little as one session of behavioral therapy.
E. Applied tension is a useful strategy for the treatment of blood phobia.

Discussion: A study by Heimberg and colleagues compared four treatments for social phobia: 1) cognitive-behavioral group treatment, 2) phenelzine, 3) supportive psychotherapy, and 4) placebo. Overall, phenelzine and cognitive-behavioral group treatment were equally effective after 12 weeks of treatment and were significantly more effective than supportive psychotherapy or placebo. Applied muscle tension is an alternative treatment to exposure therapy in the treatment of blood-injection-injury phobias. This involves repeated tensing of muscles to temporarily increase blood pressure and prevent fainting.

Pages 1051–1056, Tables 56–5 to 56–7 •

Answer C

CHAPTER

57 Obsessive-Compulsive Disorders

Michele T. Pato • Jane L. Eisen • Katharine A. Phillips

1. To make a DSM-IV diagnosis of obsessive-compulsive disorder (OCD):

A. Obsessions *or* compulsions must be present.
B. Obsessions *and* compulsions must be present.
C. Patients must always resist their symptoms.
D. The patient must recognize at all times that the behavior is unreasonable.
E. No other DSM-IV diagnosis must be present.

Discussion: The OCD diagnosis requires only that obsessions or compulsions be present. In DSM-IV, there is now the recognition that the patient may not always maintain insight into the irrational nature of his or her symptoms. In fact, DSM-IV has added a descriptor, with poor insight, to the diagnosis. In addition, although patients may sometimes resist their symptoms, at other times they may not. Many other diagnoses, such as major depression, schizophrenia, panic disorder, Tourette's disorder, and even anorexia nervosa, can be comorbid with OCD.

Page 1060 •

Answer A

2. Which of the following is true about OCD?

A. OCD is one of the rarest of psychiatric illnesses.
B. OCD is more common in girls than in boys.
C. There is no indication for a genetic predisposition for OCD.
D. OCD is among the most common psychiatric illnesses in the United States.
E. The prevalence of OCD is the same in Eastern and Western cultures.

Discussion: Epidemiological studies have shown OCD to be the fourth most common psychiatric disorder, exceeded only by phobias, substance use disorders, and major depression. Its lifetime prevalence in the United States, based on the Epidemiological Catchment Area study done in 1984, is 2.5%. Whereas this prevalence has held true in many Western cultures, lower rates have been found in India, China, and Taipei. In terms of gender distribution, it is almost equal in adults, with 52% women in one study; among children, it is more common in boys (67%).

Page 1060 •

Answer D

3. Although all the illnesses below may be comorbid with OCD, which is the most common?

A. major depression
B. Tourette's disorder
C. panic disorder
D. anorexia nervosa
E. psychotic disorders

Discussion: More than half of patients with OCD report an episode of depression (67%) at some point in their life. Fortunately, many of the medications used to treat OCD are also effective antidepressants. The prevalence of the other disorders is 7% for Tourette's disorder, 12% for panic disorder, 17% for anorexia nervosa, and as high as 14% for psychotic disorders.

Pages 1060–1062 •

Answer A

4. From a neuroanatomical point of view, which structure is likely to be involved in the neuropathological process of OCD?

A. Broca's area
B. caudate nucleus
C. substantia nigra
D. corpus callosum
E. occipital lobe

Discussion: Positron emission tomography studies show abnormalities in the caudate nucleus, cingulate gyrus, and orbitofrontal cortex. In at least one study, increased activity was shown in the caudate nucleus before treatment, with either behavioral therapy or fluoxetine leading to normalization of activity (Baxter, 1992). The other answers in the question are regions that have not been implicated in OCD and are probably not part of the frontostriatothalamofrontal loop believed to be involved in OCD.

Pages 1069–1070 •

Answer B

5. What neurochemical appears to be the most critical to the efficacy of antiobsessional agents?

A. dopamine
B. norepinephrine
C. acetylcholine
D. serotonin
E. histamine

Discussion: Whereas there are some supporting data that dopamine and noradrenergic systems may be involved in antiobsessional efficacy (Jenike, 1993; Goodman, 1993), all medications that are effective in OCD have some effect on the serotonin system, with most working as reuptake inhibitors.

Pages 1070–1071, Fig. 57–4 •

Answer D

6. Given the principles of exposure and response prevention that are critical to the success of behavioral therapy in OCD, which of the following situations is most likely to be successful in decreasing obsessions or compulsions in an OCD patient?

A. Have a patient intentionally dirty her or his hands and then wash them immediately.
B. Reassure a patient repeatedly that there is no risk of contamination from using a public bathroom.
C. Allow a patient with contamination fears to avoid sharing a bag of potato chips.
D. Prescribe a patient a central nervous system depressant during behavioral therapy so she or he will not feel so anxious.
E. Have a patient intentionally drive over bumps in the road and then refuse to let him or her go back to check whether anything was hit.

Discussion: When exposure to a feared stimulus is followed by not responding with a compulsive behavior, the subject is more likely to gradually extinguish that behavior by habituating to the anxiety that it causes. Answer A does not allow response prevention. Answer B provides reassurance to patients as a way of avoiding the anxiety they are experiencing rather than forcing them to experience the anxiety and habituate to it. Answer C uses avoidance instead of response prevention so that, again, the patient does not experience the required anxiety. Answer D uses a central nervous system depressant to block the anxiety from arising, and thus there is nothing to habituate to.

Pages 1075–1077 •

Answer E

7. Among the antiobsessional medications available, which has been the most extensively studied and may, in fact, be the most efficacious?

A. fluvoxamine
B. paroxetine
C. clomipramine
D. fluoxetine
E. sertraline

Discussion: Whereas all of these agents have some proven efficacy in OCD, the largest published multicenter trial to date is with clomipramine (The Clomipramine Collaborative Group, 1991). In addition, at least two meta-analysis studies (Jenike, 1990; Greist, 1995) seem to indicate that the largest effect size was noted in the clomipramine samples. There is, however, some controversy about the validity of such meta-analyses.

Pages 1072–1075 •

Answer C

8. OCD patients have less chance of relapse when medication is discontinued if

A. they are switched to desipramine
B. they take medication for 10 to 12 weeks
C. they receive a low dose of medication rather than a high dose
D. they have received behavioral therapy
E. they have been taking an augmenting agent

Discussion: Behavioral therapy stands out as giving good long-term efficacy, with 75% of patients continuing to do well in 1- to 6-year follow-up (O'Sullivan, 1991). Whereas there are few systematic data on the long-term treatment of OCD, most of the data on pharmacological treatment show that discontinuation of medication leads to relapse of symptoms in up to 90% of patients (Pato, 1988). In addition, when Leonard (1989, 1991) substituted desipramine for clomipramine, the study subjects experienced rapid recurrence of OCD symptoms. Because most studies available point toward higher doses being more efficacious than lower doses (Tollefson, 1994), it is unlikely that low-dose treatment would protect against relapse on discontinuation. In terms of augmenting agents, the efficacy of this approach is questionable, because no systematic study has demonstrated significant efficacy for these agents. Whereas pharmacological agents do not fare as well in discontinuation, one of the fundamental differences between pharmacological and behavioral therapies is that serum levels with pharmacological treatment disappear, but the learned behaviors taught in behavioral therapy continue to be used by the patient after treatment is finished. Thus, in successful behavioral therapy, there is never a true discontinuation of treatment.

Pages 1078–1080 •

Answer D

CHAPTER

58 Traumatic Stress Disorders

David Taylor

1. In DSM-IV, posttraumatic stress disorder (PTSD) is characterized by symptom clusters including all of the following **except**

A. persistent re-experiencing of the traumatic event
B. persistent avoidance of associated stimuli
C. persistent depressed mood
D. persistent symptoms of increased arousal

Discussion: A diagnosis of PTSD requires not only the experience of a traumatic event but also symptoms as mentioned above with the exception of depressed mood. Patients with PTSD will frequently present with symptoms that are similar to those of major depression, and in fact four of the Cluster C symptoms and three of the Cluster D symptoms overlap with symptoms of depression. It is possible for the two conditions to coexist.

Pages 1085–1086, 1089 •

Answer C

2. The new DSM-IV diagnosis of acute stress disorder is

A. just an adjustment disorder with dissociative features
B. a well-characterized syndrome
C. just like PTSD without the same duration criteria
D. diagnosed if the disturbance lasts for a minimum of 2 days and a maximum of 4 weeks and occurs within 4 weeks of the traumatic event

Discussion: A diagnosis of acute stress disorder requires the occurrence of a traumatic event, as does PTSD. This event must involve the actual threat of death or serious injury or a threat to the physical integrity of self or others; the response involves intense fear, helplessness, or horror. This distinguishes it from adjustment disorder. Whereas the occurrence of trauma is similar in PTSD and acute stress disorder, the diagnosis of acute stress disorder specifies a set of dissociative symptoms that are distinct from the PTSD symptom criteria. This is not a well-understood diagnosis given that many survivors of disasters are not interviewed for some time after the event.

Pages 1094–1098 •

Answer D

3. Epidemiological studies suggest that PTSD

A. is a chronic disorder
B. is the most common psychiatric disorder in contemporary society
C. is less common than expected in populations at risk
D. is reliably diagnosed with a variety of structured interviews

Discussion: Population-based studies of PTSD are important to avoid drawing conclusions based on unrepresentative clinical samples. Only 1 patient in 20 may seek treatment. Community-based samples yield lifetime prevalence rates ranging from 1% to 19%, whereas rates in at-risk populations range from 14% to 75%. Such a wide range of prevalence is probably related to variability in the instruments used. The original Diagnostic Interview Schedule provided unrealistically low prevalence rates. Studies suggest that PTSD often remains chronic and that recovery frequently does not occur even in nonclinical samples.

Pages 1085–1086 •

Answer A

4. Which of the following findings has **not** been reported in neuroendocrine studies of PTSD patients?

A. reduced 24-hour urinary cortisol excretion
B. supersuppression of cortisol after low-dose dexamethasone
C. blunting of adrenocorticotropic hormone response to corticotropin-releasing hormone stimulation
D. decreased numbers of glucocorticoid receptors

Discussion: The hypothalamic-pituitary-adrenal (HPA) axis has been extensively studied in PTSD. The current understanding suggests that in chronic PTSD, there is a supersuppression of the emergency HPA response to acute stress. This could be the organism's attempt to protect itself from the potentially toxic effect of high levels of corticosteroids that might occur with repeated exposure to stress or its sequelae. Other biological variables reported include heightened phasic sympathetic arousal, prolonged sleep latency, more awakenings, less sleep time, and increased rapid eye movement sleep. Pharmacological challenge studies as well as observations about treatment response have suggested roles for the noradrenergic, serotoninergic, and opioid systems.

Page 1087 •

Answer D

5. Which of the following drugs has been shown to reduce symptoms of PTSD to the greatest extent?

A. phenelzine
B. amitriptyline
C. carbamazepine
D. fluoxetine

Discussion: Tricyclic and monoamine oxidase inhibitor antidepressants are the best studied pharmacological treatments for PTSD. In double-blind placebo-controlled trials, tricyclis were effective in reducing intrusive PTSD symptoms and, to a weaker extent, avoidant symptoms. This is not thought to be related to purely antidepressant effects, and response was inversely correlated with baseline depression level in one trial. Phenelzine has been found to be the most effective drug in terms of magnitude of symptom reduction. Avoidant symptoms were improved to a greater degree than with tricyclics. Fluoxetine is also better than placebo. There is a role for antipsychotics and mood stabilizers in certain patients, particularly those with poor impulse control, mood swings, or angry and explosive outbursts.

Pages 1090–1092, Tables 58–1 to 58–3 •

Answer A

6. The goals of cognitive-behavioral therapy in PTSD include all of the following **except**

A. exposure
B. decreased conditioned anxiety
C. minimize avoidance
D. facilitate normal behaviors

Discussion: Exposure is not a goal of cognitive-behavioral therapy but one of its central techniques. These include systematic desensitization, anxiety management training, limited exposure, prolonged exposure, flooding, and cognitive restructuring.

Pages 1092–1093 •

Answer A

7. The treatment of acute traumatic states involves

A. careful review of the events
B. immediate abreaction
C. emotional first aid
D. confrontation

Discussion: The governing principles of the treatment of acute trauma are brevity, immediacy, centrality, expectancy, proximity, and simplicity. Those most highly at risk are survivors with psychiatric disorders; close relatives of traumatically bereaved people; and children and other dependent groups, such as the elderly and handicapped. In addition, rescue workers need immediate attention. Different components of treatment include information, psychological support, crisis intervention, and emotional first aid. Emotional first aid involves enhancing the acceptance of feelings, symptoms, reality, and the need for help; recognition of psychologically distressing issues; identification of resources; and acceptance of responsibility and absence of blame.

Pages 1097–1098 •

Answer C

CHAPTER

59 Generalized Anxiety Disorders

Olga Brawman-Mintzer • R. Bruce Lydiard

1. Epidemiological studies indicate that the lifetime prevalence of generalized anxiety disorder (GAD) is

A. 17.1%
B. 0.7%
C. 5.1%
D. 24.9%
E. 13.3%

Discussion: The lifetime prevalence rate for DSM-III-R GAD was dramatically lower than that for the DSM-III criteria, given the then new duration criterion of 6 months. A study by Kessler found the rate to be 5.1%, with a rate of 6.6% for women and 3.6% for men. In the Epidemiological Catchment Area study, the lifetime prevalence ranged from 4.1% to 6.6%.

Pages 1100–1101 •

Answer C

2. Which of the following symptoms is most frequently present in patients with GAD?

A. panic attacks
B. feeling a detachment and estrangement from others
C. markedly diminished interest in significant activities
D. disturbed sleep
E. fear of being home alone

Discussion: Disturbed sleep is the only symptom of GAD listed above. The criteria for GAD include excessive and uncontrollable worry, restlessness, insomnia, muscle tension, irritability, difficulty concentrating, and becoming easily fatigued. Approximately 30% of patients will have symptoms of irritable bowel syndrome.

Pages 1105–1106 •

Answer D

3. In contrast to patients with GAD, subjects with hyperthyroidism

A. experience fatigue
B. may have tachycardia
C. may complain of heat intolerance
D. present with irritability
E. always present with goiter

Discussion: The symptoms of anxiety are common to both hyperthyroidism and GAD. The overlapping symptoms include tachycardia, tremulousness, irritability, weakness, and fatigue. In GAD, however, the peripheral manifestations of excessive concentrations of circulating thyroid hormones are absent, including symptoms such as weight loss, increased appetite, warm and moist skin, heat intolerance, and dyspnea on effort. The presence of goiter makes the diagnosis of hyperthyroidism likely; however, the absence of thyroid enlargement does not exclude it.

Page 1108 •

Answer E

4. Which one of the following statements is true about comorbidity in GAD?

A. Panic disorder is the most common coexisting psychiatric disorder.
B. Approximately 25% of patients have a comorbid psychiatric disorder.
C. Major depression rarely co-occurs with GAD.
D. Borderline personality disorder is the most prevalent Axis II disorder in these patients.
E. Social phobia is the most prevalent coexisting comorbid psychiatric disorder.

Discussion: In some studies of GAD, more than 90% of GAD patients fulfilled criteria for at least one or more concurrent disorders. Among the most prevalent current comorbid diagnoses are social phobia, simple phobia, panic disorder, and depression. Social phobia is the most common. Cluster C personality disorders and alcoholism are also seen.

Pages 1101–1102, Fig. 59–1 •

Answer E

5. Which of the following statements about childhood presentation of GAD is true?

A. The disorder is uncommon in children and adolescents.
B. Ten percent of children with overanxious anxiety disorder have a comorbid psychiatric disorder.
C. They often appear overcompliant and perfectionistic.
D. They often experience significant separation anxiety.
E. They respond well to treatment with propranolol.

Discussion: Community samples of children and adolescents have found that overanxious anxiety disorder is not uncommon. In a sample of 150 adolescents, a 6-month prevalence rate of 7.3% was reported. In clinical settings, the prevalence can be as high as 52%. More than 50% of children with overanxious anxiety disorder meet criteria for at least one additional psychiatric diagnosis.

Pages 1100–1101, 1105 •

Answer C

6. Which of the compounds have demonstrated efficacy in the treatment of GAD?

A. lithium
B. tranylcypromine
C. trazodone
D. bupropion
E. pimozide

Discussion: A placebo-controlled study by Rickels compared imipramine, trazodone, and diazepam in GAD patients without comorbid depression or panic disorder. The efficacy of imipramine and trazodone compared well with that of diazepam, but the spectrum and speed of onset of action differed for the antidepressants. Diazepam was more efficacious in the first 2 weeks of treatment and controlled symptoms of hyperarousal. By 6 to 8 weeks of treatment, the antidepressants were more effective and controlled psychic symptoms of tension, apprehension, and worry.

Pages 1110–1112, Table 59–4 •

Answer C

7. Which of the following statements is true regarding the use of buspirone for GAD?

A. The onset of action is immediate, often as rapid as that of alprazolam.
B. Buspirone may be administered once a day.
C. Patients frequently report drowsiness and sedation.
D. Buspirone carries no risk of dependence or withdrawal symptoms.
E. Optimal response is usually achieved at a dose of 15 mg/d.

Discussion: Buspirone, a serotoninergic 5-HT_{1A} receptor partial agonist, has anxiolytic efficacy comparable to the benzodiazepines. There is no apparent abuse liability. There is a delayed onset of action, and doses initially recommended were probably insufficient. Doses in the range of 30 to 60 mg/d are needed. Gastrointestinal complaints are more common than complaints of drowsiness or sedation.

Page 1112 •

Answer D

8. Which of the following statements is true regarding GAD in the elderly?

A. The prevalence of GAD in the elderly is low.
B. The long-acting benzodiazepine diazepam is the preferable medication in those patients.
C. Hepatic clearance of anxiolytic medications is decreased in the elderly.
D. The use of tricyclic antidepressants is contraindicated in the elderly.
E. Elderly patients require higher doses of buspirone to achieve therapeutic effect.

Discussion: GAD is highly prevalent in the elderly and accounts for the majority of anxiety disorders in that population. If medications are needed, benzodiazepines, buspirone, and tricyclic antidepressants can be used. Because of alterations in pharmacokinetics and pharmacodynamics, doses need to be lower. Adverse side effects of benzodiazepines include sedation, falls, incoordination, and cognitive impairment. Disinhibition, aggression, and agitation are also observed. For these reasons, long-acting agents should be avoided and short half-life low-potency drugs such as oxazepam should be considered.

Pages 1114–1115 •

Answer C

CHAPTER

60 Somatoform Disorders

Ronald L. Martin • Sean H. Yutzy

1. The somatoform disorder class was created to group conditions that share

A. a common etiology
B. a similar prognosis
C. the same major diagnostic issue
D. lack of response to existing pharmacological agents

Discussion: The somatoform disorders class was created for clinical utility, not on the basis of an assumed common etiology, mechanism, or clinical course. In DSM-IV terms, it was designed to facilitate the differential diagnosis of conditions in which the first diagnostic concern is the need to "exclude occult general medical conditions or substance-induced etiologies for the body symptoms."

Pages 1119–1123, Table 60–1 •

Answer C

2. Compared with other somatoform disorders, the DSM-IV diagnostic criteria for somatization disorder are

A. focused on the patient's interpretation of symptoms rather than the symptoms themselves
B. the best validated in terms of predicting future course
C. focused on the presence of one type of symptom rather than a number of different types
D. easier for nonmedically trained interviewers to apply

Discussion: The DSM-IV criteria for somatization disorder derive from ancient descriptions of hysteria and the 19th century writings of Briquet. The Feighner criteria for hysteria, which required a given number of symptoms from a specified list to make the diagnosis, have proved to be the basis of a reliable, valid, and internally consistent psychiatric diagnosis. The clinical syndrome Feighner described was stable, with an 80% to 90% probability that the clinical picture would be the same 6 to 8 years after the diagnosis was made. The DSM-IV criteria for somatization disorder identify virtually the same patients as the Feighner criteria for hysteria.

Pages 1125–1131 •

Answer B

3. Somatization disorder is best treated by

A. insight-oriented psychotherapy
B. a pragmatic management approach
C. a combination of antianxiety and antidepressant medications
D. interpersonal psychotherapy

Discussion: A "management" rather than a "curative" strategy is recommended for somatization disorder. The goal should be to minimize distress and functional impairments associated with the multiple somatic complaints. There are three main principles of treatment. These are the establishment of a strong physician-patient relationship or bond, education of the patient, and provision of support and reassurance.

Pages 1131–1132 •

Answer B

4. DSM-IV undifferentiated somatoform disorder

A. in many ways resembles somatization disorder, although full criteria are not met
B. differs from somatoform disorder not otherwise specified in that no time requirements are included
C. is the true residual somatoform disorder
D. is less common in the general population than somatization disorder

Discussion: As defined in DSM-IV, this category includes disturbances of at least 6 months' duration with one or more nonintentional, clinically significant, medically unexplained symptoms. Somatization disorder requires a minimum of eight symptoms. It differs from somatoform disorder not otherwise specified and is less residual because of the duration criterion.

Pages 1132–1135 •

Answer A

5. DSM-IV conversion disorder

A. is characterized by disturbances in body functions
B. should be considered a "depressive equivalent"
C. often occurs before the onset of schizophrenia
D. is characterized by symptoms suggesting neurological illness

Discussion: The DSM-IV diagnosis of conversion disorder requires symptoms or deficits affecting voluntary motor or sensory function that suggest, yet are not fully explained by, a neurological or other general medical condition or the direct effect of a substance. Conversion hallucinations are considered pseudoneurological symptoms. These are not psychotic because of the absence of other psychotic symptoms and preservation of reality testing. Conversion does not occur as a prodrome to psychotic illness such as schizophrenia.

Pages 1135–1140 •

Answer D

6. DSM-IV pain disorders

A. include chronic but not acute syndromes
B. include syndromes requiring contribution by psychological factors
C. should be treated with a focus on relief of pain rather than increasing activity levels
D. should instill therapeutic nihilism

Discussion: In DSM-IV, pain disorder replaces the DSM-III-R term somatoform pain disorder, which presupposed that the psychogenicity of pain could be easily determined and separated from physical pain. The hope is for a more neutral term. Psychological factors are described as having "an important role in the onset, severity, exacerbation, or maintenance" of the pain. This is an essential feature of the definition. Acute syndromes, with duration of less than 6 months, are now diagnosable with the appropriate specifier. Treatment of pain disorders involves relief of the pain, and this usually involves breaking a cycle of negative reinforcement that consists of inactivity, medication use, and attention. Biofeedback, relaxation, and hypnosis techniques are also used.

Pages 1140–1144 •

Answer B

7. In DSM-IV, a hypochondriasis diagnosis

A. does not require the presence of a physical symptom
B. may be diagnosed if the preoccupation subsides as a result of medical evaluation and reassurance
C. does not require any particular duration
D. is not diagnosed if the preoccupation is of delusional intensity

Discussion: The DSM-IV criteria for hypochondriasis require that a person be preoccupied with fears or the idea of having a serious disease based on the misinterpretation of physical signs and sensations. Whereas such symptoms are not the predominant focus as they are in somatization disorder, conversion disorder, and pain disorder, some physical symptoms must be present. Duration must be at least 6 months. Psychotic preoccupation is generally considered delusional disorder, somatic type. However, reality testing can be difficult to determine, and so the specifier with poor insight has been included.

Pages 1144–1148 •

Answer D

8. In DSM-IV, a body dysmorphic disorder diagnosis

A. requires that there be no physical anomaly present
B. may be diagnosed if the preoccupation subsides as a result of medical evaluation and reassurance
C. does not require any particular duration
D. is not diagnosed if the preoccupation is of delusional intensity

Discussion: As defined in DSM-IV, the essential feature of this disorder is preoccupation with an imagined defect in appearance or a markedly excessive concern with a minor anomaly. The "normal-appearing person" criterion was deleted. Preoccupations persist despite reassurance. The diagnostic criteria do not include a duration requirement. As opposed to DSM-III-R, there is no longer an exclusion for psychotic preoccupation. This is because of the difficulty in determining whether a dysmorphic concern is delusional. It is thought that there is a continuum of preoccupations. This issue is far from clear, and both body dysmorphic disorder and delusional disorder, somatic type, can be diagnosed on the basis of the same symptoms in the same individual at the same time.

Pages 1148–1151 •

Answer C

9. In the treatment of somatoform disorders:

A. Hypochondriasis and body dysmorphic disorder may be approached similarly as to medication.
B. For somatization disorder and conversion disorder, a great emphasis should be placed on pharmacotherapy.
C. Conversion disorder is particularly refractory to therapy.
D. Primary care physicians should be removed from involvement in therapy as early as possible.

Discussion: Both hypochondriasis and body dysmorphic disorder have been characterized as being obsessive-compulsive spectrum disorders. These conditions are believed to have a common underlying serotoninergic dysregulation and responsiveness to selective serotonin reuptake inhibitors.

Pages 1147, 1150–1151 •

Answer A

CHAPTER

61 Dissociative Disorders

David Taylor

1. Which of the following 19th century clinicians first described what we now consider dissociative psychiatric illness?

A. Freud
B. Janet
C. Charcot
D. Breuer
E. Prince

Discussion: The French physician and psychologist Pierre Janet is credited with the initial description of this disorder, a *desagregation mentale.* This term carries with it a different nuance than the English word dissociation. It implies a separation of mental contents despite their general tendency to aggregate or be processed together. Janet described hysteria as a malady of personal synthesis. Jean Martin Charcot was interested in hypnosis and taught this to Freud. Freud and Breuer wrote of dissociative phenomena; however, Freud grew more interested in other types of psychiatric disorders. Morton Prince described the case of Sally Beauchamp, who had "alters."

Pages 1156–1157, Appendix I •

Answer B

2. Dissociation as a general model for keeping memories out of conscious awareness differs from repression in which of the following ways?

A. Memories are disguised in dissociation.
B. Retrieval of dissociated memories requires repeated trials of recall.
C. The information kept out of awareness in dissociation is organized temporally.
D. Repression is specifically tied to physical trauma.
E. The barrier to awareness of repressed memories is one of amnesia.

Discussion: Information is disguised as well as hidden in repression, whereas dissociated information is stored in a discrete and untransformed manner. Retrieval of repressed information requires translation and requires techniques such as repeated trials of recall, psychoanalysis, and interpretation; dissociated material can be recovered directly through hypnosis. The barrier to awareness in repression is due to dynamic conflict, not amnesia. Dissociation seems to be elicited as a defense most commonly after episodes of physical trauma, whereas repression is a response to warded-off fears, wishes, and other conflictual experiences.

Page 1157, Table 61–1 •

Answer C

3. Epidemiological studies of dissociative disorders have found all of the following **except**

A. These disorders are more common in women than in men.
B. The most common dissociative disorder is the not otherwise specified (NOS) category.
C. There has been a sharp rise in reported cases in recent years.
D. Dissociative disorders are seen only in Western countries.
E. One study has suggested an estimated prevalence of these disorders at 1 in 10,000 in the population.

Discussion: Women account for 90% of cases. The most common category is NOS both in the United States and in non-Western countries, where dissociative trance and possession trance are the most common diagnoses. Dissociative disorders are ubiquitous around the world. Few good epidemiological studies have been performed, and rates in clinical populations have been as high as 2%. There is controversy about overdiagnosis.

Pages 1157–1158 •

Answer D

4. Dissociative amnesia

A. involves loss of procedural as well as episodic memory
B. involves loss of episodic memory only
C. involves problems in memory storage

D. can involve loss of memory for any type of event
E. is also known as Wernicke-Korsakoff syndrome

Discussion: Dissociative amnesia is diagnosed if there are one or more episodes of inability to recall important personal information, usually of a traumatic or stressful nature. This is the classic functional disorder of episodic memory. It does not involve procedural memory or problems in memory storage and is reversible. The memory loss is for discrete periods, the memories for which have been encoded and stored but are unavailable. Unlike in Wernicke-Korsakoff syndrome, there is no problem with learning new episodic information (i.e., anterograde amnesia). Individuals with this disorder generally do not suffer disturbances in identity.

Pages 1158–1160 •

Answer B

5. Individuals with a diagnosis of depersonalization disorder

A. have hallucinations
B. frequently have a variety of other symptoms
C. are refractory to treatment
D. have impairment in reality testing
E. may also have other DSM-IV diagnoses

Discussion: Depersonalization disorder involves the occurrence of persistent feelings of unreality and detachment or estrangement from oneself or one's body, usually with the feeling that one is an outside observer of one's own mental processes. There is intact reality testing and no delusions or hallucinations. The symptom is frequently transient and may remit without formal treatment. It frequently occurs with other symptoms and in patients with other disorders, such as panic disorder or posttraumatic stress disorder, for example. The diagnosis is made when it is the predominant symptom. There are a variety of treatments for this condition.

Pages 1161–1162 •

Answer B

6. Dissociative identity disorder is often comorbid with

A. borderline personality disorder
B. schizophrenia
C. schizotypal personality disorder
D. schizoaffective disorder
E. dissociative disorder NOS

Discussion: The major comorbid psychiatric illnesses are the depressive disorders, substance use disorders, and borderline personality disorder. Such patients frequently display self-mutilative behavior, impulsiveness, and overvaluing and devaluing of relationships. Indeed, approximately a third of dissociative identity disorder patients fit criteria for borderline personality disorder as well. Comorbidity is a complex issue because many patients may also meet criteria for posttraumatic stress disorder, and many borderline personality disorder patients have a history of abuse and dissociate regularly. In addition, these patients are misdiagnosed as having schizophrenia because they may seem to have a delusion about there being more than one person in their bodies and also appear to have auditory hallucinations when one personality state speaks to or comments on the activities of another. Neuroleptics are not effective treatments for these patients.

Pages 1162–1163 •

Answer A

7. Whereas the ultimate goal of psychotherapy in the treatment of dissociative identity disorder is integration, which of the following makes that challenging?

A. Early in therapy, patients view the dissociation as protective.
B. The dissociative defense involves an identification with the aggressor.
C. The patient fears that the therapist is trying to "kill" personalities.
D. There is a tendency toward self-blame.
E. All of the above

Discussion: The patient needs to learn how to gradually control the dissociative processes in the service of working through traumatic memories. The dissociative defense represents an internalization of the abusive people in the patient's past, which makes the patient feel powerful rather than helpless. Setting aside the defense means acknowledging and bearing the helplessness of having been victimized and working through the irrational self-blame that gave such individuals a fantasy of control over events that they were in fact helpless to control.

Pages 1163–1166, Table 61–2 •

Answer E

CHAPTER

62 Sexual Disorders

Stephen B. Levine • Ellen A. Rosenblatt

1. The sexual equilibrium

A. will remain functional as long as a couple's nonsexual relationship is satisfying
B. always improves with time
C. is a predictable entity at the beginning of most relationships
D. is rooted in individual psychology, the nonsexual relationship, and the components of sexuality

Discussion: Sexual dysfunction is a two-person problem in terms of immediate effects but often in terms of cause as well. Psychiatrists should be wary when one partner is presented as normal and the other as having a problem. The ordinary interconnectivity of a couple's sexual function is referred to as the couple's sexual equilibrium. This is based on the subtle interplay of each partner's seven sexual component characteristics. These include gender identity, orientation, intention, desire, arousal, orgasm, and emotional satisfaction. In addition, a partner's opinion about an individual's particular component makeup, whether positive or negative, adds another level of understanding and affects behavior and satisfaction.

Pages 1175–1176, Table 62–4 •

Answer D

2. Possible causes of a sexual desire disorder in a person with intact sexual drive and a wish to behave sexually with a partner are

A. transference of parental attachments to the partner
B. depression
C. a secret struggle about sexual identity
D. anger, disappointment, or loss of respect for the partner
E. all of the above

Discussion: Sexual desire is manifested in a variety of ways including sexual fantasies, sexual dreams, initiation of the partner's sexual behavior, receptivity to partner-initiated sexual behavior, masturbation, genital sensations, heightened responsivity to erotic environmental cues, and heartfelt statements about wanting to behave sexually. These manifestations are the product of three intersecting mental components: *drive, motive,* and *wish.* Disorders of sexual desire can be caused by all of the above problems.

Pages 1175–1180, Tables 62–5 and 62–6 •

Answer E

3. Regarding gender identity disorders, which of the following statements is true?

A. Cross-gender–identified children prefer children of the opposite sex as their primary playmates.
B. Biological constitution seems to be the major source of an individual's gender confusion.
C. Most masculine girls (tomboys) later have a homosexual orientation.
D. Most people with cross-gender preoccupations pursue hormones and surgical alterations at some point in time.

Discussion: The organization of a stable gender identity is the first component of sexual identity to emerge during childhood. Extremely feminine young boys are presented for clinical assessment at a rate five times higher than that for masculine girls (tomboys). Cross-gender–identified children consistently demonstrate opposite-sex playmate preference. This is not typical for young children. Even though many lesbians have a history of tomboyish behavior, most tomboys have a heterosexual orientation. It is not known whether gender confusion is constitutional, adaptive, or due to some other process. The majority of individuals with gender identity disturbance do not go beyond fantasy or private cross-dressing.

Pages 1189–1194 •

Answer A

4. Paraphilia is associated with

A. unusual erotic images that are preoccupied with hostility and aggression

B. a usually normal-appearing sexual relationship with a spouse
C. a recurring intense attraction to particular pieces of clothing, body parts, or animals
D. the drive to act out fantasies that rarely interferes with day-to-day functioning
E. A and C only

Discussion: Paraphilia is characterized by a longstanding, unusual, highly arousing erotic preoccupation; a pressure to act out the fantasy; and a partner's sexual dysfunction. These are disorders of intention, the final component of sexual identity to develop. As such, they are recognized by unusual eroticism and socially destructive behaviors. The prevalence of the behaviors is likely to be far less than paraphilic imagery.

Pages 1194–1199 •

Answer E

5. All of the following are true about the female orgasm **except**

A. The concept of "normal" orgasmic attainment has broadened significantly in modern times.
B. Social and psychological beliefs may interfere with the biological ability to reach orgasm.
C. The diagnosis of female orgasmic disorder is made if a woman fails to attain orgasm at each sexual encounter.
D. A woman can overcome an orgasmic disorder by reading about orgasms in a book.
E. Hypoactive sexual desire disorder may be a sequela to persistent problems with orgasms.

Discussion: The attainment of reasonably regular orgasms with a partner is a crucial personal developmental step for young women. Orgasm is the reflexive culmination of arousal. It requires the physiological apparatus to augment and sustain arousal, the psychological willingness to be swept away by excitement, and a tenacious focus on the required physical work of augmenting arousal. The diagnosis of female orgasmic disorder is made when there is persistent psychological interference with this natural process. The judgment of dysfunction and normality is complex, given varying definitions of anorgasmy. No woman is always orgasmic. It is important to take a careful sexual history.

Pages 1184–1185 •

Answer C

6. The etiology of premature ejaculation

A. despite the years of psychiatric assumptions, remains unclarified
B. is related to anxiety about body closeness to mother
C. is a product of oedipal conflicts that have failed to resolve during adolescence
D. is now known to be due to physiological hypersensitivity in spinal cord nuclei
E. none of the above

Discussion: Premature ejaculation is a highly prevalent disorder seen primarily in heterosexuals characterized by a low threshold for the reflex sequence of orgasm. The etiology of this is not clear. In failing to develop a sense of control over the timing of his orgasm in the vagina, the man fails to meet his standards of being a satisfying sexual partner. This disruption of the sexual equilibrium is what is significant about the diagnosis, more than the actual time to orgasm.

Pages 1185–1186 •

Answer A

7. Psychogenic impotence, now known as male erectile disorder, is

A. a highly treatable problem with psychotherapy
B. a difficult to treat problem usually necessitating urological interventions
C. not known to exist after the mid-50s in men's lives
D. divisible into different prognostic categories depending on whether the problem is lifelong or acquired
E. often quickly responsive to sensate focus exercises

Discussion: What was considered psychogenic impotence is now termed, in the urological literature, adrenergic erectile dysfunction. This refers to the preponderance of sympathetic tone on the intracorporeal mechanisms that maintain flaccidity. Adrenergic dominance of the penile vasculature is created by a mind that perceives the sexual context as a dangerous, frightening, or unwanted milieu. The prevalence of erectile dysfunction rises dramatically in the sixth decade of life from less than 10% to 30%. Cardiovascular risk factors predict the most common patterns of erectile dysfunction in this age group. This creates a complex differential diagnosis, and psychogenic impotence is diagnosed if there is *selectivity* of erectile failure. There are lifelong and acquired variants.

Pages 1181–1184, Tables 62–7 to 62–9 •

Answer D

8. Fluoxetine-induced anorgasmy in a man may

A. be associated with the treatment of depression
B. be associated with the treatment of obsessive-compulsive disorder

C. wax and wane depending on the degree of sexual stimulation
D. wax and wane depending on the dose of fluoxetine
E. all of the above

Discussion: Fluoxetine and other serotoninergic agents frequently cause anorgasmy in both men and women. In men, this property of this class of medications (including the tricyclic clomipramine) has been used to treat certain conditions such as premature ejaculation and compulsive sexual acting-out behaviors seen in some paraphilias. In fact, some have considered compulsive paraphilic behaviors to be obsessive-compulsive spectrum disorders.

Pages 1186, 1199 •

Answer E

9. After the removal of the entire prostate including the capsule, an erectile disorder

A. rarely occurs because of special surgical techniques
B. uniformly occurs, characterized by episodic impotence
C. may require a separate new urological intervention to restore potency
D. will not get worse if radiation follows surgery
E. none of the above

Discussion: The autonomic innervation to the penis is usually cut when the prostatic capsule is removed in the course of a total prostatectomy. For this reason, a penile prosthesis is sometimes placed at the time of surgery.

Pages 1177–1179 •

Answer C

10. All of the following might be strongly expected to contribute to the decline of sexual desire in a 56-year-old woman **except**

A. loss of her husband's erectile reliability
B. her use of a benzodiazepine as a sleep aid periodically
C. her treatment with medroxyprogesterone (Provera) as part of hormone replacement therapy
D. normal aging effect
E. diminished erotic sensitivity of her nipples, vulva, and breasts

Discussion: In perimenopausal and postmenopausal women, arousal problems are often focused on the body as a whole. Skin insensitivity is part of this but is not the entire phenomenon. Women have concerns about estrogen replacement and consequences of menopause in terms of body image, attractiveness, fears of the partner's infidelity, and aging. Aging of the female arousal mechanisms occurs earlier than deterioration of orgasmic physiology. Women with decreasing arousal are often, therefore, still reliably orgasmic with the use of vaginal lubricants well into old age. Disturbances of the sexual equilibrium between partners can present as concerns about one partner's difficulties.

Page 1181 •

Answer B

CHAPTER

63 Eating Disorders

B. Timothy Walsh

1. Obesity is most accurately diagnosed as

A. an atypical eating disorder
B. binge-eating disorder
C. bulimia nervosa
D. a general medical condition
E. a psychiatric condition

Discussion: Obesity refers to an excess of body fat. Although obese individuals are at increased risk for a number of serious medical problems and are subject to significant social stigmatization and its psychological sequelae, empirical studies have found no more psychiatric disturbance in those who are overweight than in those who are of normal weight.

Page 1202 •

Answer D

2. To receive a diagnosis of anorexia nervosa, a patient must be

A. amenorrheic, if female
B. distressed about losing weight
C. female
D. less than 75% of ideal body weight
E. purging

Discussion: The DSM-IV criteria for anorexia nervosa require that women with the disorder be amenorrheic; patients are typically intensely distressed about *gaining* even small amounts of weight; the disorder usually, but not always, affects women, with the ratio of men to women approximately 1:10 to 1:20; DSM-IV provides a benchmark of 85% of the weight considered normal for age and height as a guideline; and individuals who purge are classed as having one of two variants of the disorder: binge-eating/purging type or restricting type.

Page 1203 •

Answer A

3. Which of the following has **not** been implicated as a general risk factor in the development of anorexia nervosa?

A. white racial background
B. dysfunctional family relationships
C. high socioeconomic status
D. history of anorexia nervosa in biological relatives
E. simple phobia for food

Discussion: Patients with anorexia nervosa severely restrict their food intake and may be extremely anxious when eating. However, they do not have a "food phobia," and phobic disorders of any type have not been implicated as risk factors in the development of anorexia nervosa. Whereas the etiology is fundamentally unknown, some risk factors have been identified, including middle- and upper-class socioeconomic status; white racial background; biological relatives with the disorder (the prevalence among relatives of patients ranges from 2% to 6%); and dysfunctional family relationships (as well as individual psychiatric illness in parents and impaired family interaction patterns).

Pages 1204–1205, Fig. 63–2 •

Answer E

4. Patients hospitalized with anorexia nervosa have a long-term mortality rate of

A. 2% to 4%
B. 5% to 10%
C. 10% to 20%
D. 25% to 35%
E. 50%

Discussion: The best data currently available suggest that 10% to 20% of patients who have been hospitalized for anorexia nervosa will, in the course of the next 10 to 30 years, die as a result of their illness. Much of the mortality is due to severe and chronic starvation, which eventually terminates in sudden death. In addition, a significant fraction of patients commits suicide.

Page 1208 •

Answer C

5. Empirical research suggests that the most effective treatment for anorexia nervosa patients whose illness started before age 18 years and who have been ill for less than 3 years is

A. antidepressant medication
B. cognitive-behavioral psychotherapy
C. family therapy
D. psychodynamic psychotherapy
E. psychoanalysis

Discussion: There is, at present, no general agreement about the most useful type of psychotherapy for treating anorexia nervosa. Although most of these treatments seem to be helpful (with the exception of traditional psychoanalytic therapy, for which most authorities see little role), the clearest empirical finding to date is that family therapy is effective for patients whose anorexia nervosa started before age 18 years and who have had the disorder for less than 3 years.

Pages 1208–1210 •

Answer C

6. The primary behavioral disturbance in bulimia nervosa is

A. binge-eating
B. compulsive exercising
C. fasting
D. laxative abuse
E. vomiting

Discussion: Episodes of binge-eating, in which the individual consumes an amount of food that is unusually large considering the circumstances under which it is eaten are the salient behavioral disturbance of bulimia nervosa. These overeating episodes, as well as a variety of compensatory behaviors, must occur at least twice a week for 3 months to merit a diagnosis of bulimia nervosa. The most common compensatory behaviors reported by patients who present to eating disorders clinics are vomiting and laxative abuse, but compulsive exercising, fasting, and diuretic misuse are also common.

Pages 1210–1211 •

Answer A

7. The percentage of young women in the United States who meet DSM-IV criteria for bulimia nervosa is

A. 0.5% to 1%
B. 1% to 4%
C. 5% to 10%
D. 10% to 15%
E. 15% to 25%

Discussion: Despite the common perception that the syndrome of bulimia nervosa has been occurring in epidemic proportions among young women in the United States, studies have found that the full-blown disorder affects only 1% to 4% of this population. Research also suggests that women born after 1960 have a higher risk for the disorder than those born before 1960.

Page 1211 •

Answer B

8. Bulimia nervosa is **not** associated with comorbid

A. anxiety disorders
B. mood disorders
C. personality disorders
D. schizophrenia
E. substance abuse

Discussion: Bulimia nervosa is associated with a number of comorbid psychiatric disorders. Among patients who are seen at eating disorders clinics, there is an increased frequency of anxiety and mood disorders, especially major depression and dysthymia; of drug and alcohol abuse; and of personality disorders. Psychotic disorders like schizophrenia are not associated with bulimia nervosa.

Page 1211 •

Answer D

9. The type of medication treatment favored by many investigators for bulimia nervosa is

A. desipramine
B. fluoxetine, 20 mg/d
C. fluoxetine, 60 mg/d
D. haloperidol
E. lithium

Discussion: The most commonly used mode of treatment that has been examined in bulimia nervosa is antidepressant medication. Fluoxetine at a dose of 60 mg/d is favored by many investigators because it has been studied in several large trials and appears to be at least as effective as and better tolerated than most other alternatives, like tricyclic antidepressants (e.g., desipramine) or fluoxetine in lower doses. Neither haloperidol nor lithium is used to treat bulimia nervosa.

Pages 1213–1214, Fig. 63–6 •

Answer C

For each numbered item, select the lettered heading most closely associated with it. Each letter may be selected once, more than once, or not at all.

A. physical abnormalities typical of anorexia nervosa

B. physical abnormalities typical of anorexia nervosa, purging subtype, and bulimia nervosa
C. physical abnormalities typical of binge-eating disorder
D. physical abnormalities typical of bulimia nervosa
E. physical abnormalities typical of obesity

____ 10. reduced bone density

Discussion: Individuals with anorexia nervosa have decreased bone density compared with age- and sex-matched peers and, as a result, are at increased risk for fractures. Low levels of estrogen, high levels of cortisol, and poor nutrition have all been cited as risk factors for the development of reduced bone density in anorexia nervosa.

Pages 1205–1207, Table 63–1 •

Answer A

____ 11. significant dental erosion

Discussion: Patients who induce vomiting for many years may have dental erosion, especially of the upper front teeth. The mechanism appears to be that stomach acid softens the enamel, which in time gradually disappears so that the teeth chip more easily and can become reduced in size. Dental erosion is most commonly associated with bulimia nervosa but also occurs in patients with anorexia nervosa, purging subtype.

Page 1212 •

Answer B

____ 12. lowered estrogen secretion

Discussion: In women with anorexia nervosa, estrogen secretion from the ovaries is markedly reduced, accounting for the occurrence of amenorrhea.

Pages 1205–1207 •

Answer A

____ 13. anemia

Discussion: Anorexia nervosa is often associated with the development of leukopenia and of a normochromic, normocytic anemia of mild to moderate severity.

Page 1206 •

Answer A

____ 14. reduced serum electrolyte levels

Discussion: The status of serum electrolytes is a reflection of the individual's salt and water intake and the nature and severity of the purging behavior. A common pattern in women with bulimia nervosa or anorexia nervosa, purging subtype, is hypokalemia, hypochloremia, and mild alkalosis resulting from frequent and persistent self-induced vomiting. Patients who lose substantial amounts of stomach acid through vomiting may become slightly alkalotic; those who abuse only laxatives may become slightly acidotic.

Pages 1206, 1212 •

Answer B

____ 15. prolonged gastric emptying time

Discussion: In patients with anorexia nervosa, the motility of the gastrointestinal tract is diminished, leading to delayed gastric emptying and contributing to complaints of "bloating" and to constipation.

Page 1206 •

Answer A

____ 16. salivary gland enlargement

Discussion: Some patients with bulimia nervosa or anorexia nervosa, purging subtype, have painless salivary gland enlargement, which is thought to represent hypertrophy resulting from the repeated episodes of binge-eating and vomiting.

Page 1212 •

Answer B

CHAPTER

64 Sleep and Sleep-Wake Disorders

David Taylor

1. The alternation of rapid eye movement (REM) and non-REM sleep is an example of

A. a circadian rhythm
B. an ultradian rhythm
C. a biorhythm
D. a Zeitgeber

Discussion: There are two major phases of sleep, REM and non-REM sleep, which alternate with each other throughout the sleep period. These phases oscillate with a cycle of about 80 to 110 minutes. This cycle is an example of an ultradian rhythm, a biological rhythm with a cycle length considerably less than 24 hours.

Pages 1217–1218 •

Answer B

2. Which of the following is **not** an example of a circadian rhythm?

A. the sleep-wake cycle
B. the hypothalamic-pituitary axis
C. core body temperature
D. glomerular filtration rate

Discussion: All of the above except the glomerular filtration rate are examples of circadian phenomena. The secretion of thyroid-stimulating hormone, melatonin, and cortisol is governed by "biological clocks" that are regulated by the suprachiasmatic nucleus (SCN) of the anterior hypothalamus. The endogenous activity rhythms of the SCN are synchronized with environment primarily by ambient light. Changes in light intensity, particularly at dawn and dusk, are important in synchronizing endogenous oscillators controlling circadian rhythms such as those listed above.

Pages 1218–1219 •

Answer D

3. Which of the following statements about the sleep-wake cycle is true?

A. REM sleep is more common in the last half of the night among those who live a conventional sleep schedule.
B. "Free-running" cycles are often seen in phase-shifted individuals.
C. Melatonin levels are an example of a Zeitgeber.
D. Lesions of the SCN cause profound somnolence.

Discussion: The propensity for, character of, and duration of sleep are closely related to the phase position of the underlying circadian oscillator. If the daily temperature curve is used to index the phase position of the biological clock, sleep in general and REM sleep in particular occur most commonly near the nadir of the temperature rhythm. Thus, in persons who live a conventional sleep schedule (11 PM to 7 AM), REM sleep is more common in the last half of the night, when core body temperature is lowest, than in the first half and more likely in morning naps than afternoon naps. Furthermore, subjects tend to awaken on the rising phase of the temperature rhythm. Bright light, a typical Zeitgeber (time giver), sets the phase position of the oscillators that control circadian temperature and melatonin. Free-running cycles occur in the absence of such environmental cues. Lesions of the SCN lead to an absence of circadian rhythms and brief bouts of sleep and wakefulness.

Pages 1218–1219 •

Answer A

4. Which of these brain regions has been implicated in the generation of REM sleep?

A. thalamus
B. visual cortex
C. dorsal tegmentum of the brain stem
D. nucleus tractus solitarius

Discussion: The non-REM–REM sleep cycle is regulated within the brain stem. Transection of the pontomesencephalic junction in cats blocks input to the pons from the forebrain. The isolated brain stem generates periodic episodes of rapid eye movements and muscle atonia, the physiological signatures of REM sleep. In contrast, on electroencephalography, the isolated forebrain of the same preparation generates alternating periods of slow waves and arousal, suggestive of non-REM sleep and wakefulness, respectively.

Pages 1220–1221, Fig. 64–3 •

Answer C

5. Which of the following is the "sleep neurotransmitter"?

A. acetylcholine
B. norepinephrine
C. histamine
D. none of the above

Discussion: No specific compound has been found to be responsible for the induction or maintenance of sleep. Acetylcholine, released from neurons originating in the dorsal tegmentum, induces REM sleep and cortical activation. Serotonin and norepinephrine, on the other hand, inhibit REM sleep, possibly by inhibition of cholinergic neurons responsible for REM sleep. These physiological mechanisms may be involved in both depression and its associated sleep disturbances. Some antidepressant medications, notably monoamine oxidase inhibitors, completely eliminate REM sleep.

Page 1221 •

Answer D

6. All-night polysomnography involves all of the following measures **except**

A. electro-oculogram
B. electroencephalogram
C. electromyogram
D. electronystagmogram

Discussion: All-night polysomnography involves all of the above except an electronystagmogram. In addition to the above, respiratory and cardiovascular functions are monitored with electrocardiography, oximetry, and a small microphone near the mouth to monitor snoring. Other specialized tests are intraesophageal pressures, nocturnal penile tumescence, and core body temperature.

Pages 1223–1224 •

Answer D

7. The differential diagnosis of primary hypersomnia includes all of the following **except**

A. narcolepsy
B. idiopathic recurring stupor
C. Klinefelter's syndrome
D. menstruation-associated hypersomnia syndrome

Discussion: Previously called non-REM narcolepsy, this disorder is relatively rare, represented by perhaps 5% to 10% of patients presenting to sleep disorders centers for the evaluation of hypersomnia. Patients present with complaints of long and nonrestorative nocturnal sleep, difficulty awakening and daytime sleepiness, and intellectual dysfunction; they do not experience the accessory symptoms of narcolepsy, such as cataplexy, sleep paralysis, and hypnagogic hallucinations, and often report frequent headaches and Raynaud's phenomenon. It must be distinguished from the above syndromes except Klinefelter's syndrome, which is a chromosomal anormality. Kleine-Levin syndrome patients, in addition to hypersomnia, often demonstrate aggressive or inappropriate sexuality, compulsive overeating, and other bizarre behaviors.

Pages 1227–1228 •

Answer C

8. In breathing-related sleep disorders, which of the following is observed?

A. prolonged sleep latency on the Multiple Sleep Latency Test
B. sleep apnea and hypopnea
C. chronic obstructive pulmonary disease
D. respiratory alkalosis

Discussion: Sleep apnea is the hallmark and major diagnostic criterion for breathing-related sleep disorder. Sleep apnea is defined as cessation of breathing lasting at least 10 seconds and an apnea index (number of apneic episodes per hour of sleep) of 5 or more. Sleep apnea can be of an obstructive, central, or mixed type. In obstructive apnea, there is a collapse of the pharyngeal airway during inspiration and compromised alveolar ventilation, hypoxemia, and hypercapnia. The resulting strenuous attempts to inspire disrupt sleep. In central apnea, there is a failure of respiratory neurons to activate the phrenic and intercostal motor neurons. This is typically associated with heart disease. Hypopnea is considered a 50% reduction in respiration. Patients with sleep apnea typically experience excessive daytime sleepiness and fall asleep almost immediately on the Multiple Sleep Latency Test. Chronic obstructive pulmonary disease disrupts sleep but for different reasons.

Pages 1223–1224, 1229–1232, 1242 •

Answer B

CHAPTER

65 Impulse-Control Disorders

Ronald M. Winchel • Yoram Yovell • Daphne Simeon

1. The following diagnoses and conditions are all exclusion criteria for the DSM-IV diagnosis of intermittent explosive disorder **except**

A. alcohol intoxication during all episodes
B. a history of impulsive behavior between episodes
C. a manic episode
D. borderline personality disorder
E. antisocial personality disorder

Discussion: Criterion C requires that a series of conditions, disorders, and states be excluded before a diagnosis of intermittent explosive disorder is made. This is because impulsive aggression is by no means specific to this disorder or even to psychiatric conditions.

Pages 1251–1252 •

Answer B

2. The following conditions have all been associated with impulsive aggression **except**

A. partial complex seizures
B. alcohol abuse
C. a central serotoninergic dysfunction
D. generalized anxiety disorder
E. diffuse slowing on the electroencephalogram

Discussion: Pure intermittent explosive disorder is a rare entity. Associated conditions, which are not exclusive of the diagnosis, include personality disorders other than borderline or antisocial, alcohol abuse but not intoxication, and nonspecific neurological findings that are not the physiological cause of the outbursts. Impulsive aggression may be related to reduced cerebrospinal fluid levels of 5-hydroxyindoleacetic acid (5-HIAA).

Pages 1252–1255 •

Answer D

3. According to DSM-IV, the diagnosis of kleptomania cannot be made in the presence of all of the following **except**

A. mania
B. antisocial motives to stealing
C. major depression and lack of memory for the event
D. stealing in response to auditory hallucinations
E. motivated by financial gain

Discussion: Kleptomania shares with all other impulse-control disorders not elsewhere classified the recurrent failure to resist impulses. It also shares a rigorous set of exclusion criteria. The theft is not motivated by financial gain or by revenge, as in antisocial behavior, and does not occur during the course of a manic or a psychotic episode.

Page 1258 •

Answer C

4. Of the following treatment combinations, select the one that is effective in kleptomania.

A. antidepressant + aversive conditioning
B. serotonin reuptake inhibitor + lithium
C. behavioral therapy + antidepressant
D. psychodynamic therapy + antidepressant
E. behavior modification + psychodynamic therapy

Discussion: The most commonly used medications in the treatment of kleptomania are the antidepressants, with a possible benefit from serotonin reuptake inhibitors in particular. A number of other medications and electroconvulsive therapy have been tried in kleptomania. Whereas the literature is limited, it appears that behavioral treatment is more efficacious than psychodynamic psychotherapy.

Page 1260–1262 •

Answer C

5. Pyromania may be characterized by which of the following statements?

A. Pyromania is a common cause of fire-setting behavior.

B. Because fire setting is often motivated by such factors as financial gain, revenge, or political expression, it is uncommon among children.
C. Although fire setting appears to be far more common among men than among women, in psychiatric samples, both men and women have similarly frequent histories of fire setting.
D. Pyromania is often associated with feelings of erotic excitement.

Discussion: Pyromania must be distinguished from non-pyromania fire-setting behavior, which can have a host of nonimpulsive motivations ranging from curiosity, financial gain, and revenge to sexual excitement. Although pyromania is rare, fire-setting behavior is common among psychiatric samples. Unlike pyromania, which is rare among women, fire-setting behavior was common in the histories of female patients (22%) as well as among male patients (28.8%).

Page 1262 •

Answer C

6. Impulsive firesetting has been associated with which biological marker?

A. abnormal dexamethasone suppression test results in 50%
B. excess central nervous system stores of the enzyme tryptophan hydroxylase
C. decreased cerebrospinal fluid concentrations of 5-HIAA
D. altered circadian patterns of growth hormone release

Discussion: As with other impulsive aggressive behaviors, there has been a finding of low cerebrospinal fluid levels of 5-HIAA in individuals with a history of fire setting. 5-HIAA is a primary serotonin metabolite.

Pages 1262–1263 •

Answer C

7. Pathological gambling may be confused with social gambling and professional gambling. Which one of the following features is helpful in distinguishing between pathological gambling and other forms of gambling?

A. The gambler identifies himself or herself as a social or professional gambler.
B. The gambler experiences a deep sense of excitement while gambling.
C. The gambler experiences significant unplanned financial losses.
D. The gambler began gambling in his or her teens.
E. More than one form of gambling is pursued (e.g., both horseracing and lottery).

Discussion: The DSM-IV definition of pathological gambling is specific about maladaptive gambling behavior. Many individuals with pathological gambling may feel that they are professional gamblers. "Chasing" behavior and unplanned losses distinguish those with a disorder.

Pages 1264–1266 •

Answer C

8. The treatment of pathological gambling resembles the treatment of substance abuse or dependence in all of the following **except**

A. Family therapy may be helpful but is not essential.
B. Treatment of a comorbid mood disorder is often required.
C. Abstinence is a prerequisite to treatment.
D. Initial dysphoria, which may progress to a full depressive episode, is to be expected shortly after abstinence is first achieved.
E. Inpatient treatment may be required in severe cases.

Discussion: The greatest difference between the treatment of pathological gambling and the treatment of other addictions is in the area of family therapy. Because relapse may be difficult to detect and because of a long history of exploitative behavior by the patient, the spouse and other family members tend to be more suspicious of and angry at the patient with pathological gambling compared with families of alcoholic patients. Frequent family sessions are often essential to offer the gambler an opportunity to make amends, learn communication skills, and deal with preexisting intimacy problems.

Pages 1269–1270 •

Answer A

9. Which of the following characterizes the typical adult patient with trichotillomania?

A. a 54-year-old woman who had recent onset after a brain injury
B. a 40-year-old man who pulls out hair about once a week
C. a 22-year-old woman with chronic schizophrenia
D. a 35-year-old woman who has been pulling out hair for more than 20 years

Discussion: Reliable data regarding the gender ratio in the general population are not yet available. It has long been suggested that women greatly outnumber men. Surveys of college students suggest a more equal ratio. The age at onset typically ranges from early childhood to young adulthood. Peak ages of presentation may be bimodal; an earlier peak occurs around age 5 to 8 years among children who have a self-limited course, whereas mean age at onset is approximately 13 years among patients who present to psychiatrists in adulthood.

Pages 1271–1272 •

Answer D

10. Which of the following is a valid statement regarding disorders that may be comorbid with trichotillomania?

A. Histories of mood disorders are common.
B. The rate of obsessive-compulsive disorder among first-degree relatives of people with trichotillomania is approximately 30%.
C. It has been estimated that a third of women with trichotillomania have a past history of or are currently experiencing an eating disorder as well.
D. The frequency of schizophrenia and schizoaffective disorder among individuals with trichotillomania is four times the frequency in the general population.

Discussion: Individuals with trichotillomania have increased risk for mood disorders and anxiety symptoms. Specific anxiety disorders, such as obsessive-compulsive disorder, may be increased as well. Although it has been suggested that trichotillomania in childhood or adolescence is associated with schizophrenia or severe disruptions of the family system, no systematically collected data support such conclusions.

Pages 1271–1274 •

Answer A

CHAPTER

66 Adjustment Disorder

James J. Strain • Jeffrey H. Newcorn

1. In differentiating an adjustment disorder from a major depressive disorder, a useful finding is

A. appetite
B. insomnia
C. guilt
D. a documented stressor
E. duration of symptoms

Discussion: Criterion A in the DSM-IV definition of adjustment disorder is that there must be a stressor. Adjustment disorder, like trauma-based disorders, substance-induced conditions, and disorders due to a general medical condition, specifies a cause. There is no such requirement for a major mood disorder, such as major depressive disorder.

Pages 1280–1281 •

Answer D

2. An adjustment disorder should not last longer than

A. 1 month
B. 3 months
C. 6 months
D. 12 months
E. indefinite time length

Discussion: In a change from DSM-III-R, the 6-month time requirement for duration of adjustment disorder was eliminated in DSM-IV to account for variable presentations and the fact that many stressors are chronic, such as serious medical illnesses like human immunodeficiency virus disease. There is no research documenting or refuting the time criterion of either onset or duration of symptoms. In any event, adjustment disorder is no longer a "transitory" diagnosis that has to change.

Pages 1280–1281, Table 66–1 •

Answer E

3. The first line of treatment for an adjustment disorder should **not** include

A. counseling
B. cognitive-behavioral therapy
C. psychotropic medications
D. interpersonal psychotherapy
E. group psychotherapy

Discussion: First-line treatment for adjustment disorder most importantly involves appropriate referral and triage because often these patients may not present to psychiatrists. Treatment may initially involve any of the modalities listed except the use of medications. The initial aim of any form of psychotherapy should be to clarify and interpret the meaning of the stressor for the patient and also to allow the patient to express affects, fears, anxieties, rage, helplessness, or hopelessness related to the stressor. Medication such as antidepressants and anxiolytics can and should be used when appropriate but should not be considered an initial treatment.

Pages 1286–1287 •

Answer C

4. Maladaptation, which is an essential symptom in the adjustment disorders, can be reflected by

A. anorexia
B. insomnia
C. anhedonia
D. inability to work
E. diminished libido

Discussion: The DSM-IV criteria for adjustment disorder specify that the "reaction is indicated either by marked distress that is in excess of what would be expected given the nature of the stressor or by significant impairment in social or occupational functioning." There is no specific symptom list with vegetative signs of depression. Obviously, the judgment about what is expectable and culturally appropriate is a highly complex one.

Pages 1284–1285 •

Answer D

5. In children and youths, in contrast to adults, those with adjustment disorder are more likely to

A. have a major mental disorder
B. have a prolonged adjustment disorder
C. respond better to medication
D. have a shorter episode of adjustment disorder
E. have a recurrence of the adjustment disorder

Discussion: In adults with adjustment disorder, the prognosis is often favorable; however, in adolescent populations, there is a different outcome. At 5 years, 43% had a major mental disorder compared with 21% of adults. School-age children actually have a better outcome and prognosis; one study showed no negative sequelae specifically attributable to adjustment disorder.

Pages 1282, 1285–1286 •

Answer A

For each numbered item, select the lettered heading most closely associated with it. Each letter may be selected once, more than once, or not at all.

6. Match the characteristic presentation with the diagnosis:

____ 1. persistent in excess of 2 years	A. major affective disorder
____ 2. stress related	B. dysthymic disorder
____ 3. at least five vegetative and ideational symptoms	C. minor depressive disorder
____ 4. manic and depressive episodes	D. adjustment disorder with depressed mood
____ 5. at least three vegetative and ideational symptoms	E. bipolar disorder

Discussion: The differential diagnosis between adjustment disorder with depressed mood and other mood disorders is most difficult with other not otherwise specified (NOS) or nearly subthreshold conditions. Minor depressive disorder is such a condition. There is a hierarchy of psychiatric conditions, which include 1) major disorders, 2) NOS disorders, 3) adjustment disorder, 4) problem-level diagnoses (other conditions that may be a focus of clinical attention), and 5) normal fluctuations of mental states. Adjustment disorder is at the margin of illness and thus is most likely to be confused with either NOS conditions or problems such as bereavement.

Pages 1280–1281, 1284–1285, Fig. 66–1 •

Answers 1, B; 2, D; 3, A; 4, E; 5, C

7. Match the treatment with the disorder:

____ 1. medication has minimal effect	A. major affective disorder
____ 2. medication is usually not indicated	B. dysthymic disorder
____ 3. lithium prophylaxis is useful	C. minor depressive disorder
____ 4. psychotherapy and chemotherapy are indicated	D. adjustment disorder with depressed mood
____ 5. may be a prodromal state of a major affective disorder	E. bipolar disorder

Discussion: The treatment of adjustment disorder compared with the treatment of major and minor mood disorders depends on the severity, duration, and response to initial treatment. Patients who do not respond to treatment for adjustment disorder should have their initial diagnosis reevaluated and, if stressors are ongoing, may need additional support. In adults, in whom there is less likelihood of development of major psychiatric disorder, this may be less of a problem than in adolescents.

Pages 1286–1288 •

Answers 1, B; 2, D; 3, E; 4, A; 5, C

CHAPTER

67 Personality Disorders

Thomas A. Widiger • Cynthia J. Sanderson

1. Which of the following personality disorders does **not** have official recognition within DSM-IV?

A. schizotypal
B. narcissistic
C. passive-aggressive
D. avoidant

Discussion: There are 10 personality disorders delineated in DSM-IV. Two additional variants are passive-aggressive (negativistic) personality disorder and depressive personality disorder, which are categorized as personality disorder not otherwise specified (NOS). Other types that have been under this designation but are no longer in DSM-IV include self-defeating personality disorder and sadistic personality disorder. Personality disorder NOS, which is also reserved for those individuals who do not meet the diagnostic criteria for any of the 10 other personality disorders, but who do have a personality disorder, is the most commonly diagnosed personality disorder category in almost every study in which it has been researched.

Pages 1291, 1293, 1313–1315 •

Answer C

2. Which personality disorder lacks empirical support for a genetic contribution to its etiology?

A. avoidant
B. borderline
C. histrionic
D. narcissistic

Discussion: The cluster of odd-eccentric personality disorders, none of which is listed above, has been studied for association with schizophrenia. The greatest empirical support has been found for schizotypal personality disorder, which is not surprising given that the diagnostic criteria were obtained from the observations of biological relatives of persons with schizophrenia. There are no data on the heritability of narcissistic personality disorder. Borderline personality disorder may breed true, and there may also be an association with mood and impulse-control disorders. Histrionic personality disorder may share a genetic disposition with antisocial personality disorder toward impulsivity or sensation seeking. Avoidant personality disorder, which is an extreme variant of the fundamental personality traits of introversion and neuroticism, may share in their substantial heritability.

Pages 1295–1296, 1297, 1302, 1305, 1307 •

Answer D

3. For which personality disorder are anhedonic deficits central to its pathological process?

A. schizoid
B. paranoid
C. schizotypal
D. borderline

Discussion: The central pathological process of schizoid personality disorder appears to be anhedonic deficits, or an excessively low ability to experience positive affectivity. A fundamental distinction in schizophrenic symptoms is between positive and negative symptoms. Whereas schizotypal personality disorder may represent subthreshold positive symptoms, schizoid personality disorder may be a muted expression of the negative symptom set.

Pages 1295–1297 •

Answer A

4. Which personality disorder is the most difficult to treat?

A. schizotypal
B. avoidant
C. dependent
D. antisocial

Discussion: Antisocial personality disorder is the most difficult personality disorder to treat. Persons with this diagnosis usually lack a motivation to change and see only the advantage of their antisocial traits and not the costs. Motivation can be forced by an external source, such as a court order, and yet in such an instance it is not sustained. Prolonged incarceration can result in eventual attenuation of behaviors with time. Community, residential, and wilderness programs with daily confrontation can be helpful. The formation of a therapeutic alliance is the most important variable in these treatments, and often a peer is most suitable to fill this role.

Pages 1300–1301 •

Answer D

5. Which personality disorder is the most prevalent within most clinical settings?

A. avoidant
B. borderline
C. schizotypal
D. dependent

Discussion: Borderline personality disorder is the most prevalent personality disorder within most clinical settings. Approximately 15% of all inpatients (51% of inpatients with a personality disorder) and 8% of all outpatients (27% of outpatients with a personality disorder) will have borderline personality disorder. Approximately 75% of the persons with borderline personality disorder will be female.

Page 1302 •

Answer B

6. For which personality disorder has the differential prevalence rate across sex (or gender) been controversial?

A. antisocial
B. narcissistic
C. obsessive-compulsive
D. histrionic

Discussion: A controversial issue in the study of histrionic personality disorder is its differential sex prevalence. Among studies of sex prevalence in the personality disorders, it has typically been found that two thirds of patients with histrionic personality disorder are female. In DSM-IV, the discussion states that the sex ratio does not significantly differ from the sex ratio in the clinical setting. This personality disorder involves to some extent maladaptive variants of stereotypically feminine traits, such as emotionality. The criteria are severe enough that a normal woman would not meet criteria. Studies have shown that psychiatrists may diagnose histrionic personality disorder in women who in fact have antisocial traits. This is because there are overlapping traits of impulsivity, sensation seeking, low frustration tolerance, and manipulativeness.

Page 1305 •

Answer D

7. Neuroleptic medications, such as low doses of thiothixene, have demonstrated an effectiveness for which personality disorder?

A. schizoid
B. paranoid
C. schizotypal
D. histrionic

Discussion: The treatment of schizotypal personality disorder involves practical advice, social skills training, and pharmacotherapy. Empirical research has focused on the use of medications. Low doses of the antipsychotic thiothixene have shown efficacy in the treatment of perceptual aberrations and social anxiousness.

Page 1298 •

Answer C

8. Which personality disorder will often result in an Axis I social phobia?

A. avoidant
B. dependent
C. borderline
D. paranoid

Discussion: The most difficult part of the differential diagnosis in avoidant personality disorder is the distinction with social phobia. Both involve an avoidance of social situations, social anxiety, and timidity, and both may be evident since late childhood or adolescence. Many persons with avoidant personality disorder actually seek treatment for social phobia. If the behavior pattern is pervasive and long-standing, the personality disorder is the better diagnosis, although of course patients may have both conditions.

Pages 1308–1310 •

Answer A

CHAPTER

68 Psychological Factors Affecting Medical Conditions

James L. Levenson

1. The diagnosis of psychological factors affecting medical conditions is suggested by all of the following **except**

A. There is a close temporal relationship between the psychological factor and the medical condition.
B. The medical condition is known to be a classic psychosomatic illness.
C. The psychological factor interferes with medical treatment.
D. The psychological factor adds to risky health behaviors.
E. Stress precipitates the medical symptoms.

Discussion: The expanded DSM-IV criteria for this diagnosis reflect the variety of ways in which specific psychological or behavioral factors can adversely affect medical conditions. In particular, psychological factors are described as potentially interfering with treatment, posing health risks, or causing stress-related pathophysiological changes. The medical condition is coded on Axis III. The psychological factor can be an Axis I or Axis II disorder, a symptom, a personality trait, a defense mechanism, a maladaptive health behavior, or a stress-related physiological response. Psychiatric illness and medical disease frequently coexist. Psychiatrists and investigators of past eras were misled by this frequent comorbidity into premature conclusions that the psychological factors were preeminent in the causation of certain medical disorders designated psychosomatic. The contemporary view is an attempt to not overvalue psychological causation in a few instances and to recognize that psychosocial factors can potentially affect any medical condition.

Pages 1318–1319, Table 68–1 •

Answer B

2. Which is the *best substantiated* effect of depression on medical illness?

A. Depression impairs immune surveillance and suppression against cancer.
B. Depression causes a hypersensitive thyroid-stimulating hormone response to thyrotropin-releasing hormone in hypothyroidism.
C. Depression is a risk factor for coronary artery disease.
D. Depression in end-stage renal disease usually results from poorly controlled uremia.
E. Human immunodeficiency virus–positive men who are depressed develop AIDS and die sooner than those without depression.

Discussion: Depression is a risk factor in coronary artery disease that is associated with increased morbidity and mortality (a fourfold increase in mortality at 6 months after myocardial infarction in one study). The mechanisms for this are unclear, although preliminary evidence suggests that depression has effects on heart rate variability, autonomic imbalance or arrhythmia, and platelet aggregation. Bereavement may result in changes in natural killer–cell activity and T-cell ratios in cancer. Depression causes a blunted, not a hypersensitive, thyroid-stimulating hormone response to thyrotropin-releasing hormone. The evidence that depression has an impact on progression of human immunodeficiency virus disease is contradictory.

Pages 1324–1329 •

Answer C

3. Irritable bowel syndrome is often accompanied by all of the following **except**

A. alcohol dependence
B. somatization
C. depression
D. panic attacks
E. history of childhood sexual abuse

Discussion: Irritable bowel syndrome is a heterogeneous condition with a high frequency of comorbid anxiety (especially panic attacks), depression, and somatization. There is no common profile of psychological symptoms or personality traits. There is an increased likelihood of a history of childhood sexual abuse but not of alcohol dependence. Whereas stress is thought by patients and their physicians to be related to exacerbations of irritable bowel syndrome, there is no evidence of a change in gastrointestinal smooth muscle response at times of stress that differs from the response of control subjects.

Page 1328 •

Answer A

4. Psychological factors are best understood to affect diabetes mellitus through each of the following mechanisms **except**

A. noncompliance with diet
B. noncompliance with insulin regimen
C. adolescents' dislike of restrictions and authority figures
D. unique diabetic personality type
E. mental stress–induced insulin resistance

Discussion: Whereas early psychosomatic literature suggested a diabetic personality type, this has not been found to be the case. There are some studies examining the relationship of personality type and glucose regulation. Psychological stress administered in the laboratory can impair glucose control in both insulin-dependent and non–insulin-dependent diabetic patients. This appears to be due to neurohormonal factors. Diabetic individuals who have psychiatric disorders have poorer glycemic control, and this can also be due to noncompliance. Diabetic adolescents in good glucose control were less likely to use primitive defenses, such as wishful thinking and avoidance, than were those in poorer control.

Page 1326 •

Answer D

5. Which statement regarding type A behavior and coronary artery disease is most accurate?

A. Type A behavior has been shown to be a more potent risk factor than hyperlipidemia, sedentary lifestyle, and diabetes.
B. Type A behavior is an inherent and unmodifiable personality pattern.
C. Type A behavior is also a proven risk factor for hypertension, stroke, and sudden death.
D. Type A behavior reduces risk for development of some forms of cancer.
E. Type A behavior is not a reliable predictor of coronary disease, but hostility may be.

Discussion: Type A behavior is one of the most studied psychological factors affecting a medical condition. Initial conviction that this is a definite risk factor for coronary artery disease has been eroded by studies that have failed to find an association between type A behavior and the extent of coronary artery disease. One long-term follow-up study found lower mortality in type A behavior patients than in type B patients. Whereas global type A behavior may not be a reliable predictor, it is possible that the component behavior of hostility may be, but this too is debatable. A few short-term studies have shown that type A behavior can be treated.

Pages 1325–1326 •

Answer E

6. Which statement is most accurate?

A. Denial is adaptive in coronary artery disease.
B. Denial is maladaptive in coronary artery disease.
C. Anxiety may be a risk factor for hypertension.
D. Biofeedback has been shown to be more effective than medication in anxious hypertensives.
E. The only evidence that psychological stressors can precipitate ventricular arrhythmias is anecdotal.

Discussion: A high level of anxiety at baseline evaluation independently predicted twice the risk for development of hypertension in middle-aged men but not in women in one study. Job strain is also a risk. There is a modest but clinically significant benefit to psychological treatments in the management of hypertension, but this is not as effective as medication, and compliance is an even greater problem. Maladaptive denial may prevent individuals with coronary artery disease from getting treatment but can be adaptive during hospitalization after an acute event and may even reduce morbidity and mortality.

Page 1326 •

Answer C

7. A 32-year-old patient with asthma reports feeling "nervous all the time." Likely explanations include all of the following **except**

A. progression to more severe asthma
B. side effect of medications for asthma
C. excess dietary caffeine
D. anticipatory anxiety about asthma attacks
E. asthma as a conversion disorder

Discussion: Although asthma was once regarded as a "classic psychosomatic disorder," it is currently viewed as a primary respiratory disorder. Respiratory distress and medications both can play a role in the development of an array of anxiety symptoms. Studies have shown that asthmatic individuals with anxiety and depression tend to have more complaints but no objective difference in measures of respiratory function.

Page 1327 •

Answer E

8. All of the following statements regarding depression and medical illness are correct **except**

A. Depression aggravates chronic pain in rheumatoid arthritis.
B. Depression is common after stroke but has little impact on outcome.
C. Depression is common in migraine but does not explain frequency of headaches.
D. Depression predicts shorter survival in end-stage renal disease.
E. There is no particular temporal relationship between inflammatory bowel disease and depression.

Discussion: Depression is frequent after stroke, particularly in the acute phase during hospitalization and the first few weeks afterward. The presence of depression is associated with poorer outcome, and functional status is improved with treatment of depression after stroke.

Page 1327 •

Answer B

CHAPTER

69 Medication-Induced Movement Disorders

Dilip V. Jeste • David Naimark

1. The most appropriate treatment for an acute neuroleptic-induced dystonia is to

A. wait 60 minutes and then administer 50 mg of oral diphenhydramine
B. wait 15 minutes and then administer 2 mg of intramuscular benztropine
C. immediately administer 50 mg of intramuscular diphenhydramine
D. immediately administer 1 mg of intramuscular lorazepam
E. call for anesthesia backup and immediately administer 4 mg of intravenous benztropine

Discussion: The treatment of acute neuroleptic-induced dystonia should involve the immediate administration of an anticholinergic or antihistaminic medication. The first dose should be 2 mg of benztropine or 50 mg of diphenhydramine or the equivalent. If there is no response within 30 minutes, this should be repeated. Oral dosing is too slow, and even mild dystonias respond more rapidly with parenteral medication. If refractory, frequent dosing intervals and intramuscular lorazepam may be necessary. If there is laryngeal or pharyngeal dystonia, 4 mg of intravenous benztropine followed by 1 to 2 mg of intravenous lorazepam is recommended; if there is a poor response, call an anesthesiologist.

Pages 1337–1338 •

Answer C

2. Neuroleptic-induced parkinsonism may be most easily confused with

A. positive-symptom schizophrenia
B. negative-symptom schizophrenia
C. panic disorder
D. bipolar disorder, manic phase
E. acute dystonia

Discussion: Neuroleptic-induced parkinsonism, a syndrome of tremor, muscle rigidity, or akinesia, develops in 10% to 15% of patients receiving neuroleptics, usually within 2 to 3 weeks of the initiation of therapy. This condition needs to be differentiated from idiopathic Parkinson's disease and other conditions causing tremor, such as cerebellar disease, strokes, tardive dyskinesia, neuroleptic malignant syndrome, and alcohol withdrawal. Neuroleptic-induced acute dystonia occurs earlier than parkinsonism (often within hours) and is usually painful. There are primary psychiatric illnesses that mimic symptoms of neuroleptic-induced parkinsonism. These include most prominently the negative symptoms of schizophrenia and depression as well as catatonia. This last may be a related condition physiologically.

Pages 1338–1340 •

Answer B

3. Neuroleptic-induced akathisia

A. is a risk factor for the development of tardive dyskinesia
B. is generally well tolerated by patients
C. most commonly occurs after at least 3 months of treatment with neuroleptic medication
D. is seen more frequently with low-potency neuroleptics
E. is the least common of the extrapyramidal side effects of neuroleptics

Discussion: Akathisia, a subjective feeling of restlessness and an intensely unpleasant need to move, is one of the most common side effects of neuroleptic treatment. It occurs within the first 4 weeks of treatment in between 20% and 75% of all patients treated with neuroleptics, especially large doses of high-potency medications. There is some suggestion in the literature that persistent acute akathisia may represent a precursor to the development of early tardive dyskinesia.

Pages 1340–1342 •

Answer A

4. Lithium-induced tremor is worsened by which one of the following factors?

A. hyperglycemia
B. hypothyroidism
C. administration of benzodiazepines

D. depression
E. alcohol withdrawal

Discussion: Lithium-induced tremor, a rhythmical action tremor usually seen in the hands and fingers, may appear as soon as treatment is initiated. The tremor is made worse by anxiety, stress, fatigue, hypoglycemia, thyrotoxicosis, pheochromocytoma, hypothermia, alcohol withdrawal, performance of voluntary movements, and concomitant administration of cyclic antidepressant medications.

Pages 1350–1352 •

Answer E

5. The most important risk factor for tardive dyskinesia is

A. female gender
B. older age
C. diabetes mellitus
D. smoking
E. organic mental syndrome

Discussion: Whereas all of the above, with the exception of smoking, are risk factors for the development of tardive dyskinesia, aging consistently appears to be the most important risk factor for its development. This may relate to the tendency of the nigrostriatal system to degenerate with age as well as to pharmacokinetic and pharmacodynamic factors. Other risk factors include mood disorder, ethnicity (e.g., possibly African-Americans > Asians), and acute and subacute neuroleptic-induced movement disorders.

Pages 1342–1343 •

Answer B

6. A 27-year-old man is hospitalized with a psychotic decompensation. He states that he is unwilling to take neuroleptic medications because "they come in green tablets, grass is green, horses eat grass, and I'm not a horse." He is not agitated and does not represent a danger to staff, other patients, or himself. What is the best course of action?

A. Administer neuroleptic immediately and then obtain informed consent from the patient once the psychosis is resolved.
B. Obtain consent from his family members and then administer neuroleptic.
C. Place patient in restraints because he is clearly having disorganized thinking and needs a controlled environment.
D. Request a legal hearing to determine whether the patient may receive electroconvulsive therapy involuntarily.
E. None of the above

Discussion: Patients who are psychotic or agitated are generally not able to consider the risks of developing a movement disorder. In such cases, any locally mandated administrative (including legal) procedures should be followed before neuroleptics are administered. It is best to initially work with the family and later to discuss issues with the patient once he or she is in better control. The discussion of this issue is not a "one-time burden" for the physician but part of an ongoing treatment alliance that will help the patient to feel more positively involved in her or his care.

Page 1335 •

Answer E

7. Which statement about neuroleptic malignant syndrome is correct?

A. It is a commonly seen neuroleptic side effect that does not require specific intervention.
B. It is often seen in hot, humid climates.
C. It tends to occur approximately 1 year after initiation of neuroleptic medication.
D. Initiation of bromocriptine and dantrolene represents the most important step in the treatment of neuroleptic malignant syndrome.
E. Once it has resolved, it typically does not recur.

Discussion: Neuroleptic malignant syndrome is a potentially fatal reaction to neuroleptic medications that is characterized clinically by muscle rigidity, fever, autonomic instability, and changes in level of consciousness. The exact incidence is unknown, but it is seen in between 0.02% and 1.9% of neuroleptic-treated patients. Risk for the development include prior episode of neuroleptic malignant syndrome, preexisting medical problems, rapid increases in neuroleptic doses, male gender, previous diagnosis of mood disorder, and hot climate. This syndrome, which usually presents in the first month of treatment, may develop at any time. The basis of treatment is quick diagnosis, speedy discontinuation of the offending agent, and supportive care in an intensive care setting. The use of dantrolene and bromocriptine has not been consistently substantiated.

Pages 1345–1350 •

Answer B

8. A possible complication of tardive dyskinesia is

A. difficulty with dentures
B. social embarrassment
C. suicidal ideation

D. vomiting and dysphagia
E. all of the above

Discussion: There are numerous physical and psychosocial complications of tardive dyskinesia. In addition to those listed above, individuals are likely to have respiratory disturbances; swallowing disorders; ulcerations of the tongue, cheek, and lips; and great subjective distress, including depressive episodes.

Page 1344 •

Answer E

CHAPTER 70 Relational Problems

John F. Clarkin • David Miklowitz

1. Expressed emotion is a term describing
   A. sibling rivalry
   B. interaction related to a general theory of family violence
   C. a type of interaction between a family member and another who has a mental illness
   D. marital interaction involving female expressivity and male withdrawal
   E. the early signs of emotional uncontrol

Discussion: One problem with estimating the frequency of relational disorders in the general population is that some measures, such as expressed emotion, were developed for the study of families in which there was an index family member with a psychiatric disorder. One way in which this has been generalized to other groups is the analysis of the Five-Minute Speech Sample. In one such study, parents of inner-city preadolescents met criteria for expressed emotion in 22% of cases, compared with 40% of parents of children with psychiatric disorders.

Page 1356 •

Answer C

2. Relational problems are placed in the DSM-IV section
   A. Axis I
   B. Axis II
   C. Axis IV
   D. other conditions that may be a focus of clinical attention
   E. V codes

Discussion: Relational problems are placed in the section entitled Other Conditions That May Be a Focus of Clinical Attention. Five specific problems are listed: relational problem related to a mental disorder of general medical condition; parent-child relational problem; partner relational problem; sibling relational problem; and relational problem not otherwise specified. The last involves extrafamily relational problems, such as problems with coworkers.

Pages 1355–1356 •

Answer D

3. Because the frequency of divorce is 40% to 50%, and family violence is present in 12% to 33% of couples, the prevalence of relational disorders is
   A. still unknown
   B. estimated at 35%
   C. unrelated to divorce, but double that of family violence
   D. not able to be determined because of reporter bias
   E. as high as 50% in lower socioeconomic classes

Discussion: Factors such as divorce or violence are best thought of as relational events rather than relational disorders. A single incident of marital violence would not necessarily signal the presence of a family relational disorder, unless there were other pertinent data. Divorce likewise may not suggest a relational disorder between a spousal couple but is highly suggestive of a level of dysfunction.

Page 1356 •

Answer A

4. The construct of coercive process is used to explain
   A. relational disorders in siblings
   B. relational disorders in couples in which violence is present
   C. a type of countertransference by marital therapists
   D. the reinforcement by parents of a child's behavior problems
   E. family violence

Discussion: Coercive process is a construct developed to describe parent-child interaction. It involves the shaping of the behavior of parents by negative behavior on the part of the child and is similar to negative escalation in couples.

Pages 1356–1357, 1358, 1361, Table 70–1 •

Answer D

5. Distressed spouses typically consider their partner's undesired communication behavior to be

A. due to mental illness
B. due to faulty genes
C. global and stable
D. related to character
E. something they can change

Discussion: The amount of quality of verbal communication have differentiated distressed and nondistressed couples. Whereas both groups are relatively inaccurate observers of their own interactional behavior, the distressed couples are comparatively less reliable. A distressed spouse tends to consider the partner's undesired communication behavior to be global and stable. Positive events are ignored, and the partner is blamed for his or her negative behavior, which is seen as intentional, global, stable, and originating from internal factors.

Pages 1357–1358 •

Answer C

6. The key ingredient to a "coercive entrapment" in a family is

A. negative reinforcement
B. positive reinforcement
C. intermittent reinforcement
D. projective reinforcement
E. defensive splitting

Discussion: When two individuals within a family (i.e., a parent and child) are controlling each other's behavior through aversive stimuli or responses that are perceived by these individuals as unpleasant, a coercive entrapment has developed. The key ingredient to this is negative reinforcement.

Page 1358 •

Answer A

7. Communication deviance was described in families of

A. sociopaths
B. psychopaths
C. schizophrenics
D. borderlines

Discussion: Wynne and Singer observed that the transactional processes of families of concurrently hospitalized schizophrenic patients were often unclear, amorphous, fragmented, or unintelligible. In their research, parents of schizophrenic patients were distinguished from parents of other types of patients and normal individuals by this high level of communication deviance. There may be a relationship between levels of communication deviance (a mild form of thought disorder) in parents and the appearance of schizophrenia in genetically susceptible offspring, but this is not proved.

Pages 1358–1359, 1361 •

Answer C

8. The empirical data on family therapy and eating disorders

A. suggest that Minuchin's early hypotheses were correct
B. suggest that adolescents with eating disorders need individual therapy
C. indicate that individual and family systems issues are both relevant
D. suggest that adolescents with nonchronic conditions might respond to family intervention
E. indicate that family strategies that are effective with schizophrenia also work with eating disorders

Discussion: In a study by Russell of family therapy for eating disorders, it was demonstrated that patients whose disorder was not chronic and had begun before the age of 19 years were more effectively treated with family therapy. The outcome measures were weight and menstrual functioning.

Page 1363 •

Answer D

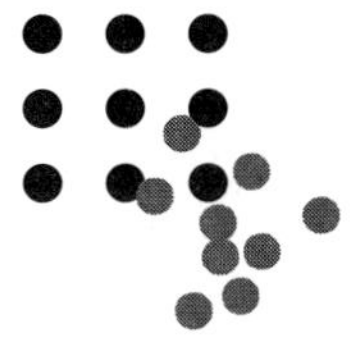

SECTION

VI

Therapeutics

CHAPTER

71 Individual Psychoanalytic Psychotherapy

David Taylor

1. The three essential operations of psychoanalytic psychotherapy are

A. limit setting, confrontation, and contracting
B. clarification, confrontation, and interpretation
C. accepting, understanding, and explaining
D. conscious, preconscious, and unconscious interventions

Discussion: The therapist in this model must engage with the patient by *accepting* the subjective experience of the patient's emotional pain and conflict. As the therapist listens to the patient, he or she will begin to *understand* the conscious and unconscious aspects of the patient's emotional problems. The therapist is then in a position to *explain* his or her understanding to the patient.

Pages 1373–1374, Table 71–1 •

Answer C

2. Which of the following is **not** an element of psychotherapy?

A. the systematic use of a human relationship for therapeutic purposes
B. the systematic use of a human relationship to profit the therapist
C. the comprehension of the patient's inner subjective world
D. the alleviation of emotional distress by effecting enduring changes in a patient's thinking, feeling, and behavior

Discussion: There are many different types of psychotherapy, which all share a core task of attempting to understand and thereby help a patient. Varieties of psychotherapy include psychoanalytically informed, cognitive-behaviorally informed, experientially informed, and strategic-systemically informed therapies.

Pages 1373–1374 •

Answer B

3. Which of the following is part of the metapsychological viewpoint that forms the foundation of all psychoanalytically informed psychotherapy?

A. the dynamic point of view
B. the repetition compulsion
C. the universality of transference
D. the defense mechanisms

Discussion: Freudian psychology is one that is based on the idea that humans are constantly defending against strong, unconscious, biologically based intrapsychic needs and desires. There are five metapsychological viewpoints, which include dynamic, topographical, structural, economic, and genetic points of view. The pattern of repetition as well as the phenomena of defenses and transference are the building blocks of the metapsychological edifice. The economic point of view, for instance, attempts to explain the nature of psychic energy as it relates to the expression of feelings and ideas and is helpful in understanding defense mechanisms.

Pages 1374–1375 •

Answer A

4. A patient's report of positive and warm associations after a first session with a psychotherapist is an example of which of the following phenomena?

A. abstinence
B. neutrality
C. transference
D. resistance

Discussion: If such a response on the part of the patient is found to be associated with a recollection of an important person in the patient's past, it can be considered transference. Transference is therefore defined as those perceptions of and responses to a person in the here and now that more appropriately reflect past feelings or responses to important people earlier in one's life. In psychoanalysis, the transference neurosis is developed by the formal characteristics of the psychoanalytic treatment, such as the abstinent position of the analyst and the use of a couch. Transference and resistance are essential qualities of psychoanalytic psychotherapy, although the transference may not become as intense. The analysis of transference by the repeated interpretation of resistance is the primary activity of the psychoanalyst or psychoanalytic psychotherapist.

Pages 1375–1377 •

Answer C

5. Research on the outcome of psychoanalytic psychotherapy has suggested that

A. working through is the most important phase of treatment
B. the therapeutic alliance is probably the most important variable
C. the length of treatment is the most important variable
D. transference distortions in the initial phase of treatment have major prognostic implications

Discussion: Research has suggested that the therapeutic alliance (in addition to the patient's and therapist's characteristics) is important in outcome. Increasing appreciation for the role of supportive factors, such as the rapport between the patient and therapist that constitutes the therapeutic relationship, has balanced the earlier, more narrowly defined position that attributed therapeutic success exclusively to insight resulting from the analyst's specific interpretive activity. This has led therapists to pay greater attention to the initial phase of engagement in treatment.

Pages 1378–1379 •

Answer B

6. Which of the following criteria is **not** a contraindication to psychoanalytic psychotherapy?

A. poor impulse control
B. severely dysfunctional interpersonal relationships
C. little ability to tolerate frustration, anxiety, or depression
D. personality disorder

Discussion: Personality disorder, with the exception of antisocial personality disorder, is one of the primary indications for this type of therapy. The listed contraindications are for the expressive end of the expressive-supportive continuum of psychoanalytic psychotherapy. A significant lack of introspective capacity and cognitive deficits are also serious concerns in consideration of psychoanalytically based treatments.

Pages 1383–1384, Table 71–10 •

Answer D

7. Supportive psychotherapy

A. had no impact on survival in breast cancer, leukemia, lymphoma, and malignant melanoma patients
B. is no better than counseling for opiate-dependent patients
C. was found to be efficacious in the Menninger Psychotherapy Research Project
D. is easier to conduct, operationalize, and study

Discussion: Supportive psychotherapy involves shoring up a patient's defenses and enhancing his or her ability to cope with the trials of illness. An important finding in the Menninger study was the unanticipated efficacy of this modality. All psychotherapy research is complicated to perform. Expressive-supportive therapies have been studied and were found to prolong survival in breast cancer patients for 18 months longer than in control subjects. Patients with leukemia, lymphoma, and malignant melanoma fared better with their illnesses. This type of treatment is superior to counseling with opiate-dependent patients in a community methadone maintenance program. This type of therapy can produce significant and lasting behavioral change through the reinforcement of health-promoting behaviors, increased capacity for self-reflection, anxiety reduction, and development of new defenses such as intellectualization.

Pages 1384–1385, Table 71–11 •

Answer C

CHAPTER

72 Group Psychotherapy

Walter N. Stone

1. Group developmental processes include **all but one** of the following:

A. determination of the limits of emotional safety
B. capacity to tolerate intense affects
C. traversal of phases for therapy to take place
D. symbolic overthrow of the therapist
E. responses to termination

Discussion: It is unnecessary for every phase to be traversed. Considerable learning takes place in the early developmental phases, particularly in relation to joining, dependence, personal boundaries, and trust, which may be invaluable for many patients with early developmental deficits. Emotional safety is necessary at all phases; in general, capacity to tolerate intense affects is characteristic of the more mature phase; and appropriate management of termination enables members to learn about responses to separation and loss.

Pages 1391–1393 •

Answer C

2. Nonspecific therapeutic factors in groups include **all but one** of the following:

A. opportunities to tell one's story (catharsis)
B. sharing of experiences (universalization)
C. seeing others change (provision of hope)
D. learning about the sources of interpersonal disturbances (insight)
E. presence of a nonjudgmental atmosphere (elements of cohesion)

Discussion: Nonspecific therapeutic factors can be considered generic components of well-conducted dynamic groups. They are present in varying combinations in all "therapeutic" groups. They can serve to stabilize many individuals and represent many elements in the early phases of group treatment. Insight (broadly defined) is a more specific therapeutic element and may accrue at any developmental phase but is more likely in the later phases.

Pages 1393–1394 •

Answer D

3. In recruiting members for a group, the optimal way of obtaining members is

A. through written announcements of a new group
B. from one's own caseload
C. by discussing plans with a colleague
D. by transfers from other therapists when a patient's insurance runs out
E. from intake workers who perform initial screening

Discussion: Recruiting group members from one's own caseload increases the likelihood of having established a therapeutic alliance and having an opportunity to work with the group agreement, which will help the prospective member gain an understanding of her or his goals and anxieties in entering a group. Careful preparation enhances the patient's potential for traversing the anxieties associated with emotionally exposing himself or herself to a group of strangers. In many situations, referrals from the therapist's own caseload are insufficient to form a group, and answers C and E are good alternatives. Answer D has the potential drawback of patients' feeling dumped into a group. If funds for individual sessions are insufficient and opportunities to address the change in treatment modalities are unavailable, the likelihood for premature termination is increased. Written announcements are generally of minimal success in recruiting group members.

Pages 1395–1396 •

Answer B

4. All of the following tasks **except one** are important in screening and preparing patients to enter a group:

A. Determine the person's goals for entering a group.
B. Let the patient address anxieties about entering a group.
C. Determine that the person will add unique characteristics to the group.
D. Establish an alliance with the patient.
E. Review the group agreement.

Discussion: Each person brings unique aspects of himself or herself to the group. Group composition optimally should be such that there is no member with "obvious" differences (i.e., a minority, a physically handicapped person). However, group therapists have learned that dealing with differences may contribute greatly to helping members understand themselves and their interpersonal and intrapsychic difficulties. For example, in the preparation process with a handicapped person, exploration of the individual's characteristic responses to strangers and others to him or her would help alert the patient and the therapist to interactions likely to occur during group tenure.

Pages 1395–1396 •

Answer C

5. In beginning a group session, **all but one** of the following themes are common:

A. dependency
B. trust
C. safety
D. aggression
E. sexuality

Discussion: Sexual conflicts and attractions are infrequently mentioned early in the life of a group, although they may be present and in conscious awareness of the members. The major emotional tasks that individuals address are those of trust and safety. Dependency, in part, is a product of having an initial linkage to the therapist and a wish for guidance in an unknown enterprise. Aggression and hostility are variably present and can arise from several initial dynamics: such as a protection against intimacy or loss of self or as a way of defining the self as empowered, in contrast to a sense of confusion and helplessness in the ill-defined initial phases of a dynamic group.

Pages 1397–1399 •

Answer E

6. All but one of the following are true about group roles:

A. They are determined solely by group process.
B. They can be understood with the concept of projective identification.
C. They can be filled by the therapist.
D. They can be used to express whole-group emotions.
E. They are useful in stabilizing affect-laden interactions.

Discussion: Roles arise from a confluence of the group's "needs" and patients' characteristics. They can be understood as stabilizing the group's emotions and promoting or inhibiting work. One person may express an idea or contain a feeling for the entire group. The therapist is not immune to being thrust in such a role. For example, when a group is struggling with an intermember conflict, members may shift attention to the leader and attribute specific characteristics of the leader as the source of the conflict. The leader might then serve the "container" role until the emotional heat diminishes sufficiently for members to gain understanding. The characteristics that members locate in the therapist probably represent aspects of themselves that they wish to disavow.

Page 1397 •

Answer A

7. Cotherapy is useful for **all but one** of the following reasons:

A. to provide support for therapists
B. for leading groups of chronically mentally ill persons
C. to recreate family dynamics
D. because it simplifies the therapist's work
E. as an arena for the patient's splitting

Discussion: Effective cotherapy is a product of considerable work done by cotherapists on their own interactions and feelings. They need to explore their responses to the patients and to one another in an ongoing fashion. This can be a significant added responsibility, and in most instances it is time-consuming. However, there are considerable personal emotional rewards in gaining a deeper understanding of one's own style and in mastering difficult therapeutic problems that emerge from a successful cotherapy relationship. Members often recreate a family atmosphere in the group, and thus in the transferences, cotherapists may be experienced as parents, with splitting and other dynamic constellations. Cotherapy is useful in groups for the chronically ill because this leadership model provides for mutual support of the therapists and greater continuity for the patients.

Page 1400 •

Answer D

8. Combining pharmacotherapy and group psychotherapy is true for **all but one** of the following:

A. It is done only by psychiatrists.
B. It is valuable for patients with mood disorders.
C. It exposes negative attitudes about use of psychotropic medications.
D. It may cause a split among members.
E. It may be a source of friction between prescribing physicians and group therapists.

Discussion: Almost all therapists include patients receiving psychotropic medications in their groups. Like any other element in the therapeutic setting, discussion of medication can expose unaddressed attitudes and conflicts among the members. Frequently, a bias emerges against medication: it interferes with gaining selfunderstanding; it implies "dependency"; or it might mean a special relationship, which may be a source of friction. These and many other attitudes can be productively explored when members acknowledge that they are taking psychotropic medications. Patients with mood and anxiety disorders are most commonly included in groups. Attention needs to be paid to communication between therapists when a person other than the group therapist is prescribing.

Page 1401 •

Answer A

9. Time-limited dynamic groups are best structured in **all but one** of the following ways:

A. frequently around a single focus
B. with careful selection of patients
C. generally with the therapist's having greater activity
D. for addressing issues of separation and loss
E. for patients with limited psychological mindedness

Discussion: Patients with limited psychological mindedness may gain some symptomatic relief as a result of the nonspecific supportive factors concomitant with any effective group treatment. However, the best therapeutic results are obtained when patients have been carefully selected and prepared. The therapist's increased activity (in comparison with extended treatment) helps patients work on their problems and keeps the group focused. Forming groups around a single focus leads to more rapid identification and a sense of belonging among members, which is useful in accomplishing therapeutic tasks in a timely manner.

Page 1401 •

Answer E

10. Outpatient groups for chronically mentally ill persons can be organized in **all but one** of the following ways:

A. They may serve as opportunities for members to discuss hallucinations.
B. They can readily accommodate a wide range of patients' impairments.
C. They are generally conducted with sessions of shorter duration than traditional outpatient groups.
D. They may focus on barriers to satisfactory social relations.
E. They can be focused on problems of adaptation to everyday living.

Discussion: Patients in the seriously and persistently mentally ill population are best served by working with individuals who suffer from similar levels of impairments. Thus, persons with different diagnoses but similar levels of disability can be accommodated in groups for this population. Too great a range in patients' capacity to form satisfactory relationships (i.e., some well-functioning schizophrenic patients or those with a bipolar illness) or in effective role fulfillment (work) interferes with group formation and members' opportunities to identify with each other. The effect is to interfere with, although not eliminate, supportive therapeutic elements inherent in group treatment. In most circumstances, groups are conducted for 45 to 75 minutes in keeping with patients' capacity to engage. Answers A, D, and E are appropriate goals. By accepting discussion of hallucinations as part of the treatment milieu, therapists decrease members' need to hide aspects of themselves, which contributes to global sense of isolation.

Page 1401 •

Answer B

CHAPTER 73

Time-Limited Psychotherapy

Holly A. Swartz • John C. Markowitz

1. The "active ingredients" or "common factors" of most psychotherapies include provision of all of the following **except**

A. an affectively significant, confiding relationship
B. an explanation for the patient's distress
C. success experiences
D. resolution of childhood conflict
E. hope

Discussion: The common factors of psychotherapy are those nonspecific, putatively "curative" elements shared by all forms of psychotherapy, including time-limited therapies. According to Jerome Frank in 1971, these factors include provision of alternative ways of coping with problems; facilitation of emotional involvement in the process; and answers A, B, C, and E. Answer D is incorrect because the model of understanding a patient's current problems as a product of childhood experiences is specific to psychodynamically derived psychotherapies but not to psychotherapy in general.

Page 1406 •

Answer D

2. Which of the following statements best characterizes time-limited therapy?

A. Time-limited therapies are defined as therapies that are completed in fewer than 25 sessions.
B. Time-limited therapies are prescribed for a circumscribed period specified at the outset of treatment.
C. Time-limited therapies emphasize the importance of understanding and interpreting the transference relationship in as short a time as possible.
D. The key element of time-limited therapy is the brief, 30-minute session.
E. All of the above.

Discussion: Time-limited therapy implies that treatment is administered for a circumscribed period, usually defined at the outset of treatment. Answer A is incorrect because the time-limited therapies are not defined by a specific number of sessions, although they typically last 12 to 20 sessions. The duration of the individual sessions may vary also, but sessions typically last 45 to 50 minutes. Interpretation of the transference is a technique specific to psychoanalytically derived treatments and is not characteristic of many time-limited therapies.

Pages 1406–1407 •

Answer B

3. Interpersonal psychotherapy has demonstrated likely efficacy for treatment of all of the following disorders **except**

A. major depression in men seropositive for human immunodeficiency virus (HIV) infection
B. bulimia
C. opiate dependence
D. recurrent major depression
E. dysthymia

Discussion: Interpersonal psychotherapy has demonstrated clear efficacy for the treatment of recurrent major depression and bulimia in randomized, controlled clinical trials. Data from pilot studies treating patients with dysthymia and HIV-seropositive men for depression with interpersonal psychotherapy are promising. Interpersonal psychotherapy was not found to be helpful for the treatment of opiate and cocaine abusers in clinical trials.

Pages 1406–1410 •

Answer C

4. Which of the following best describes the role of the therapist in time-limited therapy?

A. The therapist's stance, like that of an analyst, is neutral and not active.
B. The therapist must maintain a discrete focus throughout treatment.
C. The therapist requires an additional certificate of qualification to treat patients with time-limited therapy.

D. The therapist can change a long-term therapy into a time-limited treatment by shortening the duration of treatment.
E. The therapist rarely prescribes medication while administering time-limited therapy because the two models are incompatible.

Discussion: The therapist maintains a treatment focus that is often explicitly selected by patient and therapist at the beginning of treatment. The other statements are incorrect. In time-limited therapy, the therapist is an active, non-neutral participant and can easily prescribe medication if indicated because the two modalities seem to complement each other well. Time-limited therapies are characterized by specific techniques and paradigms; therefore, they are distinct from truncated long-term approaches. Therapists need additional training to learn each specific time-limited modality but do not require additional professional credentials to treat patients with time-limited therapy.

Page 1407 •

Answer B

For each numbered technique, select the lettered description most closely associated with it. Each letter may be selected once, more than once, or not at all.

5. Match the technique with the correct description:

____ 1. important theorists include Malan, Sifneos, and Davanloo
____ 2. draws parallels among current problems, past relationships, and the relationship with the therapist
____ 3. explicitly defines depression for the patient as a medical illness
____ 4. has been used in a randomized clinical trial to treat parasuicidal behaviors in patients with borderline personality disorder

A. interpersonal psychotherapy
B. cognitive-behavioral therapy
C. brief psychodynamic psychotherapy
D. dialectical behavioral therapy
E. brief eclectic psychotherapy

Discussion: Interpersonal therapy, cognitive-behavioral therapy, and dialectical behavioral therapy have all been rigorously tested in randomized, well-controlled trials. (Dialectical behavioral therapy is not a short-term treatment.) Brief psychodynamic psychotherapy, although well established, is less well tested.

Pages 1408–1414, Table 73–1 •

Answers 1, C; 2, C; 3, A; 4, D

CHAPTER

74 Cognitive and Behavioral Therapies

Michael E. Thase • Jesse H. Wright

1. The cognitive and behavioral therapies share each of the following elements **except**

A. psychoeducation
B. homework
C. objective assessment
D. schema modification
E. prescriptive interventions

Discussion: Schema modification is a goal of Beck's model of cognitive-behavioral therapy (CBT), but it is not a part of most other therapies of this class.

Pages 1418–1420 •

Answer D

2. Most controlled studies indicate that cognitive and behavioral therapies are as effective as relevant pharmacotherapies for treatment of

A. bipolar depression
B. panic disorder
C. severe major depression
D. schizophrenia
E. double depression

Discussion: Only studies of panic disorder have consistently found pharmacotherapy and CBT to be equivalent. Cognitive and behavioral therapies are probably helpful in combination with pharmacotherapy for bipolar depression and schizophrenia; however, they are not considered alternatives to pharmacotherapy. Some patients with severe major depression are responsive to cognitive and behavioral therapies, although controlled evidence is mixed vis-à-vis comparability with pharmacotherapy. There are, to date, no controlled studies of double depression directly comparing CBT with pharmacotherapy.

Pages 1432–1434 •

Answer B

3. For outpatient treatment of nonpsychotic major depressive disorder, Beck's model of therapy is

A. contraindicated
B. superior to interpersonal therapy
C. about as effective as pharmacotherapy
D. more susceptible to relapse than pharmacotherapy
E. typically conducted for a period of 9 to 12 months

Discussion: Beck's model of CBT is the best studied psychotherapy for treatment of nonpsychotic major depression; however, most evidence indicates that it is equivalent to other credible acute phase treatments. Therapy is typically conducted for a 3- to 6-month period. Relapse rates tend to be *lower* for the subsequent year compared with those of patients who received pharmacotherapy.

Pages 1432–1433 •

Answer C

4. Cognitive and behavioral treatments of anxiety disorders generally emphasize **all but one** of the following:

A. increasing exposure to feared situations
B. increasing one's awareness of physiological cues
C. increasing the patient's repertoire of coping strategies
D. reducing escape or avoidance behaviors
E. monitoring of change by objective assessment measures

Discussion: Many people susceptible to pathological anxiety have increased awareness of physiological cues to anxiety. Cognitive and behavioral therapies typically help patients to *decrease* their sensitivity and responsivity to such cues.

Pages 1428, 1430 •

Answer B

5. Desensitization and flooding procedures are

A. conceptually distinct methods that increase exposure
B. widely incorporated in CBT of depression
C. reflect humane and inhumane strategies, respectively

D. historically important but outmoded strategies
E. the center points of Linehan's dialectical behavioral therapy

Discussion: Although desensitization and flooding are based on theoretically distinct models of anxiety reduction, both methods result in the same functional goal: increased exposure. Further, whereas the theoretical underpinning of these strategies is outmoded, both methods are still used for treatment of anxiety disorders. However, neither has much to do with contemporary cognitive-behavioral approaches to depression or borderline personality disorder.

Page 1429 •

Answer A

6. Most contemporary cognitive and behavioral therapies

A. explicitly use operant schedules of reinforcement
B. explicitly use classical conditioning strategies
C. draw heavily on psychodynamic theories of motivation
D. emphasize the transference relationship as the vehicle of change
E. none of the above

Discussion: Most contemporary cognitive and behavioral therapists *implicitly* draw on operant and classical principles but do *not* emphasize use of explicit reinforcement schedules (e.g., tokens or contingency contracts) or counterconditioning paradigms. Neither psychodynamic theories of motivation nor analysis of the transference relationships is central to these therapies.

Pages 1418, 1422, 1428–1429 •

Answer E

7. All but one of the following statements about automatic negative thoughts are true:

A. They may be grouped by themes to infer schemas.
B. The "triad" refers to thoughts about persons, places, and things.
C. They are typically associated with increased dysphoric arousal.
D. They are not inherently pathological.
E. Their frequency is usually decreased by effective treatment.

Discussion: The triad refers to a grouping of automatic negative thoughts on the basis of themes about one's self, world, and future. The other statements are correct.

Pages 1419–1420, Figure 74–2, Table 74–1 •

Answer B

8. Combinations of pharmacotherapy and cognitive or behavioral therapies have been shown to result in **all but one** of the following:

A. improved cost-efficiency of acute phase therapy
B. improved medication compliance of bipolar patients
C. improved posthospital course of depressed patients
D. decreased relapse of panic after withdrawal of medication
E. enhanced social skills of chronic schizophrenic patients

Discussion: Despite the great potential for additive benefits of combined treatment strategies, improved cost-efficiency has not been shown, particularly during acute phase therapy.

Pages 1432–1434 •

Answer A

CHAPTER

75 Family Therapy

Loren R. Mosher • Judith L. Schreiber

1. Development and use of family therapy as a treatment technique in psychiatry occurred in the early 1950s when

A. research established family therapy's unique contributions to treatment
B. pioneer psychiatrists became disappointed with the therapeutic effectiveness of psychoanalysis and sought a means of reducing failure rates of other modalities then in use
C. social workers and child guidance clinics began to move away from family involvement
D. insurance became available for family treatment

Discussion: It is important to understand family therapy's early origins in disappointment with other therapies, especially psychoanalysis.

Pages 1439–1440 •

Answer B

2. Double-bind, undifferentiated family mass, pseudomutuality, and mystification are

A. examples of etiological theories common to the second phase of family therapy's development
B. experiences cited by patients as contributing to their difficulties
C. alternative formulations of previously delineated treatment systems
D. research areas in family therapy

Discussion: These are important constructs that came out of family therapy's etiological heyday.

Page 1440 •

Answer A

3. By the 1970s, the study of the family produced a movement in psychiatry away from

A. the conceptualization of "mental illness" as permeating and perhaps issuing from the family as well as from the wider social milieu
B. a focus on individual intrapsychic illness
C. the consideration of family context as relevant to treatment
D. the consideration of "communication deviance" as a possible etiological agent

Discussion: This focuses on what is arguably family therapy's greatest contribution to contemporary psychiatric thinking.

Page 1440 •

Answer B

4. A present dilemma facing the field of family therapy is

A. the inclusion of family therapy concepts in DSM-IV
B. the absence of an agreed on typology of family disorders
C. the increasing preeminence of family therapy concepts in popular culture
D. rejection of a strictly medical model of mental illness

Discussion: This relates the world of DSM-IV to family therapy.

Page 1440 •

Answer B

5. In conceptualizing family interaction, family systems theory adopts constructs based on a model that is

A. antithetical to cybernetics and circular processes
B. similar to the medical model of mental illness
C. vertically causal
D. nonlinear

Discussion: This question focuses attention on a unique contribution of family therapy.

Pages 1441–1443 •

Answer D

6. In communication theory, metacommunication refers to

A. the exchange of information concerning a given subject matter

B. the concurrent message regarding the relationship between interactional partners that is contained in an exchange of information
C. congruity of affect and expression
D. unhealthy complementarity

Discussion: Metacommunication is a critical descriptive and therapeutic construct in family therapy.

Page 1442 •

Answer B

7. Researchers have concerns about the evaluation of family therapy's efficacy because of

A. increasing numbers of family therapists outside the medical field
B. lack of long-term controlled studies of family therapy of schizophrenia
C. methodological limitations
D. difficulty in measuring the effects of behavioral family management

Discussion: This illustrates the complexities of real-world research in the area of family therapy.

Pages 1443–1445 •

Answer C

8. Family therapy outcome research with children

A. is broader in scope than with adults
B. is more limited than with adults
C. has focused primarily on conduct-disordered children
D. has shown child management training to be the most effective type of intervention

Discussion: It is important to highlight the relative dearth of family research with children.

Pages 1445–1446 •

Answer B

9. In the initial interview with a family, it is recommended that

A. circular questioning techniques be used
B. the identified patient be excluded
C. the therapist spend no time in small talk
D. the therapist offer a hypothesis outlining the origin of the family problem

Discussion: The technique of circular questioning, in addition to providing a useful method of gathering information, provides the beginning therapist with an anxiety-relieving paradigm.

Pages 1446–1450 •

Answer A

10. Careful observation of the interview *process* during the course of important content questions

A. seldom yields useful information in comparison to direct questioning
B. provides information about relationship dynamics, power, and communication in the family
C. interferes with the therapeutic process
D. causes anxiety in the family

Discussion: For students, it is important to emphasize the *how* rather than the easier *what* question.

Pages 1446–1450 •

Answer B

CHAPTER

76 Couples Therapy

Eric Gortner • Jackie Gollan • Neil Jacobson

For each numbered item, select the lettered heading most closely associated with it. Each letter may be selected once, more than once, or not at all.

1. Match each couples therapy model with the therapeutic goal most closely associated with it.

A. discover leading-edge feelings and create joint platform
B. change positive to negative exchange ratio and remedy skills deficits
C. acknowledge and actively experience unaddressed emotional needs
D. alter couple's emotional boundaries
E. explore couple's patterns of defense and work through underlying anxiety

____ 1. behavioral marital therapy
____ 2. object relations couples therapy
____ 3. ego analytical couples therapy
____ 4. emotionally focused therapy
____ 5. structural couples therapy

Discussion: See Chapter 76 for a complete discussion of the types of couples therapy.

Pages 1453–1457, 1459–1461, Table 76–1 •

Answers 1, B; 2, E; 3, A; 4, C; 5, D

2. All of the following are important principles of ego analytical couples therapy **except**

A. unconscious complementarity principle
B. hidden validity principle
C. leading-edge feelings principle
D. joint platform principle
E. victims principle

Discussion: The unconscious complementarity principle is used in object relations couples therapy. The ego analytical position is a more significant theoretical departure from traditional analytical thought than the object relations perspective. The central tenet of ego analytical therapy is that a major portion of distress stems from the patient's intolerance and invalidation of his or her sensitivities and problem. Hidden validity, leading-edge feelings, joint platform, and victims principles are all used in ego analytical couples therapy.

Pages 1454–1455 •

Answer A

3. Which of the following is the feature that most distinguishes the premarital relationship enhancement program (PREP) approach from other behavioral models?

A. PREP's focus on behavioral techniques
B. PREP's commitment to empirical investigation of treatment methods
C. PREP's use of communication and problem-solving skills training
D. PREP's main focus on couples that are currently functioning well
E. PREP's willingness to engage in nontraditional behavioral models, such as paradoxical interventions

Discussion: The difference between PREP and other behavioral models is that PREP focuses on couples that are currently functioning well. Like behavioral marital therapy, PREP uses behavioral techniques and tests data empirically. The main goal of PREP is to teach effective communication and problem-solving skills.

Pages 1458–1459 •

Answer D

4. According to research to date, which of the following statements best approximates current estimates regarding the effectiveness of most marital therapies?

A. Approximately 25% of couples entering therapy can expect to conclude in the nondistressed range of relational functioning.
B. Approximately 75% of couples entering therapy can expect to conclude in the nondistressed range of relational functioning.
C. Approximately 50% of couples entering therapy can expect to conclude in the nondistressed range of relational functioning.

D. On average, less than 30% of couples entering therapy will conclude in the nondistressed range of relational functioning.
E. Virtually all couples who enter therapy can expect significant clinical improvement by the end of therapy.

Discussion: Approximately 50% of couples entering therapy can expect to conclude in the nondistressed range of relational functioning. In clinical research, patients in treatment groups consistently show better outcomes at posttest than do patients in waiting list control groups.

Page 1468

Answer C

5. In predicting who will benefit from couples therapy, which statement is **not** supported by the available literature to date?

A. Younger couples tend to respond better to marital therapy than older couples do.
B. Emotional disengagement tends to predict poorer therapy outcomes.
C. Other concurrent psychiatric illness tends to relate to poorer therapy outcomes.
D. Higher pretherapy distress levels tend to predict better response to therapy.
E. Educational and socioeconomic status have tended to show inconsistent results in terms of predicting therapy outcomes.

Discussion: In evaluating outcome of couples therapy, emotional disengagement, higher pretherapy distress levels, and concurrent individual psychiatric illness are all negative prognostic signs. Some types of individual psychopathology, such as characterological problems, are more likely to cause poor outcome compared with clinical depression. Demographical variables other than age are of limited usefulness in predicting outcome.

Pages 1468–1469 •

Answer D

6. Which of the following therapeutic interventions would be the **least** consistent with a behavioral approach to couples therapy?

A. behavior exchanges
B. communication and problem-solving skills training
C. formation of a collaborative set
D. homework assignments
E. emotional validation training

Discussion: Behavioral marital therapy is a highly structured form of therapy. Homework assignments are a central and necessary component of this therapy. A "collaborative set" is developed initially. This refers to the mutual sense of commitment, cooperation, and hope that improves engagement of the couple in therapy. Behavior exchange is a technique of behavioral marital therapy.

Pages 1455–1457 •

Answer E

7. The most significant difference between traditional behavioral marital therapy and integrative behavioral couples therapy is integrative behavioral couples therapy's

A. reluctance in using behavior exchange procedures
B. emphasis on communication and problem-solving skills training
C. integration of change and acceptance strategies
D. focus on structured homework assignments
E. use of arbitrary reinforcement techniques

Discussion: The majority of therapeutic attention in behavioral marital therapy is devoted toward changing couples' behavioral patterns and having each partner better accommodate the other's demands for change. Integrative behavioral couples therapy focuses on and introduces the idea that couples will benefit if these change demands are balanced with acceptance and appreciation of some of the core differences between partners.

Pages 1457–1458 •

Answer C

8. According to object relations couples therapy, a couple's distress is best understood as resulting from

A. the individual's failure to "pass" from the latent to libidinal stages of development
B. inwardly directed hostility that is outwardly projected
C. unconscious defenses against intimacy and nurturance
D. problems in the fit of each partner's unconscious needs and their object choice
E. overly expressed emotional needs

Discussion: This object relations view suggests that couples connect not only on a conscious level but, more important, also on an unconscious one. There is an "unconscious complementariness" to couples, which refers to the fit of each partner's unconscious needs and their object choice. In this sense, through a process of mutual projection and introjection, couples are unconsciously "colluding" to reduce anxiety. A couple's distress occurs when these projective and introjective processes are not mutually gratifying.

Pages 1453–1454 •

Answer D

9. The primary therapeutic target in ego analytical couples therapy is

A. repressed needs and desires toward the partner
B. self-reproach and condemnation regarding the presence of difficulties
C. resistance toward the very process of therapy
D. self-defeating, unconscious patterns of need gratification
E. unexpressed emotional needs and feelings

Discussion: Ego analytical couples therapy proposes that self-reproach, evidenced as shame and guilt, plays a major role in the patient's feelings of unentitlement. A central goal of ego analytical therapy is to free patients from this self-reproach and condemnation about having problems. This freedom allows them to devote resources toward thinking, talking, and problem solving.

Pages 1454–1455 •

Answer B

For each numbered item, select the lettered heading most closely associated with it. Each letter may be selected once, more than once, or not at all.

10. Match each couples therapy model with the therapist's stance or technique most closely associated with it.

A. assignment of homework and instructor of skills
B. creation of a holding environment and interpretation of defenses
C. uncovering hidden self-blame and invalidation
D. facilitation of experiencing unacknowledged feelings
E. paradoxical interventions

____ 1. strategic couples therapy
____ 2. emotionally focused therapy
____ 3. object relations couples therapy
____ 4. behavioral marital therapy
____ 5. ego analytical couples therapy

Discussion: For discussion of these techniques, see text of Chapter 76.

Pages 1453–1457 •

Answers 1, E; 2, D; 3, B; 4, A; 5, C

CHAPTER

77 Hypnosis

José R. Maldonado • David Spiegel

1. Hypnosis is a psychophysiological state characterized by

A. absorption
B. dissociation
C. suggestibility
D. all of the above
E. none of the above

Discussion: Hypnosis is a natural state of attentive, focused concentration. It is a psychophysiological state that is characterized by *absorption,* the tendency to engage in self-altering and highly focused attention with complete immersion; *dissociation,* which permits keeping out of conscious awareness many routine experiences that would ordinarily be conscious; and suggestibility, a heightened responsiveness to social cues.

Pages 1477–1478 •

Answer D

2. The term *trance logic* implies that

A. hypnotized individuals are more logical under trance than when they are in their normal awake state
B. while under hypnosis, the subject's thinking pattern does not obey the rules of "normal" logical processes
C. hypnotized individuals are not capable of logical thinking while under trance
D. while under hypnosis, subjects are incapable of differentiating between moral and immoral acts suggested by the therapist
E. none of the above

Discussion: Trance logic is an aspect of absorption. This term implies a thinking pattern that does not obey the rules of normal logical processes. For instance, a highly hypnotizable subject may hallucinate an experience of sustaining a conversation with a person who is not present in the room at the suggestion of the hypnotherapist.

Page 1477 •

Answer B

3. Which of the following statements about hypnosis is **not** true?

A. Hypnotizability is a stable and measurable trait.
B. All hypnosis is self-hypnosis.
C. Women are more hypnotizable than men.
D. Hypnosis is not intrinsically dangerous.
E. Hypnosis is not therapy.

Discussion: All of the above statements are true except that there are no gender differences in hypnotizability; men and women are equally hypnotizable.

Pages 1478–1479 •

Answer C

4. The following psychiatric disorders are associated with high hypnotizability scores **except**

A. schizophrenia
B. posttraumatic stress disorder
C. dissociative identity disorder
D. phobias
E. eating disorders

Discussion: Hypnotizability scores are useful in clinical screening of hypnotic capacity as well as for discriminating among different psychiatric disorders. Patients with psychosis, suffering from delusions, loosening of associations, and hallucinations, might be expected to do poorly in tests requiring attention and concentration. Hypnosis represents a state of heightened concentration and focused attention. Severely psychotic patients, or people afflicted with schizophrenia, would not be hypnotizable. Several other psychiatric syndromes (generalized anxiety disorder and, to a lesser extent, major affective disorder) have been found to be associated with generally lower hypnotic responsiveness.

Pages 1481–1482 •

Answer A

5. The stages in the uses of hypnosis for the treatment of traumatic disorders include **all but**
   A. condensation of the traumatic memories
   B. consolation by the therapist
   C. control over the access to traumatic memories
   D. confession of feelings and experiences never before acknowledged
   E. confrontation of the perpetrator in court

Discussion: The use of hypnosis in the treatment of posttraumatic stress disorder and dissociative disorders can be conceptualized as having two major goals, which can be achieved by the use of six different techniques. The goals are to bring into *consciousness* previously repressed memories and to develop a sense of *congruence* between memories associated with the traumatic experience and current self-images. By making conscious previously repressed memories, the patient has the opportunity to understand, accept, and restructure them. These goals are achieved by working through the following six treatment stages: confrontation, condensation, confession, consolation, concentration, and control. Confrontation means confronting the trauma.

Pages 1487–1488 •

Answer E

6. When using hypnosis in the treatment of trauma victims, therapists must look for the following pitfalls:
   A. the creation of confabulated memories
   B. the development of traumatic transference
   C. inappropriate expressions of anger toward the therapist
   D. all of the above
   E. none of the above

Discussion: The strength of transference during the psychotherapy of trauma victims is enormous. The use of hypnosis does not prevent development of a transference reaction; it actually may facilitate its emergence earlier than in regular therapy because of the intensity with which the material is expressed and memories are recovered. This kind of traumatic transference between a therapist and the victim of sexual assault is different in the sense that the feelings transferred are related not so much to early object relationships but to abuser or circumstances that are associated with the trauma.

Pages 1487–1488 •

Answer D

7. When used for the treatment of pain, hypnosis
   A. can facilitate an alteration in the *subjective* experience of pain
   B. promotes physical relaxation, which decreases the patient's perception of pain
   C. facilitates neurophysiological changes in information processing that translate into analgesia
   D. all of the above
   E. none of the above

Discussion: Hypnosis, when used for treatment of pain, has been shown to facilitate an alteration in the subjective experience of pain, promote physical relaxation (decreasing the perception of pain), and facilitate neurophysiological changes in information processing that translate into analgesia.

Pages 1489–1491 •

Answer D

8. "Psychosomatic" disorders that respond well to hypnotic manipulation include **all but**
   A. peptic ulcers
   B. warts
   C. irritable bowel syndrome
   D. bronchial asthma
   E. all of the above

Discussion: Most patients with high hypnotizability also have an unusual capacity for psychological control over somatic function as evidenced in the treatment of conditions that have a psychosomatic component. Hypnosis is useful in both the diagnosis and treatment of "psychosomatic illnesses" such as peptic ulcers, warts, irritable bowel syndrome, and bronchial asthma.

Pages 1490–1491 •

Answer E

9. Which of the following statements about the forensic uses of hypnosis is true?
   A. The use of hypnosis might open the possibility of challenge to witnesses' credibility or even to the admissibility of a witness in a court of law.
   B. The victim should be guided through the experience by using leading questions to avoid generating excessive anxiety in the patient.
   C. Hypnosis is as good as a truth serum; therefore, the memories recovered by a trained therapist will seldom be challenged in court.
   D. Owing to issues of confidentiality, it is not advised to caution attorneys that hypnosis will be used to enhance the patient's recollection.
   E. When a subject is acting in good faith, hypnosis always will amplify the truth and avoid falsehood.

Discussion: See Chapter 77 for explanation.

Pages 1492–1493, Table 77–10 •

Answer A

10. Hypnosis has been associated with changes in the following tests or measures **except**

A. neurotransmitters
B. event-related potentials
C. magnetic nuclear resonance imaging
D. all of the above
E. none of the above

Discussion: Hypnotic analgesia involves neurophysiological changes. Studies have suggested that highly hypnotizable individuals diminish the P100 and P300 components of their event-related response to a somatosensory stimulus by focusing on a hallucinated image, which blocks their perception of pain. Endogenous opiates may be involved as well, but studies of naloxone administration have been at best equivocal.

Pages 1493–1496, Figures 77–4, 77–5, Table 77–11 •

Answer C

CHAPTER

78 Behavioral Medicine

Mark A. Slater • Anne L. Weickgenant •
Joel E. Dimsdale

1. Of the three leading causes of death identified by McGinnis and Foege (1993), how many are the result of behavioral choices?

A. 0
B. 1
C. 2
D. 3

Discussion: Of the three leading causes of death—heart disease, cancer, and stroke—factors that are causally related include tobacco, diet, lack of exercise, and alcohol. These are all activities that are the result of behavioral choices. Cigarette smoking is a proven risk for heart disease, malignant neoplasms, and stroke. Sedentary lifestyle has been implicated as a risk factor for many major diseases including coronary heart disease and diabetes. Poor dietary habits and obesity are associated with diabetes, hypertension, and coronary heart disease. Excessive alcohol consumption is associated with liver disease, dementia, and more.

Pages 1502–1503, Table 78–2 •

Answer D

2. Which therapy is most effective for smoking cessation?

A. nicotine replacement
B. behavioral management
C. combination of nicotine replacement and behavioral management
D. neither nicotine replacement nor behavioral management

Discussion: A comprehensive review of the research literature found that success rates for smoking cessation were significantly higher when nicotine replacement was incorporated into a comprehensive behavioral treatment package.

Page 1507, See also Chapter 48 •

Answer C

3. In the Prochaska and DiClemente stages of change model, which stage comes between the contemplation and action stages?

A. preparation
B. precontemplation
C. maintenance
D. motivation

Discussion: In delineating stages of readiness to quit smoking, the preparation phase involves the smoker's making a "firm decision to quit in the next 6 months."

Page 1504, Table 78–3 •

Answer A

4. Prochaska and DiClemente's emphasis on the maintenance stage has been associated with which focus in behavioral medicine?

A. prolonged treatment
B. relapse prevention
C. medication tapering
D. intensive therapies

Discussion: The maintenance phase, which lasts for the 6 months after the behavioral change, is analogous to relapse prevention. The core assumption in behavioral smoking interventions and relapse prevention is that participants who learn, practice, and use behavioral and cognitive coping skills for managing cravings and smoking triggers will be more successful at quitting.

Pages 1504, 1507 •

Answer B

5. Which behavioral arousal control method requires specialized equipment?

A. progressive muscle relaxation
B. autogenic training
C. biofeedback
D. diaphragmatic breathing

Discussion: Biofeedback as a tool for the treatment of tension dates to the early 1970s and has been used to provide information on physiology that was once thought involuntary. With repeated training, patients can produce and detect physiological changes to bring under control many aspects of autonomic arousal, such as blood pressure, heart rate, musculoskeletal tension, and peripheral vascular blood flow.

Page 1508 •

Answer C

6. Behavioral medicine is characterized by

A. the integration of behavioral and biomedical sciences
B. a focus on medical disorders rather than psychiatric illness
C. an emphasis on health and illness
D. all of the above

Discussion: Behavioral medicine is an interdisciplinary endeavor. Most importantly, it is focused on medical disorders rather than psychiatric or behavioral problems. It differs from consultation liaison psychiatry and psychosomatic medicine and arose to fill a need that was not being addressed in psychiatry or medicine.

Pages 1501–1502, Table 78–1 •

Answer D

CHAPTER

79 Psychosocial Rehabilitation

Alex Kopelowicz • Charles J. Wallace •
Patrick W. Corrigan • Robert Paul Liberman

1. Which therapeutic modality has been demonstrated to decrease relapse rates in patients with schizophrenia?

A. antidepressant medication
B. psychiatric rehabilitation
C. partial hospitalization programs
D. illicit drug use
E. none of the above

Discussion: In a study conducted in Vermont, individuals who had been living in a psychiatric hospital with serious symptoms of schizophrenia were followed up 30 years later with interviews and observations of their functioning in communities throughout the state. In the intervening years, these patients had all been involved in some form of psychiatric rehabilitation. The authors found that 82% of these people had not been hospitalized for psychiatric reasons in the previous year; two thirds were functioning in the normal range of the Global Assessment of Functioning Scale, had close friends, and reported living full lives, including having some job or being actively involved in their daily lives. Furthermore, only 25% required daily maintenance antipsychotic medication.

Page 1515 •

Answer B

2. According to the authors, which of these factors has **not** contributed to the feasibility of illness self-management?

A. mental health consumerism movement
B. emergence of skills training technology
C. destigmatization of mental illness
D. optimistic long-term outcome data
E. increasing homelessness of the mentally ill

Discussion: Biopsychosocial rehabilitation is not enhanced by severe disruptions, such as homelessness; in fact, homelessness and substance abuse are obstacles to illness self-management.

Pages 1513–1514 •

Answer E

3. According to the authors' model of illness stages, unemployment is considered

A. a symptom
B. an impairment
C. a disability
D. a handicap
E. none of the above

Discussion: The biopsychosocial model makes careful distinctions among various elements or aspects of an illness, any part of which can contribute to symptomatic impairment. In this construct, unemployment is considered a social role handicap. An individual with schizophrenia may have negative and positive symptoms (impairments) that are associated with the disability of poor work capacity.

Pages 1513–1515, Table 79–2 •

Answer D

4. The main source of enduring financial and social support of patients with schizophrenia is

A. the federal government
B. the state hospital
C. the family
D. the community mental health center
E. none of the above

Discussion: Families are an essential resource and support for many patients participating in rehabilitation programs. The support of families and the preservation and cultivation of their vital role are goals of psychosocial rehabilitation.

Page 1517 •

Answer C

5. Long-term outcome studies, conducted in areas where continuous treatment has been accessible, have shown that the percentage of schizophrenic patients functioning fairly well 20 to 40 years after their first psychiatric hospitalization is

A. less than 5%
B. 10% to 15%
C. 25% to 30%
D. about 50%
E. more than 75%

Discussion: Outcome studies from the United States, Europe, and Japan have repeatedly demonstrated that when people with severe forms of schizophrenia are evaluated 20 to 40 years after the most disabling period of their illness, more than half are functioning in a reasonably normal way.

Page 1515 •

Answer D

6. The first step in the process of biopsychosocial treatment and rehabilitation is

A. pay the psychiatrist's fee
B. vocational rehabilitation
C. medication compliance
D. patient hospitalization
E. successful engagement in a treatment alliance

Discussion: Successful engagement in a therapeutic relationship is the first step in the process of biopsychosocial treatment and rehabilitation. The task is to build a collaborative relationship with patients and their families.

Pages 1515–1516 •

Answer E

7. Meta-analytical studies of social skills training with schizophrenic patients have found

A. no benefits compared with customary care
B. no benefits compared with individual psychotherapy
C. improved social adjustment compared with customary care
D. increased relapse rates compared with group therapy
E. no difference in skills acquisition compared with a group receiving antipsychotic medications

Discussion: Two meta-analyses of more than 35 studies of social skills training with schizophrenic patients found significant effect sizes on discharge rates from hospitals; relapse rates; acquisition, durability, and generalization of skills; and social adjustment.

Pages 1522–1523 •

Answer C

8. Programs that use a psychosocial model to treat the severely mentally ill include

A. Fairweather Lodge
B. Fountain House
C. training in community living
D. none of the above
E. all of the above

Discussion: Fountain House uses a transitional employment model with a "job bank" stocked with a variety of employment opportunities that match the heterogeneity of individuals' skills and interests.

Pages 1526–1527 •

Answer E

9. The Client Assessment of Strengths, Interests, and Goals (CASIG)

A. assumes a biologically based etiology for severe mental illness
B. must be conducted by a psychiatrist
C. does not take into account the patient's preferences for treatment
D. considers the goals and needs of all the relevant stakeholders
E. focuses exclusively on the patient's symptoms

Discussion: CASIG is a set of assessments and forms that help mental health workers plan, document, and evaluate biopsychosocial rehabilitation. CASIG is based on the biopsychosocial model with the additional assumption that the plan must integrate the goals, needs, and constraints of all the relevant stakeholders—the patient, his or her significant others, individuals in the living environment, and the payers.

Pages 1519–1521, Figures 79–3, 79–4, 79–5 •

Answer D

CHAPTER

80 Electroconvulsive Therapy

Matthew V. Rudorfer • Michael E. Henry
• Harold A. Sackeim

1. The first electroconvulsive treatment of humans was done by

A. Ladislas Meduna
B. Julius Wagner von Juaregg
C. Ugo Cerletti and Lucio Bini
D. Egas Moniz

Discussion: Cerletti and Bini in 1938, after demonstrating the safety of electrically induced seizures in animals, applied the technique to a wandering incoherent man who recovered. Meduna demonstrated that convulsive therapy could improve schizophrenic patients. He induced seizures chemically with camphor and later with pentylenetetrazol (Metrazole). Wagner von Juaregg won the Nobel Prize in 1927, the only one ever given in psychiatry, for the introduction of malarial treatment of general paresis. Moniz first described and popularized leukotomy as a treatment.

Pages 1535–1536, Table 80–1 •

Answer C

2. Which of the following statements regarding electroconvulsive therapy (ECT) use in the United States is true?

A. ECT use is more common in the public mental health sector.
B. ECT use increased in the 1980s.
C. ECT use increased in the 1970s.
D. ECT is more commonly used in the treatment of African-American patients.

Discussion: ECT use declined in the 1970s according to National Institute of Mental Health data. However, ECT use began to stabilize and increased slightly in the 1980s. In the United States, this treatment is now primarily offered in private general and psychiatric hospitals, which is a change from historical patterns in the United States and also differs from the English experience. ECT is most often used with female patients with a diagnosis of mood disorder. African-American patients were grossly underrepresented in a survey of inpatients. One third of ECT patients were at least 65 years old, a fourfold greater representation than among the psychiatric inpatient population.

Pages 1536–1537 •

Answer B

3. Neurophysiological investigation has suggested all of the following effects of ECT **except**

A. The seizure threshold rises throughout the course of ECT.
B. A small anticonvulsant protein is found in the cerebrospinal fluid of animals after electroconvulsive shock.
C. Electroconvulsive shock is GABAergic.
D. Bilateral ECT produces changes in cerebral blood flow, but unilateral ECT does not.

Discussion: Both unilateral and bilateral ECT produce changes in regional cerebral blood flow. Although cerebral blood flow is often reduced in untreated depression, successful ECT results in further generalized and regional (primarily frontal) decreases, in both depression and mania. The extent of cerebral blood flow decline is correlated with degree of clinical improvement, and the cerebral blood flow changes are localized to the side of electrode placement with unilateral ECT. The latency of response and a correlation with the efficacy of anticonvulsants in mood disorders are both findings related to the slow rise in seizure threshold and the GABAergic properties of experimental electroconvulsive shock.

Pages 1538–1540, Figure 80–1 •

Answer D

4. Studies of the use of ECT in the treatment of depression have found

A. ECT is as efficacious as other modalities of treatment, such as medications.
B. Melancholia and suicidal ideation predict response to ECT.
C. Dexamethasone suppression test predicts response to ECT.

D. History of antidepressant medication failure predicts ECT nonresponse.

Discussion: ECT is not likely to be successful in pharmacotherapy-resistant depressed patients. This finding challenges decades of generally retrospective case series. A prospective trial of bilateral ECT was administered to 53 patients with major depression, yielding only a 50% clinical response rate in the 24 patients who previously had failed to respond to adequate pharmacotherapy. In contrast, 86% of patients who did not have histories of medication nonresponse responded to ECT. In a meta-analysis of comparison studies, ECT was found to be more efficacious than all other treatments. Psychosis and psychomotor retardation are predictors of response, and melancholia and suicidal ideation are not. The dexamethasone suppression test is not helpful in prediction of response.

Pages 1540–1541 •

Answer D

5. One predictor of a positive response to ECT is

A. hypersomnia
B. grief
C. antisocial personality disorder
D. delusions of guilt
E. chronic pain

Discussion: Controlled trials have demonstrated the presence of mood-congruent delusions as one of the few consistent predictors of ECT response; indeed, psychotic depression is a major indication for ECT as a treatment of first choice. In contrast, specific symptoms or apparent causes of depression are unrelated to responsiveness to ECT. Convulsive therapy may be effective for secondary depression in the presence of a medical or other psychiatric disorder, but if anything, a concomitant personality disorder has been associated with poor outcome to ECT.

Pages 1540–1541 •

Answer D

6. An absolute contraindication to ECT is

A. pregnancy
B. aortic aneurysm
C. intracranial mass
D. status 6 weeks after myocardial infarction
E. none of the above

Discussion: There are no *absolute* contraindications to the use of ECT. The typical rise in intracranial and peripheral blood pressure and the possibility of cardiac arrhythmias associated with each ECT session render structural neurological and cardiovascular disease relative higher risk factors for convulsive therapy. This additional risk can be tempered by premedication (e.g., with antiarrhythmic or antihypertensive drugs) at the time of ECT. Moreover, the time-limited and intensively monitored nature of ECT is often associated with a superior benefit/risk ratio in the medically ill or pregnant patient compared with alternative pharmacological treatments.

Pages 1545, 1548–1549 •

Answer E

7. Which statement correctly describes the appropriate role of ECT in the treatment of bipolar disorder?

A. ECT is effective in bipolar depression but not in mania.
B. ECT is effective either in bipolar depression or in mania.
C. In bipolar patients, ECT should be used only in combination with lithium to prevent switches into mania or rapid cycling.
D. With the development of anticonvulsant medications for use in lithium-resistant bipolar patients, the use of ECT for this indication has been terminated.

Discussion: Bipolar and unipolar depressions are equally responsive to ECT. Less commonly appreciated is the typically favorable response of acute mania to ECT. Although convulsive therapy has been used for half a century in the treatment of mania, only in the past decade has the equivalent efficacy of ECT and lithium in acutely manic patients been demonstrated in prospective, controlled trials. Advances in pharmacotherapy have lessened, but not eliminated, the need for ECT in mania. ECT is most commonly reserved for instances of medication resistance, medically complicated cases, or extreme presentations of mania (e.g., in the context of severe medical illness, pregnancy, or manic delirium). As with all efficacious antidepressant treatments, ECT can trigger manic or hypomanic switches in vulnerable depressed patients; however, lithium is regarded as relatively contraindicated in combination with ECT because of the increased risk for neurotoxic effects.

Pages 1541–1542, 1549 •

Answer B

8. The administered electrical stimulus dose relative to the patient's seizure threshold

A. is always irrelevant as long as a generalized seizure is produced
B. has no relationship to adverse effects of ECT

C. may be more relevant for clinical response to unilateral than to bilateral ECT
D. must be sufficiently great at the first treatment such that a missed seizure never occurs

Discussion: Electrical stimulation of the brain in convulsive therapy must exceed the seizure threshold such that a therapeutic generalized seizure occurs, but if excessive, it will aggravate treatment-associated confusion and memory deficits. Therefore, current practice typically involves determination of seizure threshold at the first treatment. Generalized seizures of adequate duration are necessary and sufficient to effect clinical response to *bilateral* ECT. However, recent data demonstrate that *unilateral* ECT of relatively low dose, using electrical stimulation only slightly greater than seizure threshold, is ineffective in the treatment of depression, despite the production of seemingly adequate generalized seizures.

Pages 1547–1548 •

Answer C

9. Choose the **incorrect** statement regarding ECT and seizures.

A. Seizure monitoring in unilateral ECT can be effected by use of a blood pressure cuff inflated above systolic pressure in an extremity contralateral to the electrode's placement.
B. Seizure threshold increases with age.
C. The brief-pulse electrical waveform is more efficient at producing seizures than the sine wave.
D. As an ECT course proceeds, electrical dosage may need to be increased because of the progressive rise in seizure threshold.

Discussion: Seizure threshold is commonly greater in older individuals and in men and tends to rise during a course of ECT. The sharply demarcated and repetitive "on" and "off" electrical stimulus delivered by the new generation of brief-pulse ECT devices enables generalized seizure induction with considerable less stimulus intensity than was the case with the older sine wave devices. Optimal seizure monitoring during ECT incorporates both the electroencephalogram recording and visual observation of unmodified motor convulsive activity through the "cuff" technique; use of the cuff on an extremity *ipsilateral* to the electrical stimulation in unilateral ECT demonstrates the desired spread of seizure activity to the cerebral hemisphere contralateral to the electrode's placement.

Pages 1546–1548 •

Answer A

10. Which of the following is **not** used as an ECT premedication?

A. succinylcholine
B. atropine
C. methohexital
D. glycopyrrolate
E. scopolamine
F. caffeine

Discussion: The introduction of general anesthesia and muscle relaxation to the ECT protocol significantly enhanced the safety of the procedure, rendering obsolete formerly common adverse effects such as compression fractures of the spine. Most modern ECT is conducted after intravenous administration of a short-acting barbiturate anesthetic (e.g., methohexital or thiopental). Once the patient is asleep, succinylcholine is infused through the intravenous line for muscle relaxation before the actual seizure induction. An optional medication often introduced before the anesthetic is an anticholinergic agent, either atropine or glycopyrrolate, to dry secretions and prevent the bradycardia that may result from the initial parasympathetic surge that follows application of the electrical stimulus. On an individual basis, additional premedications that may be used include compounds to lessen or prevent ECT-associated blood pressure rise or arrhythmias (e.g., β-blockers, nifedipine).

Pages 1546–1548 •

Answer E

11. Which of the following medications raises seizure threshold?

A. fluoxetine
B. clonazepam
C. theophylline
D. haloperidol
E. caffeine

Discussion: An important source of potential interactions between ECT and other treatments is the effect of the medication on seizure threshold, which can influence the efficacy of ECT. The best studied example of this potentially subtle but serious interaction is benzodiazepines. Some members of this family of minor tranquilizers, such as clonazepam or alprazolam, are used fairly often in patients with mood disorders; in addition, long half-life benzodiazepine hypnotics may remain present in significant concentrations the morning after dosing. The anticonvulsant effect of such routine benzodiazepine use may impair the efficacy of concurrent ECT. In contrast, some drugs used for other medical conditions, such as theophylline, *lower* seizure threshold and may lead to prolonged seizures or status epilepticus during

ECT. The desire to increase seizure duration has led to the development of intravenous caffeine as an adjunctive ECT premedication in cases of inadequate seizure production. Most psychotropic medications, such as haloperidol, have little effect on seizure threshold at therapeutic doses. Although occasional cases of prolonged seizures during ECT have been reported in patients receiving one of the newer antidepressant drugs (e.g., fluoxetine), this is not a consistent finding and requires systematic investigation.

Page 1549 •

Answer B

12. Which statement about ECT and cardiovascular function is **incorrect?**

A. Transient arrhythmias immediately after the seizure are common and typically benign.
B. Esmolol may be administered prophylactically to hypertensive patients just before ECT.
C. Subconvulsive electrical stimulation administered in the absence of anticholinergic premedication may be associated with asystole.
D. Depressed patients with heart disease should be treated with antidepressant medications and avoid ECT.

Discussion: A two-stage acute physiological response to ECT has been described. An initial parasympathetic discharge is soon followed, with the onset of seizure activity, by the more familiar sympathetic outflow with accompanying increases in heart rate and blood pressure and transient, self-limited cardiac rhythm disturbances. In the absence of a seizure (i.e., after a subthreshold electrical stimulation), the parasympathetic-driven bradycardia may progress to asystole if an anticholinergic premedication, generally atropine or glycopyrrolate, has not been given. In individuals with preexisting hypertension or other cardiac disease or risk factors, antihypertensive or antiarrhythmic premedication may be used to blunt the extent of the expected elevation in blood pressure and to prevent serious arrhythmias; esmolol, an ultrashort-acting β-blocker, is often used to temper the acute cardiovascular changes associated with ECT. Given the opportunity for close cardiac monitoring and prophylactic intervention and the time-limited nature of the period of increased risk, ECT often enjoys a benefit/risk ratio superior to that of antidepressant medications for patients with heart disease; this is especially true of older, potentially cardiotoxic drugs, such as the tricyclic antidepressants.

Pages 1545, 1548–1549 •

Answer D

13. Memory difficulties after ECT have been related to which parameters of treatment administration?

A. electrode placement
B. electrical waveform
C. electrical dosage of the ECT stimulus
D. number of treatments
E. frequency of treatment sessions
F. all of the above

Discussion: Standard ECT of one or two generations ago, consisting of a series of bilateral, sine wave stimulations at high intensity, was associated with a low frequency of missed seizures and good efficacy, but often at the expense of considerable cognitive adverse effects. Refinements in technique, by attending to a host of treatment parameters under the control of the treatment team now permit substantial reduction in adverse memory effects while ECT efficacy is maintained. Thus, memory problems may be minimized with the use of nondominant, right unilateral electrode placement and brief-pulse electrical stimulation; brief-pulse devices are now routine in most ECT. Seizure threshold determination and avoidance of excessively suprathreshold stimulation are also advantageous, with the caveat that minimally suprathreshold stimulation is not therapeutic in conjunction with unilateral electrode placement. Although the number of ECT sessions must be determined on an individual basis, the increased risk of cognitive adverse effects with increasing length of the treatment course should be considered. Finally, there is evidence that twice-weekly ECT, such as is standard in Europe, is associated with fewer treatment-associated memory difficulties than are seen with the conventional American-standard three-times-weekly schedule; however, the rate of antidepressant response to twice-weekly treatments may be slower.

Pages 1546–1549 •

Answer F

14. Follow-up of patients who have responded to ECT reveals that:

A. With continuation of antidepressant pharmacotherapy after completion of ECT, relapse in a 1-year period approaches zero.
B. After recovery, most patients indicate that they would refuse to undergo ECT again in the future.
C. Risk of relapse in the first year after ECT correlates with a history of failure to respond to an adequate antidepressant medication trial before undergoing ECT.
D. Controlled clinical trials support the efficacy of continuation and maintenance ECT after recovery from a depressive episode with a standard course of ECT.

Discussion: Given that ECT is the only treatment of severe mental disorders that is withdrawn once it has proved effective, a serious risk for relapse after treatment response perhaps is not surprising. Early data showing a substantial preventive effect of continuation of antidepressant medication after completion of a successful course of ECT have not been borne out in later studies. These suggest that relapse rates of 50% or greater are not uncommon in the first 6 to 12 months after ECT, even in medicated patients, and are highest in those with a history of poor response to seemingly adequate antidepressant pharmacotherapy before the index course of ECT. Although the effectiveness of weekly to monthly (or even less frequent) continuation and maintenance ECT in preventing relapse after a successful course of ECT has been documented in case series for several decades, controlled clinical trials of this empirical treatment strategy are lacking. An often overlooked aspect of the long-term course of convulsive therapy is the high rate of patients' satisfaction, leading the majority of individuals who have undergone successful ECT to compare the experience favorably with a trip to the dentist and to agree in principle to follow a hypothetical future recommendation for a repeated course of ECT in the event of a relapse (and, according to some patients, failure to respond to medication).

Pages 1549–1550 •

Answer C

15. Choose the **incorrect** statement about informed consent for ECT.

A. Because of the severity of illness of candidates for ECT, their consent is not required before initiation of treatment.
B. Informed consent for ECT is a process that continues throughout the course of treatments.
C. In addition to discussion between physician and patient, the informed consent procedure for ECT typically includes involvement of family or significant others and use of supplementary written or video information.
D. Permission for administration of *involuntary* ECT must be granted by a judge.

Discussion: As with any modern medical procedure, administration of ECT to voluntary patients requires their informed consent. This entails not only an explanation of the treatment but a complete discussion of the potential benefits and risks of ECT and of all treatments available for the patient's condition. Although severely ill, most candidates for ECT are capable of rendering decisions regarding their treatment, including signing themselves into the hospital and granting consent for somatic therapy. It is considered good practice to include relatives and friends significant to the patient in the discussions of issues related to informed consent to help ensure that the patient fully understands what is being presented. The necessity to proceed with ECT in the absence of the patient's consent requires *legal,* not medical, decisions, although input from the medical team (e.g., regarding the presence of catatonia, inanition, or other life-threatening conditions) is generally taken seriously in judicial proceedings. Consent for ECT may be withdrawn by the patient at any time during the usual 3 or 4 weeks of treatment. Repeated discussion of the pros and cons of continuing ECT during and, in some cases, after the acute series is necessary, given possible changes in both the patient's condition and memory status. In the event of continuation or maintenance ECT for a prolonged time, repeated formal informed consent every 6 months is recommended.

Page 1546 •

Answer A

CHAPTER

81 Psychosurgery for Obsessive-Compulsive Disorder

David Taylor

1. Which of the following is **not** a prerequisite for psychosurgery for patients with obsessive-compulsive disorder (OCD)?

A. 10-week trial of clomipramine
B. adequate trial of behavioral therapy
C. carefully documented "obsessional psychosis"
D. Patient's full comprehension of the risks and benefits

Discussion: Patients with OCD must be correctly diagnosed, because severe or malignant OCD may be mistaken for a psychotic illness. Candidates must have had at least 5 years of treatment for OCD with medication trials of at least 10 weeks' duration of clomipramine, paroxetine, fluoxetine, fluvoxamine, sertraline, and a monoamine oxidase inhibitor as well as augmentation at least once with lithium, a low-dose neuroleptic, or buspirone. All must have had an adequate trial of behavioral therapy. In practice, this means that the illness, if correctly diagnosed, is refractory. Independent review boards usually evaluate each patient.

Pages 1557–1558, Table 81–1 •

Answer C

2. Which of the following is a commonly used neurosurgical procedure for the treatment of OCD?

A. hypophysectomy
B. cingulotomy
C. temporal lobectomy
D. thalamotomy

Discussion: Cingulotomy and capsulotomy are commonly performed procedures for this indication. Other procedures are subcaudate tractotomy and limbic leukotomy. All techniques include the use of stereotactic apparatus. Lesions are made with a radiofrequency thermolesion, the placement of β-radioactive yttrium 90 rods, or with a radiosurgical gamma capsulotomy technique. Details of these procedures are given in the text.

Pages 1558–1560 •

Answer B

3. Which of the following neural circuits has been implicated in the neuroanatomy of OCD?

A. frontostriatal-pallidothalamic-frontal loops
B. amygdalofugal pathway
C. medial forebrain bundle
D. arcuate fasciculus

Discussion: A model of dysfunction in OCD has been based on the existence of abnormal activity in frontostriatal-pallidothalamic-frontal loops. These loops between the basal ganglia, limbic system, and frontal lobes pass through the anterior limb of the internal capsule. It has been suggested that there may be two important components of the neuroanatomy of OCD: the above-mentioned loop; and the Papez circuit, which includes the cingulum. The former is hypothesized to mediate the obsessive-compulsive component, and the latter the anxiety component.

Pages 1560–1562 •

Answer A

4. In the study of neurosurgical interventions for OCD, the use of sham operations

A. is forbidden by the Nuremberg rules
B. is considered acceptable by the Canadian Psychiatric Association
C. has been approved by institutional review boards in the United States
D. was done in the United Kingdom in 1975

Discussion: A serious ethical, methodological, and historically problematical area is the use of sham operations to demonstrate, with a true control group, whether there is any benefit to these interventions. Such a trial was proposed but not funded in the United Kingdom in 1975, and the Canadian Psychiatric Association has advised against the use of sham operations. With the advent of new technology, such as the gamma knife, which does not necessitate opening of the cranium, a controlled trial is feasible. A study has been proposed and approved in New England that would involve 48 patients (24 to receive sham procedure). Patients and investigators are blinded to surgical condition, and evaluations preoperatively and postoperatively are conducted with structured interviews, neuroimaging techniques, and neuropsychological testing.

Pages 1562–1563 •

Answer C

5. Which of the following is a documented risk of neurosurgery for OCD?

A. weight loss
B. cognitive impairment
C. personality change
D. suicide

Discussion: Suicide may well be a complication of such procedures, especially when they are performed among depressed OCD patients. Four of 33 patients who had undergone cingulotomy for OCD had died by suicide in long-term follow-up. These patients were all suicidal preoperatively, and no OCD patients who were not suicidal became suicidal postoperatively. Weight gain has been reported after capsulotomy. Cognitive impairment has not been noted in studies; indeed, patients often achieve better test results after surgery because they may not be as medicated. Studies of personality have not documented postoperative deterioration; symptoms may be improved, or this may be a function of taking the tests more than once.

Pages 1564–1565 •

Answer D

CHAPTER

82 Antipsychotic Drugs

Stephen R. Marder

1. Which of the following populations of patients with schizophrenia should **not** be considered candidates for treatment with clozapine?

A. patients with a history of seizures
B. patients with illnesses that are refractory to conventional drugs
C. patients with disabling tardive dyskinesia
D. patients with a high sensitivity to extrapyramidal symptoms

Discussion: Clozapine has been demonstrated to be effective in a majority of patients who are refractory to other antipsychotics. Because it causes fewer extrapyramidal symptoms than conventional drugs do, it should be considered for patients who are difficult to treat with other antipsychotics because of development of extrapyramidal symptoms at drug doses that are needed to treat their psychosis. Clozapine is less likely to cause tardive dyskinesia than are other antipsychotics, and it appears to be an effective treatment for many patients with tardive dyskinesia. Clozapine is more likely to induce seizures than other antipsychotics. As a result, it should be used cautiously in patients with seizure disorders.

Pages 1576–1577 •

Answer A

2. Which of the following side effects of conventional antipsychotics is most common?

A. parkinsonism
B. akathisia
C. tardive dyskinesia
D. dystonia

Discussion: Akathisia, usually manifest as a subjective feeling of restlessness with increased restless movements, is the most common form of extrapyramidal symptoms from antipsychotic medications. The proportion of patients with akathisia has been estimated to be as high as 50% to 75% of patients treated with antipsychotics. Drug-induced parkinsonism, with stiffness, tremor, and shuffling gait, affects about 30% of patients who are chronically treated with traditional antipsychotics. Dystonias are the most dramatic form of acute extrapyramidal symptoms but also the least common. Prevalence surveys indicate that tardive dyskinesia affects approximately 20% of patients who are chronically treated with conventional antipsychotics.

Pages 1579–1580 •

Answer B

3. Which of the following new antipsychotic drugs has clearly demonstrated that it is effective in patients who are refractory to conventional antipsychotics?

A. thioridazine
B. sertindole
C. risperidone
D. clozapine

Discussion: Clozapine is the only antipsychotic that has been studied in patients who are carefully defined as treatment refractory. In the multicenter study that led to clozapine's approval in the United States, clozapine was compared with chlorpromazine and benztropine in a group of patients who had demonstrated that they were resistant to treatment with at least three other antipsychotics. In this study, clozapine was more effective on a number of measures of positive and negative symptoms. Although there are some preliminary reports indicating that risperidone may be effective in this population, none has been a well-controlled trial.

Pages 1574–1575 •

Answer D

4. Which of the following statements about the dose of antipsychotics for schizophrenia is true?

A. The practice of treating patients with high doses of intramuscular antipsychotic during the first days of treatment (rapid neuroleptization) has been supported by controlled trials.
B. Patients who are assigned to higher doses, such as more than 2000 mg of chlorpromazine or

40 mg of haloperidol, improve more rapidly than those assigned to lower doses.
C. Most patients demonstrate an optimal response at 300 to 1000 mg/d of chlorpromazine or 5 to 20 mg/d of haloperidol.
D. Patients should be administered the maximal dose of antipsychotic that they can tolerate without severe side effects.

Discussion: Most patients with schizophrenia will respond at doses of 300 to 1000 mg/d of chlorpromazine or 5 to 20 mg/d of haloperidol. Higher doses are likely to cause more side effects without additional clinical benefit. Studies have evaluated the usefulness of rapid neuroleptization and higher doses compared with more moderate doses. In both cases, the more moderate doses were just as effective and resulted in fewer side effects. In addition, there is some evidence that higher doses may increase the vulnerability to tardive dyskinesia.

Pages 1575–1576 •

Answer C

5. Antipsychotics are effective for managing which of the following?

A. organic mental syndromes with psychosis
B. bipolar disorder with psychosis
C. schizoaffective disorder
D. all of the above

Discussion: Antipsychotics are effective in reducing psychotic symptoms in nearly every illness that causes psychosis. In bipolar disorder, antipsychotics are frequently an effective adjunct to mood-stabilizing drugs. They are also effective in illness with a clear organic cause, such as steroid-induced psychosis and Huntington's disease.

Pages 1570–1572 •

Answer D

6. Which of the following statements about the effect of antipsychotics on the long-term outcome of schizophrenia is true?

A. Patients who receive antipsychotics during long-term therapy demonstrate less cognitive impairment than patients who are untreated.
B. Delaying antipsychotic treatment can result in a worse long-term outcome.
C. Long-term treatment with antipsychotics leads to cognitive decline.
D. Reliable predictors are available to assist psychiatrists in deciding which patients will respond to an antipsychotic.

Discussion: A review by Wyatt indicated that early intervention with antipsychotics reduced long-term morbidity and decreased the number of rehospitalizations. These findings suggest that patients may pay a long-term price if psychiatrists delay the introduction of drug treament. There is no evidence that antipsychotics either cause cognitive impairment or are an effective treatment for it. Reviewers have concluded that the contribution of controlled research to helping predict which patients should or should not receive antipsychotic drugs has been disappointing.

Pages 1570–1571 •

Answer B

7. High-potency antipsychotics are **not** preferable to low-potency drugs for which of the following conditions?

A. seizure history
B. pregnancy
C. Parkinson's disease
D. compromised hepatic function

Discussion: High-potency antipsychotics are more antidopaminergic than low-potency drugs. As a result, they are more likely to cause extrapyramidal symptoms and to worsen Parkinson's disease. Because low-potency antipsychotics tend to lower the seizure threshold more than high-potency drugs, high-potency antipsychotics are preferred for patients with a seizure history. If patients have compromised hepatic function, a lower dose of a high-potency drug should be prescribed. High-potency drugs are also preferable during pregnancy because they are less likely to cause sedation, hypotension, and gastrointestinal slowing.

Pages 1574–1575, 1578–1579 •

Answer C

8. Which of the following statements about oral antipsychotics is true?

A. Oral drugs are extensively metabolized during the first pass through the liver and gut.
B. Most oral antipsychotics should be administered at least twice daily.
C. Oral antipsychotics are more bioavailable than depot drugs.
D. Antipsychotics administered by the oral route have a more rapid onset than intramuscular antipsychotics.

Discussion: Antipsychotics are less bioavailable orally than when they are administered parenterally. This is because these agents may not be completely absorbed in the gastrointestinal tract, and they are extensively metabolized during the first pass through the liver and gut. Intramuscular antipsychotics reach a maximal plasma concentration before oral drugs do, giving them a somewhat more rapid onset of clinical effects. Nearly all antipsychotics have long elimination half-lives. As a result, they can be administered as a single daily dose.

Pages 1573–1574 •

Answer A

CHAPTER

83 Mood Stabilizers

Alan J. Gelenberg • Heather Stone Hopkins • Pedro L. Delgado

1. To avoid lithium intoxication, plasma lithium concentrations should not exceed

A. 0.6 mEq/L
B. 0.8 mEq/L
C. 1.3 mEq/L
D. 1.5 mEq/L
E. 2.0 mEq/L

Discussion: In the treatment of acute mania, lithium doses should be adjusted to achieve a 12-hour plasma concentration between 0.8 and 1.3 mEq/L at steady state. In the maintenance treatment of bipolar disorder, between 0.8 and 1.0 mEq/L appears to be the optimal range of levels to protect against recurrent episodes. Levels above 1.5 mEq/L have led to toxic effects of lithium.

Page 1588 •

Answer D

2. Which of the following is true about the kinetics of lithium?

A. It is almost completely excreted unchanged by the kidneys.
B. It is highly lipophilic.
C. It is highly protein bound.
D. It is metabolized by the liver.
E. It is poorly absorbed from the gastrointestinal tract.

Discussion: Lithium is rapidly and completely absorbed after oral administration. It is not protein bound, does not undergo metabolism, and is not lipophilic. Ninety-five percent of the drug is excreted by the kidneys.

Page 1588 •

Answer A

3. A patient suffering from a first acute episode of primary mania (without psychosis) should be treated first with which of the following?

A. carbamazepine
B. electroconvulsive therapy
C. lithium
D. psychotherapy
E. valproate

Discussion: Although some trials suggest that valproate and carbamazepine are efficacious in the treatment of acute mania, lithium has the most clearly established efficacy in this condition. Neuroleptics are often used alone or in combination with lithium in psychotic manic patients because they have a more rapid onset of action, but it has not been proved that there is any advantage to using the combination rather than lithium alone in the first weeks of treatment in nonpsychotic patients. Electroconvulsive therapy has also been shown to be effective but is generally considered for patients who are unresponsive to or intolerant of medication. Psychotherapy is beneficial during maintenance treatment, usually in conjunction with medication, but it is not effective alone for treating an acute episode.

Pages 1589–1594 •

Answer C

4. Carbamazepine dosage may have to be increased 2 to 4 months after treatment initiation because

A. carbamazepine's active metabolite has a short half-life
B. carbamazepine's induction of hepatic enzymes increases its own metabolism
C. 80% of plasma carbamazepine is protein bound
D. intolerable side effects will occur if therapeutic doses are achieved too early in treatment
E. patients develop tolerance to medication

Discussion: Carbamazepine induces the hepatic P-450 cytochrome system, thereby increasing its own metabolism over time in some patients. In patients in whom clearance increases as a result of autoinduction, steady state may not be achieved until 3 to 4 weeks after treatment initiation.

Pages 1591–1592 •

Answer B

5. Which of the following conditions has been associated with the onset of rapid cycling in bipolar disorders?

A. agranulocytosis
B. diabetes
C. diminished renal concentrating capacity
D. gastrointestinal upset
E. hypothyroidism

Discussion: Several studies have evaluated thyroid function in patients with bipolar disorder and found a correlation between hypothyroidism and rapid cycling. Results from these studies suggest that thyroid hormone supplementation may slow the occurrence of affective episodes.

Pages 1599–1600 •

Answer E

6. Antidepressants should be used cautiously during maintenance treatment of bipolar disorder because

A. there is no evidence that they work
B. they can paradoxically worsen depression
C. they may cause long-term cardiac damage
D. they may interact with lithium
E. they may trigger a manic episode

Discussion: There is a widespread clinical impression that administering an antidepressant to a bipolar patient can trigger a switch into mania. If symptoms of depression are mild and short-lived, some psychiatrists may consider watchful waiting while maintaining close contact to detect any more severe deterioration before prescribing an antidepressant. If an antidepressant is used, it should be tapered and discontinued in a period of weeks once symptoms of depression have completely remitted and the patient has returned to euthymic state.

Pages 1593–1594 •

Answer E

7. Concomitant administration of valproate and carbamazepine in the treatment of an acute manic episode may lead to

A. a depressive episode
B. valproate intoxication
C. decreased plasma levels of carbamazepine
D. decreased plasma levels of valproate
E. rapid cycling

Discussion: Valproate is metabolized by the hepatic P-450IID6 system. Unlike carbamazepine, it does not induce its own metabolism in general, but it does appear to inhibit the degradation of other drugs metabolized in the liver. Therefore, coadministration of carbamazepine and valproate would cause increased plasma levels of carbamazepine and decreased plasma levels of valproate.

Pages 1590–1591 •

Answer D

8. Which of the following has **not** been associated with the use of psychosocial intervention, as an adjunct to pharmacotherapy, in the treatment of patients with bipolar disorder?

A. decreased need for medication
B. increased medication compliance
C. increased social functioning
D. reduced frequency of hospitalization
E. reduced length of hospitalization

Discussion: Numerous studies of various forms of psychotherapy have shown that it can increase medication compliance and social functioning and reduce the length and frequency of hospitalization for patients with bipolar disorder. However, all of these studies employed psychotherapy in addition to medication treatment, and no one has shown that psychotherapy decreases the need for medication.

Page 1601 •

Answer A

CHAPTER

84 Antidepressants

Martin B. Keller • Robert J. Boland

1. The monoamine hypothesis of depression is supported by the fact that:

A. Decreased monoamine levels are consistently found in depressed patients.
B. Antidepressants generally take several weeks for therapeutic effect.
C. All tricyclic and many newer agents can block reserpine-induced hypothermia, antagonize reserpine-induced ptosis, and potentiate yohimbine lethality.
D. Chronic antidepressant administration appears to be associated with down-regulation of the β-adrenoreceptor, up-regulation of the central α-adrenoreceptor, and up-regulation of central serotonin receptors.
E. Both bupropion and nomifensine seem to exert their primary action on the dopamine system.

Discussion: According to the monoamine hypothesis of depression, the essential feature of an antidepressant is the ability to enhance either norepinephrine or serotonin. Evidence for the monoamine hypothesis includes the observation that reserpine can cause depression.

Page 1606 •

Answer C

2. All of the following statements are true **except**

A. In double-blind, placebo-controlled trials, all available tricyclic antidepressants have been found to be either superior to placebo or equal to imipramine in antidepressant therapeutic effect.
B. In double-blind, placebo-controlled trials, all available serotonin reuptake inhibitors have been found to be either superior to placebo or equal to imipramine in antidepressant therapeutic effect.
C. In double-blind, placebo-controlled trials, trazodone, although superior to placebo, has been found to be less effective than such standard antidepressants as imipramine.
D. There is preliminary evidence to suggest that the atypical agent bupropion may have a specific efficacy in patients who do not respond to tricyclic antidepressants.
E. All antidepressants, on average, appear to be equivalent in their ability to treat depression.

Discussion: Tricyclics, serotonin reuptake inhibitors, trazodone, and bupropion are all more effective than placebo and roughly equivalent in their ability to treat depression. Despite numerous double-blind comparisons of trazodone and tricyclics, there is a clinical impression that trazodone is less effective as a treatment of depression. This may result from improper dosing or the requirement to use divided doses.

Page 1607 •

Answer C

3. In addition to depression, certain antidepressants have been shown useful in the treatment of all of the following **except**

A. panic disorder
B. obsessive-compulsive disorder
C. childhood enuresis
D. bradyarrhythmia
E. migraine headaches

Discussion: Although the quinidine-like effect of tricyclic antidepressants makes them plausible antiarrhythmics, these medications are rarely used for this indication. Bradyarrhythmia would not be treated by such agents in any event.

Pages 1609–1612 •

Answer D

4. In assessing the need for antidepressant treatment, the psychiatrist should give the *least* consideration to

A. the course and duration of previous episodes of depression
B. the severity of symptoms
C. whether the depression appears to be "endogenous" or "exogenous" in etiology

D. whether the depression meets certain subtypes, such as atypical or melancholic depression
E. the degree of functional impairment caused by the illness

Discussion: A number of symptoms have been suggested as predictors of good and poor response. In the past, depressive illness was distinguished by whether it was endogenous or exogenous. The former was thought to be biological and the latter reactive. It was assumed that endogenous depression would respond better to somatic therapies. Such a distinction was excessively simplistic and lacked construct validity with retrospective bias as a primary problem. Other distinctions, which avoid etiological inference but attempt to identify subtypes such as atypical or melancholic depression, are more useful and valid.

Pages 1612–1614 •

Answer C

5. In choosing a *particular* antidepressant, the psychiatrist should consider

A. a personal or family history of good response to a particular antidepressant
B. a history of symptoms that suggests a minor variant of mania
C. a history of such physical disorders as epilepsy, prostatic hypertrophy, or conduction abnormality
D. the cost of an agent
E. all of the above

Discussion: Even though antidepressants are equally efficacious, different patients will have preferential responses to one agent or a class of agents. Cross-sectional factors, such as physical and laboratory findings, history of medical contraindication, or risk of lethal overdose during the present episode, influence choice of medication. Longitudinal factors, such as past or family history of medication response, need to be considered.

Pages 1614–1616 •

Answer E

6. All of the following statements concerning the pharmacokinetics of antidepressants are true **except**

A. Most antidepressants are highly protein bound.
B. For monoamine oxidase inhibitors, consideration of their metabolism is probably less important than an appreciation of how monoamine oxidase itself is synthesized.
C. Because all antidepressants have relatively long half-lives (between 10 and 40 hours), they can be given in single daily doses. Multiple daily doses should be considered only in the light of side effects.
D. All serotonin reuptake inhibitors are potent inhibitors of the cytochrome P-450IID6 enzymes, which is the basis for many of their drug-drug interactions.
E. Despite significant differences in half-lives and active metabolites, the serotonin reuptake inhibitors have curiously similar onsets of action.

Discussion: Trazodone has a half-life of 3 to 9 hours as well as a lack of active metabolites; therefore, it has variable levels throughout the day and must be given in divided doses. Nefazodone and venlafaxine also require multiple daily doses because of half-life considerations. The other statements about the pharmacokinetics of antidepressants are true.

Page 1615 •

Answer C

7. All of the following statements about the influence of gender on antidepressant action are true **except**

A. Women may have slower gastrointestinal absorption than men, because they have less gastric acid and slower gastric emptying.
B. Water retention associated with the menstrual cycle may affect the volume of distribution.
C. Current evidence suggests that there are clear pharmacological differences between men and women, and such differences should guide our selection of agents and doses.
D. Oral contraceptives can alter the hepatic metabolism of tricyclic antidepressants.
E. In women, the volume of distribution can differ from that of men of similar weight and height, given the increased ratio of adipose tissue to lean body mass.

Discussion: Few clinical studies specifically look at the pharmacology of antidepressants in women. There are not enough data to determine whether gender can significantly influence the pharmacokinetics and pharmacodynamics of antidepressants. Conflicting conclusions from studies of drug levels have been confounded by the use of oral contraceptives. Similarly, whereas anecdotal evidence suggests that there are distinct gender responses to individual antidepressants, this has not been adequately investigated.

Pages 1615–1616 •

Answer C

8. Regarding side effects of antidepressants:

A. Muscarinic blockade is responsible for increased peristalsis, which in turn can cause vomiting and

diarrhea in some patients receiving antidepressants.
B. Antidepressants that are potent muscarinic blockers should be avoided in all persons with glaucoma.
C. Histamine tends to work in a fashion contrary to other receptor effects—for example, it can lessen the orthostatic hypotension caused by adrenergic blockade, and it can lessen the cognitive impairment associated with muscarinic blockade.
D. Although blockade of the noradrenergic α-receptor can cause observable postural hypotension on physical examination, this is rarely a clinically significant effect.
E. Serotonin reuptake blockade can cause akathisia and even extrapyramidal symptoms, although it is not clear whether this is a direct or indirect effect.

Discussion: Muscarinic blockade is responsible for decreased peristalsis; parasympathetically mediated accommodation reflex; and precipitation of acute narrow-angle glaucoma, although this is rare as an iatrogenic complication of antidepressant use. Histamine causes orthostatic hypotension, weight gain, and cognitive impairment. Noradrenergic α-receptor blockade causes falls in the elderly.

Pages 1616–1619, Table 84–2 •

Answer E

9. Which statement is **incorrect?**

A. Although a number of pressor amines, such as levodopa, can cause a hypertensive crisis in patients taking monoamine oxidase inhibitors, tyramine is most commonly associated, because it is a natural fermentation product in many foods.
B. For patients receiving monoamine oxidase inhibitors, all alcoholic beverages, particularly beer and wine, should be avoided.
C. Hypertensive episodes in patients taking monoamine oxidase inhibitors can occur even in the absence of a tyramine-type reaction.
D. Only monoamine oxidase type A is responsible for oxidation of tyramine.
E. B and D are incorrect.

Discussion: The dietary restrictions for monoamine oxidase inhibitor antidepressants need to be understood in terms of the data in support of a likely reaction. For instance, whereas bananas, especially if they are overripe, have a high tyramine content (particularly the peel), the recommendation for avoding bananas is based on a single case report in which the individual also ate the peel. Chianti wine and vermouth have high tyramine content and should be avoided, but small quantities of other alcoholic beverages are probably allowable. Both monoamine oxidase type B and type A are involved in tyramine metabolism.

Pages 1619–1622, Table 84–3 •

Answer E

10. In considering drug-drug interactions of antidepressants, which of the following statements is **incorrect?**

A. Specific substances reported to increase tricyclic levels include fluoxetine, antipsychotic medications, methylphenidate, and cimetidine.
B. The elimination of lithium is primarily dependent on its renal excretion; thus, lithium levels are unaffected by the addition of a serotonin reuptake inhibitor such as fluoxetine.
C. Phenobarbital, carbamazepine, and nicotine can all lower the levels of tricyclic antidepressants through the induction of metabolic enzymes.
D. Guanethidine is contraindicated with tricyclic antidepressants, because it relies on intracellular reuptake for its antihypertensive effect.
E. The "serotonin syndrome" can occur when a serotonin reuptake inhibitor is combined with such serotoninergic potentiators as the monoamine oxidase inhibitors, pentazocine, and L-tryptophan as well as less obvious serotoninergic drugs, such as lithium.

Discussion: Fluoxetine has been reported to raise lithium levels. The mechanism for this is not clear, because lithium is primarily excreted through the kidneys.

Page 1625 •

Answer B

11. In considering the use of an antidepressant for a person with cardiovascular disease, what factors should be considered?

A. The most common cardiovascular side effect of tricyclic antidepressants is orthostatic hypotension.
B. Data suggest that antiarrhythmic drugs can increase the risk for mortality among patients with ventricular arrhythmias and atrial fibrillation.
C. Bupropion remains the only nontricyclic antidepressant specifically investigated in patients with preexisting heart disease.
D. The serotonin reuptake inhibitors do not prolong the PR or QRS interval. Thus, they probably lack any of the proarrhythmic and

antiarrhythmic activities of tricyclic antidepressants.

E. All of the above

Discussion: Tricyclic antidepressants are type 1A antiarrhythmics with effects similar to quinidine and procainamide. Patients with either bundle branch block or a significant intraventricular conduction defect (QRS > 0.11 seconds) are at greatest risk. Findings from a multicenter trial suggested that type 1A drugs can cause increased mortality in patients with ventricular arrhythmias, which has led some to suggest caution in prescribing tricyclics to patients with ischemic heart disease. Fluoxetine has been reported to cause bradycardia especially in combination with other agents.

Pages 1625–1626 •

Answer E

12. In considering antidepressant use in elderly patients, which statement is **not correct?**

A. The elderly show decreased efficiency of the hepatic microoxidase system, resulting in the slower metabolism of antidepressants.

B. The elderly have a decreased muscle to fat ratio, resulting in an alteration of the volume of distribution for a substance and a wider distribution of antidepressants in the elderly body.

C. The elderly are likely to have a greater frequency of side effects from antidepressants.

D. Elderly patients require lower blood levels of antidepressant medication for therapeutic effect.

E. With the possible exception of paroxetine, the half-lives and steady-state concentrations of the serotonin reuptake inhibitors are only minimally affected by age.

Discussion: The pharmacokinetic parameters relating to hepatic metabolism and volume of distribution in the elderly are important. Pharmacodynamics are less well understood. Despite numerous reported changes in the density and numbers of various receptors, the clinical significance of these changes is not clear. Whereas pharmacokinetic concerns may require lower dosing, the assumption that lower blood levels are sufficient in the elderly is not correct. Plasma levels are comparable to young adult levels.

Page 1626 •

Answer D

13. Which of the following statements about dosing strategies for antidepressants is true?

A. Because tricyclics take several weeks to achieve steady state, it is preferable to begin at a high dose (e.g., 150 mg of imipramine) and increase by 50-mg increments (every other day) to a target dose of 400 mg.

B. Although trazodone is often given in multiple daily doses, it may be preferable to give the medication in a single nightly dose for depressed patients with insomnia.

C. Of available blood levels, the best established are for nortriptyline, desipramine, and venlafaxine.

D. The dose-response curve of such serotonin reuptake inhibitors as fluoxetine is poorly understood.

E. Given the relatively safe therapeutic index of the serotonin reuptake inhibitors, it is reasonable to quickly increase the dose to hasten the drug response.

Discussion: The issue of dosage for fluoxetine remains complicated. Some studies have suggested that fluoxetine may not have a linear dose-response curve; some patients may respond to lower doses of medication, such as 10 mg. Other studies have documented responses to fluoxetine at incredible doses and blood levels, such as 320 mg/d and more than 2000 ng/mL, respectively, without adverse effects.

Pages 1629–1630 •

Answer D

14. Which statement about the time course of antidepressant response is **not correct?**

A. Few patients show a significant response before 2 weeks.

B. It may take 6 weeks or longer for an antidepressant response.

C. Patients who show a partial response to antidepressant treatment may be more likely to benefit from augmentation (with agents such as lithium carbonate, thyroid hormone, or a stimulant) than those who show no response at all.

D. There is reasonable evidence to suggest that patients who fail a trial of fluoxetine may respond to a change to another agent such as sertraline or paroxetine.

E. There is a high risk for relapse if treatment is discontinued immediately after the acute response. Thus, the American Psychiatric Association recommends a minimum of 16 to 20 weeks of treatment after the full remission of symptoms.

Discussion: There is little benefit in making treatment changes before 3 weeks except to mitigate side effects. Whereas there is little reason to try an agent from the same class of antidepressant if there is nonresponse, one must distinguish true nonresponse from intolerance of the drug. In the latter instance, a change to a similar agent with a different side effect profile may be indicated.

Pages 1630–1631 •

Answer D

15. Which features may predict that a patient will be a good candidate for treament discontinuation?

A. single episode of acute depression
B. onset of depression before age 21 years
C. an exogenous subtype of depression
D. those who are 40 years or older at the first episode of depression and have had at least one subsequent recurrence
E. those who are 50 years or older at the time of the first depressive episode

Discussion: After a continuation period of treatment that follows remission of at least 16 to 20 weeks, somatic therapy is usually discontinued in the patient with a single episode of major depression.

Pages 1632–1633 •

Answer A

CHAPTER

85 Anxiolytic Drugs

David Taylor

1. Which of the following is **not** true regarding the use of benzodiazepines in the treatment of anxiety disorders?

A. strong anxiolytic effect
B. rapid onset of action
C. increased risk for interaction with other medications
D. lack of tolerance for anxiolytic effect

Discussion: The efficacy of benzodiazepines in relieving anxiety symptoms has been amply demonstrated in many clinical trials. Their advantages include all of the above except the statement about drug interactions. Benzodiazepines generally have a low risk for interaction with other medications. However, those that are oxidatively metabolized by the liver can interact with other psychotropic drugs, which can inhibit hepatic microsomal enzymes. Whereas there is a fairly rapid development of tolerance for sedative side effects, there is a lack of tolerance for anxiolytic effects.

Page 1641 •

Answer C

2. Alprazolam is

A. the first psychotherapeutic drug approved by the Food and Drug Administration for a DSM-III diagnosis
B. approved for generalized anxiety disorder
C. more effective than other benzodiazepines in the treatment of panic attacks
D. four times as potent as lorazepam

Discussion: Alprazolam was found to be more effective than placebo in the treatment of panic attacks in large trials. Panic was initially not thought to respond to benzodiazepine treatment until high-potency medications such as alprazolam were investigated. Subsequent studies have shown that panic attacks can be blocked by lorazepam, diazepam, and clonazepam at therapeutically equivalent doses. However, at the doses required, such medications may be more likely to cause excessive sedation, psychomotor impairment, and ataxia. Alprazolam is twice as potent as lorazepam.

Pages 1641–1642, Table 85–1 (1643) •

Answer A

3. Which of the following syndromes is **not** responsive to benzodiazepine treatment?

A. catatonia
B. Parkinson's disease
C. chronic dystonia
D. akathisia

Discussion: Benzodiazepines are useful for the treatment of acute rigidity, such as that seen in catatonia and neuroleptic malignant syndrome. Although not useful in acute dystonias, they can alleviate the discomfort of chronic dystonia. Tremor may respond, but essential tremor and Parkinson's disease are less likely to be sensitive to this type of treatment.

Page 1642 •

Answer B

4. Withdrawal from benzodiazepines is frequently associated with

A. psychosis
B. seizures
C. rebound anxiety
D. lacrimation

Discussion: Rebound anxiety is defined as a prompt, brief recurrence, after sudden discontinuation of anxiolytic medication, of the same anxiety symptoms that brought the patient to treatment, but at a level of severity higher than at baseline. This is part of a withdrawal syndrome that has a set of other features including confusion, clouded sensorium, muscle cramps and twitches, diarrhea, and weight loss but not lacrimation. Abrupt discontinuation has been reported to result in psychotic symptoms and seizures, but this is usually associated with high doses, extended duration of use, preexisting seizure disorder, or concomitant use of drugs that lower the seizure threshold. Thus, these severe events are rare.

Page 1645 •

Answer C

5. Which of the following statements about the abuse potential of benzodiazepines is true?

A. Most recovering alcoholic patients have been found to increase benzodiazepine dosage during a year of treatment.
B. Animal models suggest that these are drugs with high abuse liability.
C. Normal humans always prefer benzodiazepines to placebo.
D. Most physicians have encountered patients with benzodiazepine abuse.

Discussion: Given the fact that physicians frequently encounter patients who have a benzodiazepine use disorder, it is surprising that research data suggest that these drugs are not as likely to be abused as one might expect. Studies of the reinforcing effects of benzodiazepines in animal models indicate that it is significantly more difficult to establish and maintain consistent self-administration of these compounds than classic drugs of abuse. Normal humans, with few exceptions, prefer placebo to benzodiazepines, given a choice after initial exposures to both substances. Substance abusers, however, do prefer benzodiazepines to placebo. Even among patients recovering from alcohol dependence who were treated for up to a year with benzodiazepines, no more than 5% showed a tendency to increase their dosage.

Pages 1645–1646 •

Answer D

6. The use of buspirone is

A. rarely successful
B. indicated for panic disorder
C. successful for patients who previously responded to benzodiazepines
D. especially indicated in the treatment of anxious alcoholic individuals

Discussion: Buspirone, which is not a benzodiazepine, has been found to be helpful in the treatment of generalized anxiety disorder and among anxious alcoholic individuals. It is ineffective in panic disorder, according to three controlled trials, but there appear to have been methodological problems in these studies. Patients who have used benzodiazepines may not respond to buspirone or may need extra support to maintain compliance.

Page 1646 •

Answer D

CHAPTER

86 Sedative-Hypnotics

David Taylor

1. In general, elderly individuals report that

A. they spend less time in bed than younger adults
B. they are better rested with less sleep than younger adults
C. they are easily aroused from sleep
D. noise is less disruptive to them

Discussion: The elderly generally spend more time in bed than younger adults, but not all of this time is spent asleep. Actual average total sleep time increases slightly after age 65 years, but this mainly reflects an increasing number of long-sleepers and increased daytime napping; short-sleepers increase in number as well. The elderly are more easily aroused and spend less time in stage 4 sleep. Their overall pattern reveals sleep that is fragmented by periods of wakefulness. The ability to tolerate noise diminishes with age.

Page 1652 •

Answer C

2. Which of the following is **not** an ingredient of herbal sleep remedies available in the United States?

A. valerian root
B. barley
C. chamomile
D. mad-dog skullcap

Discussion: Whereas some herbal sleep remedies contain hops and oats, barley is not a constituent. Although not as frequently used in the United States, *Valeriana officinalis* is still a popular over-the-counter hypnotic in Europe, particularly in teas, tinctures, and extracts. Other ingredients include passion flower and various minerals. A major problem is that many such remedies contain toxic ingredients.

Page 1653, Table 86–5 •

Answer B

3. Commonly available over-the-counter sleep aids are associated with

A. histamine H_2 receptor blockade
B. greater efficacy than benzodiazepines
C. greater compliance than with prescribed hypnotics
D. less efficacy if combined with an analgesic

Discussion: Most over-the-counter sleeping pills are histamine H_1 receptor antagonists with sedating properties. These agents have not been studied in carefully controlled trials so that their efficacy could be established. One telephone survey found that 17% of over-the-counter users reported that the pills were helpful as opposed to 32% to 42% of those using benzodiazepines as hypnotics. Compliance in general is higher with these agents. Diphenhydramine combined with aspirin was compared in one study with placebo and each agent alone. The combination was found to be superior to placebo provided that there were complaints of pain accompanying the sleep disturbance. If not, there was no difference between the four interventions.

Pages 1653–1654, Table 85–6 •

Answer C

4. Benzodiazepine hypnotics have all of the following effects on sleep architecture **except**

A. decrease of sleep latency
B. decrease of stage 1 sleep
C. decrease of stage 2 sleep
D. decrease of time in slow-wave sleep (stage 4)

Discussion: Benzodiazepines shorten sleep latency, decrease stage 1 sleep, *increase* stage 2 sleep, and generally reduce time in stage 4 sleep. Patients feel that their sleep is more restorative.

Pages 1654–1655 •

Answer C

5. Which of the following statements regarding benzodiazepine hypnotics is true?

A. The marketed benzodiazepines do not differ in terms of efficacy and safety.
B. Their method of action is not well understood.

C. Only benzodiazepines marketed as hypnotics are effective for that purpose.
D. Rebound insomnia is rarely a problem with shorter half-life benzodiazepines.

Discussion: Any benzodiazepine could be used to induce sleep provided that an appropriate dose is chosen. The basic issues are rapidity of absorption from the gastrointestinal tract, rapid uptake into the brain, adequate duration of action, duration of activity of any active metabolites, and elimination at a rate that significantly reduces brain concentrations before awakening the next morning. The five benzodiazepines marketed as hypnotics do not differ in terms of efficacy and safety. Shorter half-life agents cause marked rebound insomnia, but this is rarely a persistent phenomenon. Benzodiazepines are central nervous system depressants with a mechanism of action that is thought to be related to their ability to augment the opening of neuronal γ-aminobutyric acid receptor–related chloride channels.

Pages 1654–1655 •

Answer A

6. Which of the following statements is true regarding anterograde amnesia occurring with benzodiazepines marketed as hypnotics?

A. It is uncommon.
B. It is more likely to occur among those using triazolam.
C. It occurs only in the setting of concomitant alcohol abuse.
D. It is more commonly seen in phase-shifted persons.

Discussion: Anterograde amnesia is not uncommon, particularly with triazolam or in phase-shifted persons. No rigorous data support the assertion that triazolam is more risky in this regard. One large Canadian study comparing more than 48,000 triazolam users with more than 160,000 users of other benzodiazepines and more than 97,000 nonbenzodiazepine-using control patients concluded that triazolam users had outcomes comparable to the other benzodiazepine-treated patients.

Page 1655 •

Answer D

7. Zolpidem is **not**

A. a benzodiazepine
B. active at central benzodiazepine receptors
C. at all associated with tolerance, withdrawal, or abuse
D. antagonized by flumazenil

Discussion: Zolpidem is marketed as a nonbenzodiazepine alternative to benzodiazepine hypnotics. However, it is a central (omega) benzodiazepine receptor agonist, and its actions are reversible by the antagonist flumazenil. There may be a slightly reduced likelihood of producing tolerance and withdrawal.

Page 1656 •

Answer A

8. Which of the following medications is **not** metabolized by cytochrome P-4503A4?

A. triazolam
B. temazepam
C. estazolam
D. alprazolam

Discussion: All currently available triazolobenzodiazepines are 3A4 substrates. Triazolam is a high hepatic clearance drug that depends on this particular enzyme for its metabolism. The selective serotonin reuptake inhibitors and nefazodone inhibit a variety of hepatic microsomal enzymes, and if they are used with triazolam, higher peak concentrations in blood and brain are likely to occur. Temazepam is not in the same family as triazolam and the other compounds listed and is primarily metabolized by glucuronidation; therefore, it is not affected by inhibitors of oxidative metabolism.

Pages 1656–1657, Table 86–10 •

Answer B

CHAPTER

87 Psychostimulants

Laurence L. Greenhill • Jeffrey Halperin • John S. March

1. Evidence for the role of the catecholamines dopamine and norepinephrine in attention-deficit/hyperactivity disorder (ADHD) is suggested by

A. pharmacological treatment studies
B. electroencephalography
C. reduced cerebrospinal fluid 5-hydroxyindoleacetic acid (5-HIAA) levels in disruptive boys
D. molecular structure of psychostimulant medications

Discussion: The molecular structure of the various isomers of methylphenidate and amphetamine has been implicated in differential efficacy and onset of action. The basis of the neurochemical hypothesis for this disorder is the finding that all three major stimulant medications—dextroamphetamine, methylphenidate, and pemoline—have their primary effects on these two neurotransmitter systems. Furthermore, the more selective norepinephrine-acting tricyclic medications, such as desipramine and imipramine, as well as the α-adrenergic agonist clonidine, have all been found to reduce the symptoms of ADHD children. Neuroimaging studies have focused on the dopamine-rich caudate and striatum in this population. Whereas there are findings of reduced cerebrospinal fluid 5-HIAA levels in disruptive boys, that compound is a metabolite of serotonin, a noncatecholamine biogenic amine.

Pages 1660–1661 •

Answer A

2. All of the following are true of methylphenidate pharmacokinetics **except**

A. Bioavailability is about 30%.
B. It is not highly protein bound.
C. Central nervous system concentrations are half of plasma levels.
D. It is metabolized by hydrolysis and oxidation in the liver.

Discussion: Low plasma concentrations of methylphenidate are effective in part because of its low plasma protein binding, which makes it highly available to cross the blood-brain barrier. This creates a favorable brain-plasma partition, with a higher concentration in the central nervous system than in plasma.

Page 1662 •

Answer C

3. Unlike other clinical instruments, such as rating scales and interviews, a Continuous Performance Test (CPT) purportedly generates an objective measure of

A. aggressive behavior
B. social skills
C. attentional functioning
D. activity level

Discussion: Most investigators consider the number of missed targets or omission errors on a CPT to reflect inattention. Although aggressive behavior may be correlated with certain types of CPT errors (i.e., those related to impulsivity), aggressive behavior is incorrect because the test does not evaluate aggression. Similarly, activity level may correlate with aspects of CPT performance, but it is not directly measured. There is no evidence to suggest that CPT performance relates to social skills.

Pages 1663–1664 •

Answer C

4. Which of the following statements about the effects of stimulants on growth is true?

A. It is a common adverse event.
B. Untreated ADHD children also have decreased growth.
C. Sixty-five children observed to age 18 years showed an initial growth loss during methylphenidate treatment but "caught up" during adolescence and reached heights predicted from their parents' heights.
D. Research studies of 13 children treated for 18 months with dextroamphetamine showed consistent changes in growth hormone release.

Discussion: Growth suppression, in particular of height velocity, is a rare phenomenon. Changes in weight velocity may be related to appetite suppression. Studies have found no independent effect of ADHD itself, no consistent changes in growth hormone levels, and minimal overall effects due to a "catch-up" phenomenon in adolescence.

Pages 1673–1674 •

Answer C

5. Most investigators interpret commission errors on the CPT as reflecting problems with

A. attention
B. impulse control
C. hyperactivity
D. aggression

Discussion: Commission errors are incorrect responses or false alarms that are believed by many to reflect the subject's inability to withhold a response. Attention is more commonly believed to be reflected by omission errors. The CPT does not directly measure hyperactivity or aggression.

Pages 1663–1664 •

Answer B

6. Clinical utility of the CPT has **not** been evaluated with regard to

A. its ability to diagnose ADHD
B. its ability to monitor treatment response
C. its ability to predict treatment response
D. its ability to predict long-term outcome in ADHD children

Discussion: Although findings have been mostly disappointing, several studies have examined the usefulness of the CPT for diagnosing ADHD, monitoring treatment response, and predicting treatment response. The relationship of CPT performance to long-term outcome has not been systematically examined.

Pages 1663–1664 •

Answer D

CHAPTER

88 Cognitive Enhancers for Alzheimer's Disease

David Taylor

1. The Food and Drug Administration requires that new antidementia agents be efficacious as measured by

A. improved performance on a complete neuropsychological test battery
B. improved Mini-Mental State Examination and Global Assessment of Functioning Scale
C. improved performance on scales for behavior and activities of daily living
D. improved score on Alzheimer's Disease Assessment Scale and the Clinical Global Impression of Change
E. all of the above

Discussion: The standard rating instruments used in clinical trials in studies of these agents are the Alzheimer's Disease Assessment Scale, an index of cognitive and neuropsychological change, and the Clinical Global Impression of Change, a global clinical measure. Whereas improvements in day-to-day functioning and behavior are important variables, these are not the primary measures of efficacy used in the evaluations of antidementia drugs. The Mini-Mental State Examination is used as a secondary measure in clinical trials.

Pages 1685–1686 •

Answer D

2. Which of the following are typical inclusion criteria for patients in Alzheimer's disease clinical trials?

A. good physical health
B. normal blood pressure
C. computed tomography and magnetic resonance imaging studies without significant focal lesions
D. none of the above
E. A to C are correct

Discussion: In addition to having a diagnosis of probable Alzheimer's disease by established criteria, a Mini-Mental State Examination score of 10 to 26, and a score of less than 4 on the Modified Hachinski Scale, patients must meet all of the above inclusion criteria. Subjects must also be English speaking and have a reliable caregiver. Exclusion criteria typically consist of a history of other psychiatric or neurological disorders, a stroke or evidence of a stroke on computed tomography or magnetic resonance imaging, significant concurrent physical illness, or abnormal laboratory findings. These rigorous criteria allow only a minority of Alzheimer's disease patients to enter clinical trials; hence, results may not be generalizable to the Alzheimer's disease population as a whole.

Page 1686 •

Answer E

3. Which of the following is **not** an appropriate first step in the treatment of behavioral symptoms of Alzheimer's disease, such as agitation?

A. medical evaluation
B. psychiatric evaluation
C. environmental evaluation
D. hospital admission or use of neuroleptics
E. administration of specific antidementia medication, such as tacrine

Discussion: All of the above except the use of tacrine are appropriate initial approaches to the management of agitation in Alzheimer's disease. Admission and use of neuroleptics are reserved for severe and acute problems. Many agitated patients have concomitant or preexisting medical or psychiatric disorders. Careful attention to environmental issues, such as routines, sensory stimulation, or recent disruptions, is necessary. Noninvasive and helpful supportive measures, such as psychotherapy and education of caregivers, are often sufficient treatment. Medications such as olazepine, risperidone, clozapine, carbamazepine, valproic acid, trazodone, fluoxetine, buspirone, L-deprenyl, and thiothixene are being investigated for use in treatment of behavioral symptoms.

Pages 1688–1690 •

Answer E

4. Clinical trials of tacrine have shown

A. modestly significant clinical effects
B. dramatic clinical effects
C. that response was not dose dependent
D. that treatment should continue indefinitely
E. rare transaminase elevations

Discussion: Several clinical trials have shown modestly significant clinical effects. Clinical response seems to be dose dependent. Doses of 80 to 160 mg/d are required for therapeutic effects in a minority of patients. It is not yet clear how long patients should be treated with tacrine or other cholinesterase inhibitors. Approximately 30% of patients may have transaminase levels above three times the upper limit of normal.

Pages 1691–1693 •

Answer A

5. Which of the following statements about L-deprenyl is true?

A. It selectively inhibits monoamine oxidase type B at doses of 15 to 20 mg/d.
B. It has not been found to improve cognitive function in Alzheimer's disease, but it does so in Parkinson's disease.
C. Rodents treated with L-deprenyl perform better in mazes.
D. L-Deprenyl may preserve surviving neurons.
E. The efficacy of L-deprenyl in Alzheimer's disease has been well established.

Discussion: L-Deprenyl, which selectively inhibits monoamine oxidase type B at doses of only 5 to 10 mg/d, is currently marketed for the treatment of maintaining motor function in Parkinson's disease. In three open parallel-group studies comparing L-deprenyl with acetylcarnitine, phosphatidylserine, and oxiracetam, it was reported to be superior to each in improving cognitive function in the course of 3 months. An adequate efficacy trial has not been completed. L-Deprenyl has also been reported to have beneficial effects on behavior in dementia patients in areas such as cooperativeness, anxiety, depression, and agitation. L-Deprenyl may have the potential to preserve surviving neurons; the hypothesis that chronic inhibition of monoamine oxidase may retard progression of illness is based on antitoxic mechanisms. Rodents given this medication have increased survival, and there may be some neurotrophic properties not related to monoamine oxidase inhibition.

Page 1694 •

Answer D

6. Which of the following calcium channel blockers may be valuable in Alzheimer's disease?

A. verapamil
B. diltiazem
C. nimodipine
D. nifedipine
E. none of the above

Discussion: Nimodipine has been tested in Alzheimer's disease patients. In one trial, the low-dose nimodipine group (30 mg three times daily) showed less deterioration than the placebo group on several memory tests during a 10- to 12-week treatment period. Another study found it to be superior to ergoloid mesylates (Hydergine) and placebo. It is marketed in Europe as a cognitive enhancer. A Bristol-Myers Squibb investigational compound in this class is also being studied. The process of neuron death in aging and Alzheimer's disease may be mediated by an increase in intracellular free calcium, which activates various destructive enzymes.

Page 1696 •

Answer C

CHAPTER

89 Experimental Therapeutics: Nonstandard Drug Treatments

Arthur Rifkin

More than one answer may be used in questions 1–11.

1. The Food and Drug Administration approves a drug for marketing on the basis of

A. efficacy only
B. safety only
C. both A and B
D. either A or B
E. neither of these reasons

Discussion: Under the federal Food, Drug, and Cosmetic Act, the Food and Drug Administration must find a drug both effective and safe.

Page 1703 •

Answer C

2. Several studies have shown that electroconvulsive therapy in schizophrenia

A. is effective as an adjunct to antipsychotic drugs in patients who have not responded to antipsychotic medication
B. is not effective
C. is effective if depressive symptoms are present
D. increases speed of response when it is given with antipsychotic medication

Discussion: Several studies indicated that when given with antipsychotic medication, electroconvulsive therapy is associated with a more rapid response, but the control group "caught up."

Page 1705 •

Answer D

3. A small study of methadone as an adjunct to antipsychotic medication in schizophrenia indicated that

A. it was ineffective
B. it was effective
C. it helped only those patients who had abused opioids
D. withdrawal symptoms did not occur when patients stopped methadone
E. it helped, clearly, by reducing anxiety with no effect on psychotic symptoms

Discussion: A study by Brizer and colleagues in only seven subjects showed methadone more effective than placebo as adjunctive medication for schizophrenia; and six subjects, who stoped methadone after the study, did not have withdrawal symptoms.

Page 1705 •

Answers B and D

4. According to several placebo-controlled studies, when added to an antipsychotic drug in schizophrenic patients who showed little response to the antipsychotic, lithium

A. demonstrated overall efficacy
B. demonstrated efficacy only for mood-related symptoms
C. revealed a high proportion of cases of neurotoxic effects
D. revealed a low frequency of neurotoxic effects
E. demonstrated no efficacy

Discussion: Three placebo-controlled studies assessed lithium in schizophrenic subjects who had demonstrated little response to standard treatment. These studies suggested that lithium was effective without a high frequency of neurotoxic effects.

Pages 1705–1706 •

Answers A and D

5. Carbamazepine (CBZ) has been tested in three double-blind, placebo-controlled studies as an adjunct to antipsychotic medication for schizophrenic patients. The results indicated

A. a clear-cut improvement in those given CBZ
B. a lack of clear-cut improvement in those given CBZ
C. that a substantial proportion could not tolerate CBZ
D. a superior response for manic-like symptoms in all studies

Discussion: One study found no effect of CBZ, although the sample was small. The second study also found no difference. The third study, using a large sample, found no global effect, although there was a significant result on manic symptoms (some of the sample had schizoaffective disorder). None of these studies reported any serious side effects.

Pages 1706–1707 •

Answer B

6. Studies of augmentation of antidepressants with lithium or liothyronine (T_3) showed

A. neither clearly helps
B. both clearly help
C. lithium but not T_3 helps
D. T_3 but not lithium helps
E. T_3 helps by inducing mild hyperthyroidism

Discussion: Double-blind, placebo-controlled studies indicated that both T_3 and lithium are effective in augmenting antidepressant treatment in major depression. Subjects treated with T_3 did not develop hyperthyroidism.

Pages 1707–1708 •

Answer B

7. Moclobemide differs from phenelzine and tranylcypromine in that it

A. deaminates only phenylethylamine and benzylamine (i.e., type B monoamine oxidase)
B. acts as a competitive rather than a noncompetitive inhibitor of monoamine oxidase
C. is less likely to cause a tyramine reaction
D. deaminates only serotonin and norepinephrine
E. is less effective for major depression

Discussion: Moclobemide, unlike phenelzine and tranylcypromine, is a competitive inhibitor of monoamine oxidase, so that its effect is more short-lived. It selectively deaminates serotonin and norepinephrine and does not affect phenylethylamine and benzylamine, that is, it metabolizes type A monoamine oxidase. It has only a weak tyramine reaction, requiring at least 150 mg of tyramine to raise systolic blood pressure 30 mm Hg, an amount of tyramine in excess of that in most meals.

Page 1708 •

Answers B and D

8. Combined monoamine oxidase inhibitor and tricyclic antidepressant treatment of major depression

A. is particularly dangerous and should be avoided
B. is safe if the tricyclic antidepressant is started after the monoamine oxidase inhibitor
C. is safe if the tricyclic antidepressant is started with or before the monoamine oxidase inhibitor
D. has been proved more effective than either drug given alone
E. may be more effective than either drug given alone on the basis of anecdotal reports

Discussion: The combination of these drugs was thought to be particularly dangerous for many years, an erroneous opinion based on adverse reactions that could be explained, usually, by complicating factors. More careful studies showed that adding a tricyclic antidepressant to a monoamine oxidase inhibitor *can* cause severe side effects, whereas starting both together or adding a monoamine oxidase inhibitor to a tricyclic antidepressant is safe. The advantage of combining these drugs comes from anecdotal reports, not systematic data.

Pages 1708–1709 •

Answers C and E

9. Valproate has been shown to

A. have efficacy equal to lithium for acute mania
B. have efficacy equal to antipsychotic drugs for acute mania
C. be an effective maintenance treatment to prevent mania but not depression
D. be an effective maintenance treatment to prevent both mania and depression
E. be equally effective to lithium for acute mania on the basis of several placebo-controlled studies

Discussion: There has been one study comparing valproate and lithium with placebo for acute mania, showing both significantly superior to placebo and equally effective to each other, although they had a low probability of demonstrating a clinically significant difference. Maintenance valproate treatment has not been systematically tested.

Pages 1710–1711 •

Answer A

10. High-dose levothyroxine for rapid-cycling bipolar disorder

A. is effective in patients with reduced thyroid functioning
B. has been shown effective by prospective, double-blind, placebo-controlled studies
C. has been suggested as effective on the basis of anecdotal reports
D. is given, according to the report with the largest sample size, by increases of 0.05 to 0.1 mg/d every 1 to 2 weeks
E. is used to a maximal dose of 0.25 mg/d

Discussion: The basis of using high-dose levothyroxine comes from anecdotal reports, not data from prospective, double-blind, placebo-controlled studies. The authors of the study with the largest sample used doses of 0.15 to 0.4 mg/d by increasing by 0.05 to 0.1 mg/d every 1 to 2 weeks until troublesome side effects or clinical efficacy. The mechanism of action is unknown. One group reported that rapid-cycling bipolar disorder was associated with grade I hypothyroidism, yet the previously mentioned study found that initial thyroid status did not predict outcome.

Pages 1711–1712 •

Answers C and D

11. Imipramine

A. reduces panic attacks
B. alleviates symptoms of major depression
C. probably reduces symptoms of generalized anxiety disorder
D. is less effective than alprazolam for panic disorder
E. frequently causes an overstimulatory adverse reaction in patients with major depression, but not in those with panic disorder

Discussion: Imipramine's ability to help panic disorder and major depression is well established. A study showed that it helps generalized anxiety disorder as well. Alprazolam has not been shown superior to imipramine for panic disorder. Imipramine frequently causes over-stimulation in patients with panic disorder, but not in those with major depression.

Pages 1712–1713 •

Answers A, B, and C

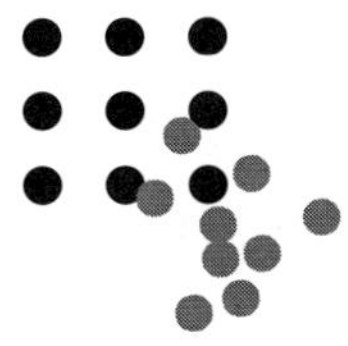

SECTION **VII**

Section Editor: Stephen M. Goldfinger

Special Clinical Settings and Problems

CHAPTER

90 The Social Context of Psychiatric Practice

Stephen M. Goldfinger • J. Arturo Silva

There are no questions for this chapter.

CHAPTER

91 Social Stabilization: Achieving Satisfactory Community Adaptation for the Disabled Mentally Ill

Phyllis Solomon • Arthur T. Meyerson

1. Case management usually includes all of the following functions **except**

A. advocating for the patient's needs
B. counseling
C. home visits
D. prescribing medication
E. educating the patient

Discussion: Whereas some physicians do case management, case managers are rarely physicians and cannot provide psychopharmacological treatment.

Pages 1728–1729 •

Answer D

2. Supported employment may involve all of the following as primary goals and functions **except**

A. symptom reduction
B. employer education
C. on-site job coaching
D. coworker education
E. training in specific job-related skills

Discussion: Symptom reduction may occur as a result of supported employment, although it is not a primary goal.

Page 1739 •

Answer A

3. The following is **not** among primary goals of psychiatric rehabilitation

A. increased capacity to deal with finances
B. vocational skills
C. increased capacity for self-care
D. decreased hallucinations and delusions
E. decreased inappropriate social behaviors

Discussion: Although decreased symptoms may occur, this is not a primary focus of rehabilitation.

Pages 1733–1735 •

Answer D

4. According to Goldman and colleagues, psychiatric disability is estimated to affect

A. 500,000 Americans
B. 1.5 to 2.5 million
C. 3 million
D. 5 to 10 million
E. more than 10 million

Discussion: Goldman and colleagues attempted to estimate the incidence and prevalence of those suffering from a severe mental disorder with moderate to severe disability of prolonged duration. Including adults only, and excluding nonpsychotic and substance abuse disorders, these authors conservatively estimated the population as between 1.7 and 2.4 million persons.

Page 1727 •

Answer B

5. Social stabilization of the disabled mentally ill person involves adaptation in the following spheres **except**

A. concentration and attention
B. socialization
C. recreation
D. housing
E. vocational-educational

Discussion: Loss of concentration and loss of attention are impairments, not disabilities.

Pages 1727–1728, 1733–1734 •

Answer A

6. Case management is necessary because of the following **except**

A. the lack of an integrated services system
B. insufficient availability of psychiatrists
C. the need for continuity of care
D. patients' difficulty in advocating for their own needs
E. the absence of patients' social support networks

Discussion: Case management does not substitute for medical care.

Pages 1728–1730 •

Answer B

7. The five core functions of case management include the following **except**

A. assessment
B. planning
C. linking
D. treating
E. advocating

Discussion: Treating is not a core function, although a case manager may also do therapy.

Pages 1728–1729, Table 91–2 •

Answer D

8. The following factors are considered either protective or decompensating in Anthony and Liberman's vulnerability-stress-coping and competence model of disabling mental illness **except**

A. antipsychotic medication as protective
B. biological vulnerability
C. social supports
D. employment
E. coping skills

Discussion: Employment may either be stressor or augment self-esteem and social networking. It is not considered a primary factor in the model, although it is a desired adaptation.

Pages 1733–1734, See also Chapter 79 •

Answer D

9. Family psychoeducation has been demonstrated to provide the following outcomes in schizophrenic patients **except**

A. reduction of family stress
B. increase in family capacity to cope with an ill relative
C. increased knowledge of the patient's illness
D. Increased vocational success among patients
E. decreased frequency of relapse and rehospitalization

Discussion: Outcome literature in family psychoeducation has focused on medication compliance, rates of rehospitalization, and changing family attitudes. Vocational outcome has not been studied.

Pages 1744–1747 •

Answer D

CHAPTER

92 From Asylums to Communities: A Historical Perspective on Changing Environments of Care

Megan Hester • David Taylor

1. Which of the following is true about early asylums or custodial care environments?

A. Public asylums were essentially large, jail-like settings where inmates were commonly chained, beaten, starved, and placed on public display for a fee.
B. The first state mental institutions were established in the 1820s.
C. In Colonial America, the mentally ill were sometimes sold for slave labor.
D. All of the above

Discussion: Whereas early custodial care settings were established for the purpose of supporting care of the mentally ill, they often served as a control for social deviants. Public asylums were jail-like and flagrantly mistreated inmates. In Colonial America, the mentally ill were housed under an early version of "foster care"; responsibility for the mentally disabled person was given over to the lowest bidder, who was then paid to board the person. The first state institutions were established in the 1820s, more than 70 years after Benjamin Franklin attempted to pass an act to develop a hospital for the reception and cure of the lunatic poor.

Pages 1751–1752 •

Answer D

2. By the 1950s, state mental hospitals

A. had improved conditions considerably owing to the exposure from Albert Deutsch's book *The Shame of the States*
B. had lost many patients and represented only one fifth of all the hospital beds in the nation
C. were "total" institutions with no regard for individual autonomy
D. none of the above

Discussion: The mental hospitals, in the 1950s, held more than 550,000 people and represented half of all hospital beds in the nation. Albert Deutsch's book *The Shame of the States* served to expose and reform Veterans Administration and psychiatric hospitals. State hospitals were often dirty, and gang showers and mass feedings were common. "Batch living," where inmates were addressed en masse and activities were conducted in groups, occurred in state mental hospitals, and many inmates felt that privacy was lacking. Violations of privacy included forced treatments and forced medication. In addition, inmates were forced into social contact with other inmates; deference to staff was enforced through punitive means.

Pages 1752–1753 •

Answer C

3. Remedies created by Benjamin Rush, the father of American psychiatry, for mentally ill patients include all **except**

A. bloodletting
B. use of emetics
C. blistering
D. high-dose alcohol
E. warm and cold baths

Discussion: Rush believed that insanity was seated primarily in the blood vessels of the brain, so he created a set of remedies for various mental conditions. These remedies included bloodletting, use of emetics, blistering, warm and cold baths, and purging. He also invented "the gyrator," a circular swing that affected blood flow to the brain, which also included a wooden chair with heavy straps to use as restraints. Rush's primitive treatments helped form the beginnings of the idea that the mentally ill should be treated, not just boarded.

Page 1753 •

Answer D

4. Nonhospital alternatives for acute psychosis included all **except**

A. Fountain House
B. R. D. Laing's Kingsley Hall
C. Soteria House
D. Windhorse's therapeutic household

Discussion: Laing founded Kingsley Hall in 1965 as a "psychic commune" for psychotic people. Through seminars, open meetings, teach-ins, and performances by counterculture musicians, artists, and poets, Laing sought to help residents reemerge into the ego-bound world. Kingsley Hall was closed in 1971 but spawned the development of other similar centers. Soteria House was a similar living arrnagement, but staff was predominantly same-age peers. Low-dose medication strategies were used, and the program was found to result in a relatively good outcome and less social disability. Windhorse drew from Buddhist meditation practice. Each individual is served by a team of people whose primary focus is to orient the person to the present moment. The individual may receive low doses of psychiatric medication and intensive psychotherapy several times a week. The model is based on the idea that psychosis is a disruption of the balance of mind-body-environment and that recovery is possible within the context of a compassionate, caring community. Fountain House is a clubhouse model rehabilitation center.

Pages 1754, 1763–1764 •

Answer A

5. The behaviorists Paul and Lentz studied schizophrenic inpatients and found

A. that the patients in a token economy did not have reduced bizarre behavior
B. that the patients in a milieu therapy–therapeutic community approach developed specific skills
C. that patients in the social learning group were able to reduce or eliminate bizarre behavior
D. none of the above

Discussion: The study by Paul and Lentz, which divided patients into two groups—social learning group (token economy), and milieu therapy–therapeutic community approach—found that the token economy group not only was successful in reducing bizarre behavior but also was effective in overcoming skill deficits with significant improvements in all the individuals. Whereas milieu therapy significantly reduced all but one type of bizarre behavior, it was less effective in helping people develop specific skills. However, both programs had a meaningful impact on the community tenure of those leaving the institution versus control subjects.

Page 1756 •

Answer C

6. Problems with the linear residential continuum model include

A. continuity of care suffers.
B. standardized programming does not match individual needs.
C. lengths of stay are often unrealistic.
D. moves are stressful.
E. all of the above

Discussion: Many people in the target population require a high degree of continuity of care, and the lack of residential stability inherent in transitional programs and the demand for independent living can lead to recidivism to expensive inpatient services. Moving people from a most intensive setting to independent living is often stressful, and the individual does not adjust and must return to the more intensive residential settings. Lengths of stay are often unrealistic because of pressure placed on psychiatrists to discharge inpatients sooner. Preset levels of service or programming and standardized, mechanistic expectation of change do not fit the needs of this population.

Pages 1757–1758 •

Answer E

7. In the 1960s and 1970s, federal courts mandated levels of treatment and provided funding for state hospitals as a result of

A. public reaction to exposure, by the media, of previous treatment practices
B. class-action lawsuits
C. accreditation standards under the Joint Commission on Accreditation of Hospitals
D. answers B and C
E. answers A and C

Discussion: In the 1960s and 1970s, federal courts began to set mandated levels of active treatment in right-to-treatment class-action lawsuits, such as *Wyatt v Stickney* in Alabama. Federal funding later became contingent on accreditation standards set by the Joint Commission on Accreditation of Hospitals. Many states introduced licensure standards for community treatment facilities as well.

Page 1754 •

Answer D

8. All of the following are true about Fairweather Lodge **except**

A. Those who leave the lodge take the share of assets that they earned.
B. Recidivism is cut by 75%, and most participants stay out of the hospital and achieve employment.
C. The model begins on an inpatient psychiatric ward.
D. Work roles have a hierarchical structure so that people can advance to positions with greater responsibilities.
E. More than 100 Fairweather Lodges exist today.

Discussion: Fairweather Lodge is based on the idea that status, role, and resource deficits are the basis of chronicity and that communal groups and normal social roles could overcome these problems. The model begins in an inpatient psychiatric ward where patients participate in exercises in which they make decisions and form a functional group. The group is then responsible for establishing rules of their business and helping the household run. Work rules have a hierarchical structure, giving people a chance to advance. However, those who leave the lodge do not take a share of the assets produced; instead, new members are recruited from the expatient population. Outcome findings show that recidivism is cut by 75%, and most patients stay out of the hospital and achieve employment. More than 100 Fairweather Lodges exist today, and a few states are continuing to develop this model.

Page 1756 •

Answer A

9. Supportive housing

A. promotes social segregation and homogeneous grouping
B. emphasizes social integration
C. provides support services and conducts skills teaching before the program is begun with other individuals
D. is similar to traditional residential treatment

Discussion: Social housing does not promote social segregation and homogeneous grouping; rather, it emphasizes social integration by having disabled people live in typical neighborhoods dispersed throughout the community. Support services are provided flexibly, on an as needed basis, to help engender a fit between the person and his or her environment. This differs from traditional residential treatment in that traditional residential treatment is often preprogrammed and links a standardized level or intensity of services to a particular place. The supportive housing model recognizes that people with severe disabilities do not become completely self-sufficient and require long-term assistance.

Pages 1759–1762 •

Answer B

10. A supported housing demonstration in Eugene, Oregon, found all of the following true **except**

A. In the first year, a fairly high proportion of at-risk clients continued to lead chaotic lives and experience a high degree of homelessness.
B. In the first year, recidivism was not reduced.
C. In long-term follow-up, participants began to achieve more residential stability.
D. In long-term follow-up, participants were much better able to stay out of trouble with the law.

Discussion: In the first year, although a high proportion of at-risk clients continued to lead chaotic lives and experience a high degree of homelessness, recidivism was reduced. Participants' use of state hospital beds dropped from 1106 days in the 6 months before admission to the program to 370 days in the first 6 months after entry. In long-term follow-up, participants began to achieve more residential stability and were much better able to stay out of trouble with the law.

Page 1760 •

Answer B

CHAPTER

93 Advocacy, Self-help, and Consumer-Operated Services

Harriet P. Lefley

1. The government agency that has been most instrumental in the growth of mental health advocacy groups is

A. Community Support Program
B. Joint Commission for Community Mental Health
C. Office of Knowledge Exchange
D. Office of Demonstration Programs
E. National Institute for Psychosocial Rehabilitation

Discussion: The Community Support Program, founded by the federal government in 1978 to help cope with deinstitutionalization, has aided in the development of local self-help and advocacy groups. This has taken place in Learning Community Conferences together with substantial grant support for organization development.

Page 1776 •

Answer A

2. Select the organization that has been most active in promoting a role for patients-consumers in planning and service delivery:

A. American Orthopsychiatric Association
B. National Council of Community Mental Health Centers
C. American Association of Community Psychiatrists
D. National Association of State Mental Health Program Directors
E. National Mental Health Association

Discussion: The National Association of State Mental Health Program Directors (NASMHPD) developed a position paper in 1989 that specifically outlined the role of expatients–consumers in state mental health systems. "Their contribution should be valued and sought in areas of program development, policy formation, program evaluation, quality assurance, system design, education of mental health service providers, and the provision of direct services (as employees of the provider system)." A 1993 NASMHPD survey indicated that 65.5% of state mental health agencies financially supported consumer and family-run programs.

Page 1776 •

Answer D

3. NARSAD is an organization devoted primarily to

A. protection of patients' civil rights
B. research
C. consumer-operated job placement
D. rehabilitative services
E. legislative lobbying

Discussion: The National Alliance for Research on Schizophrenia and Depression (NARSAD) was cofounded by the National Alliance for the Mentally Ill (NAMI) in 1985 to fund basic research in psychiatric disease. Many young researchers are rewarded through their generous grant programs.

Page 1774 •

Answer B

4. The Bazelon Center is

A. a self-help organization for manic-depressives
B. a center for mental health law
C. a model psychiatric rehabilitation program
D. a model consumer drop-in center
E. a university-based center for mental health research

Discussion: The Judge David L. Bazelon Center for Mental Health Law, fomerly the Mental Health Law Project, was organized in 1972 to halt abuse and neglect in state mental hospitals and training schools for persons with mental and developmental disabilities and to prevent exclusion of disabled children from publicly funded education. Its current agenda includes provision of legal resources to combat exclusionary zoning and rental policies, promotion of access to health care, social services, and income support.

Page 1772 •

Answer B

5. Consumerism in mental health refers to

A. patients as purchasers of services
B. patient-physician relationships
C. patients' participation in service delivery
D. patients' influence with managed care companies
E. patients' ability to bring malpractice suits

Discussion: Consumerism as applied to mental illness is the doctrine that service recipients have essential contributions to make to mental health planning, service delivery, and research. Consumer is only one of several terms now in use for psychiatric patients. Of these self-defining terms, consumer is the most widely accepted.

Pages 1771–1772 •

Answer C

6. A former National Institute of Mental Health director has described this as "the single most positive event in the history of mental illness":

A. the discovery of thorazine
B. the National Mental Health Consumers Association
C. *A Mind That Found Itself*
D. the National Alliance for the Mentally Ill (NAMI)
E. Deinstitutionalization

Discussion: Herbert Pardes, M.D., a former National Institute of Mental Health director, is a powerful ally of the family movement. In 1979 in Wisconsin, 284 family members convened at the University of Wisconsin, Madison, to form the national organization NAMI. Currently, NAMI has about 150,000 members and more than 1000 affiliates in all 50 states.

Page 1774 •

Answer D

7. Alternatives Conferences refer to

A. annual meetings of present and former patients
B. think tank meetings for creative psychiatric service models
C. professional meetings of community mental health center directors
D. meetings focusing on managed care outcomes
E. educational meetings for family lobbyists

Discussion: Annual national Alternatives Conferences, which are funded by the Community Support Program and other federal agencies, bring together consumers from all over the country for organizational skill-building and knowledge sharing.

Page 1776 •

Answer A

8. MacFarlane's psychoeducational research with families showed the superiority of

A. individual family therapy
B. multiple family groups
C. family therapy without the patient present
D. the family systems approach
E. family therapy with the patient present

Discussion: MacFarlane's findings lend tangential empirical backing to the efficacy of social support sharing of experiences by family members in a self-help format. His research revealed the value of psychoeducational multiple family groups in preventing relapse in schizophrenia.

Page 1777 •

Answer B

9. According to research, which is the most likely conclusion regarding relations of professionals and self-help groups?

A. Self-help groups function best on their own without professional help.
B. Most self-help group leaders are relieved when professionals offer their services.
C. Professionals attending self-help group meetings should limit their participation.
D. Professionals help by adding formal structure to often disorganized meetings.
E. There is more disclosure and information exchange when professionals help lead support groups.

Discussion: A study of professional involvement with members of GROW found no difference in member outcomes but significant differences in perceptions and behaviors. Members of groups led by professionals showed fewer agreements and self-disclosures, had less small talk and information giving, and rated their groups lower in cohesion and higher in leader control than did members of groups with indigenous leaders.

Page 1778 •

Answer A

10. Recovery, Inc. and GROW are examples of

A. the consumer empowerment model
B. the bootstraps model
C. the political advocacy model
D. the therapeutic insight model
E. the therapeutic support group model

Discussion: Recovery, Inc., founded in 1937, has 850 chapters nationally and offers "a self-help method of will training; a system of techniques for controlling temperamental behavior and changing attitudes toward nervous symptoms and fears." GROW is an international organization founded in Australia in 1957. There are more than 100 groups in the United States. The basis is a 12-step program to provide skills for avoiding and recovering from a breakdown.

Pages 1774–1775 •

Answer E

11. NAMI's efforts have been influential in **all but one** of the following areas:

A. attaining needed legislation
B. changing clinical training
C. destigmatizing mental illness
D. protection and advocacy for patients
E. changing mental health grant review policies

Discussion: NAMI has been influential in many areas, including public education, resource development, anti-stigma campaigns, lobbying, and advocacy. NAMI sponsors publications and national conferences and has been instrumental in raising research dollars for mental illness.

Page 1774 •

Answer E

12. In the California Well-Being Survey, the percentage of psychiatric patients who reported that their hospitalization had been totally helpful was more than

A. 25%
B. 40%
C. 50%
D. 60%
E. 75%

Discussion: In the California Well-Being Survey, a study of psychiatric patients designed and conducted by consumers and directed by a professional research-consumer, more than 50% of the respondents felt that their hospitalization had been helpful, 22% reported both positive and negative aspects, and only 20% found hospitalization harmful.

Page 1775 •

Answer C

CHAPTER

94 Organization and Financing of Mental Health Care

Michael F. Hogan

1. The stigma of mental illness is largely derived from historical treatment patterns. Which of the following approaches was **not** a European forerunner of modern psychiatric care?

A. leprosy facilities
B. the ship of fools
C. psychopathic hospitals
D. Poor Laws

Discussion: The psychopathic hospital was an American innovation during the era of "mental hygiene" reform around 1900. All of the other approaches were used in Europe in the Middle Ages or later; leprosy facilities converted to hospitals, the ship of fools was used to ostracize the insane, and the English Poor Laws created a safety net that is the antecedent of today's welfare system.

Pages 1781–1784 •

Answer C

2. The founders of the American Psychiatric Association were

A. private practitioners
B. general hospital psychiatrists
C. physicians in the military
D. state hospital superintendents

Discussion: The forerunner of the American Psychiatric Association was the Association of Medical Superintendents of American Institutions for the Insane, founded in 1844.

Pages 1782–1783 •

Answer D

3. Which mental health reform movement was **not** primarily predicated on improving acute care?

A. Dorothea Dix and the founding of asylums
B. Adolph Meyer and the mental hygiene movement
C. the community mental health movement
D. the Community Support Program

Discussion: Each of these reforms except the Community Support Program approach was oriented toward improving acute care in different ways, consistent with values and science of its day. Therefore, each failed the persistently mentally ill population, who require titrated long-term care.

Pages 1782–1790 •

Answer D

4. How rapidly did the American mental health system expand between 1955 and 1975, measured in total annual episodes of care?

A. 400%
B. 200%
C. 100%
D. 50%

Discussion: The total annual episodes of care measured by the National Institute of Mental Health grew from 1.7 million in 1955 to 6.9 million in 1975. Most of this increase was in outpatient care; episodes of care increased from 400,000 to almost 5 million during this period.

Page 1787, Figure 94–1 •

Answer A

5. Which approaches to modifying insurance coverage have been a problem for psychiatric patients?

A. experience rating
B. benefit limits
C. high copayments
D. all of the above

Discussion: Each of these approaches has caused problems for mental health care. Experience rating leads to high insurance costs for people who need and use care. Benefit limits prevent access to care or encourage use of more expensive inpatient care, which is often better covered, and have led to higher copayments for outpatient treatment.

Pages 1795–1796 •

Answer D

6. Which American president championed the use of health maintenance organizations (HMOs)?

A. Franklin Delano Roosevelt
B. John F. Kennedy
C. Richard M. Nixon
D. Lyndon B. Johnson

Discussion: The Home Act of 1973 was enacted during President Nixon's administration as a vehicle to improve and expand care while controlling costs.

Page 1798 •

Answer C

7. What is the typical level of mental health treatment expenditures as a percentage of overall health care costs, generally and in HMOs?

Generally	**HMOs**
A. 5% of all costs	5%
B. 10%	3%
C. 2%	2%
D. 5%	10%

Discussion: Overall expenditures for mental health are estimated at about 10% of all health care treatment costs, but expenses in HMOs have been much lower and are estimated at about 3% of all costs.

Page 1798 •

Answer B

8. Which is the most accurate statement about the efficacy of psychiatric treatments, based on current research?

A. Mental health diagnoses and treatments are less reliable, and treatment is in general less effective than in other areas of medicine.
B. Psychiatric treatment for less serious disorders is effective, but treatment effectiveness for schizophrenia and major depression is far worse than the efficacy of treatment in other areas of medicine.
C. Psychiatric treatment is generally more effective than treatment in other areas of medicine.
D. The efficacy of psychiatric treatment is generally equal to or superior to treatment in other areas of medicine, despite that gaps exist in demonstrating which interventions work for which conditions.

Discussion: Although psychiatry, like other medical disciplines, suffers from uneven use of the most modern treatments, the effectiveness of treatment is generally comparable or superior to that in other areas of medicine. At the same time, the data do not yet support clear links between interventions and particular conditions. Clinical judgment thus remains an essential ingredient in treatment and care management.

Pages 1799–1800 •

Answer C

9. Which characteristic represents the most significant discrepancy between psychiatric care and health care in general?

A. the effectiveness of available treatments
B. the use of managed care techniques
C. the existence of a large public sector system coupled with poor private insurance coverage
D. all of the above

Discussion: This question illustrates the dilemmas of mental health policy, financing, and practice. Treatment efficacy rates are increasingly well established in psychiatry, and managed care methods are used as frequently as in other areas of health care, yet mental health remains the only sector of health care with a substantial public role focused on care of poor and disabled patients without commercial health care insurance.

Pages 1801–1802 •

Answer C

CHAPTER

95 Interface with the Legal System

Ken Duckworth • Michael Kahn

1. The "due process of law" clause of the U.S. constitution is found in which amendment?

A. First
B. Sixth
C. Eighth
D. Fourteenth

Discussion: The Fourteenth Amendment specifically states: "No State shall make or enforce any law which shall abridge the privileges or immunities of citizens of the United States; nor shall any state deprive person of life, liberty, or property, without due process of law; nor deny to any person within its jurisdiction the equal protection of the law."

Pages 1803–1804 •

Answer D

2. "Beyond a reasonable doubt" is the standard for burden of proof in

A. criminal cases
B. civil cases
C. criminal and civil cases
D. psychiatric commitment cases

Discussion: The law has different standards for the burden of proof that the party bringing a matter to court must meet to prevail. They are as follows: beyond a reasonable doubt, which is thought to represent greater than 90% certainty; clear and convincing evidence, which is less than 90% but greater than preponderance of the evidence, which is 51%. In general, in civil actions, the last standard applies; in criminal cases, the first and most rigorous standard applies because the liberty and possibly the life of the defendant are at stake.

Page 1804 •

Answer A

3. Which of the following statements regarding the *Rennie v Klein* case is **not true?**

A. uses *Belchertown* and *Roe* as precedent
B. represents the treatment-driven model
C. deferred to professional judgment
D. used *Romeo* as precedent

Discussion: Applebaum has described two broad models of treatment refusal. The rights-driven model seeks to maximize the patient's autonomy. In this model, there is decision-making by the courts or guardians. The treatment-driven model tends to view treatment as an essential element of commitment to a hospital. In this model, the emphasis is on providing treatment of the patient, and the psychiatrist has more autonomy in making decisions for the patient. *Belchertown* and *Roe* are examples of rights-driven cases as opposed to *Rennie,* which held that New Jersey's procedures for reviewing the administration of antipsychotics to an unwilling patient were consistent with due process: the "decision to administer such drugs against a patient's will must be based on accepted professional judgment."

Pages 1805–1806 •

Answer A

4. With regard to civil commitment, which of the following is **not true?**

A. A standard is uniform across all states.
B. The burden of proof as set by the Supreme Court is "clear and convincing."
C. It includes *parens patriae* and police power.
D. Some states require judicial hearings.

Discussion: Whereas it is generally agreed in mental health circles that patients have a theoretical right to be treated "in the least restrictive setting," there are times when a person's mental illness compels ethical and legal issues about where a person may be hospitalized involuntarily. Each state has different provisions for short-term emergency commitment. Many states have removed this process from the judicial setting; some states, however, require a "probable cause" hearing. Long-term commitment requires a separate proceeding according to statutory procedure. The U.S. Supreme

Court has not ruled on a substantive standard of commitability; states determine this individually.

Pages 1806–1807 •

Answer A

5. In *Lake v Cameron,* Judge Bazelon established the concept of

A. hospitalization for the homeless
B. treatment or hospitalization quid pro quo
C. least restrictive alternative
D. libertarian commitment

Discussion: In *Lake v Cameron,* the District of Columbia Court of Appeals held that a 60-year-old demented homeless woman could not be involuntarily hospitalized if there were other alternatives. Judge Bazelon wrote, "Deprivation of liberty solely because of danger to the ill persons themselves should not go beyond what is necessary for their protection." This case is most famous for the concept of least restrictive alternative because it focused on the place of confinement as well as the fact of confinement.

Page 1807 •

Answer C

6. Which of the following is **not** an accepted exception to confidentiality?

A. patient's request for release of records
B. emergencies
C. professional society presentations
D. mandatory reporting statutes

Discussion: Major exceptions to confidentiality in addition to the above include the duty to protect or warn; court-ordered evaluations; and patient-initiated litigation.

Pages 1808–1810 •

Answer C

7. With respect to informed consent, which of the following is **not true?**

A. Voluntariness is one of its components.
B. It can be useful in the therapeutic alliance.
C. It has evolved to a more "patient-based" standard.
D. In general, it is a "one-time" procedure.

Discussion: The doctrine of informed consent has evolved considerably in the past several decades to a more patient-based model. Psychiatrists are well served in documenting the process of informed consent with the patient or guardian. The idea of informed consent as a *process* is an essential element to good psychiatric care. The physician-patient relationship continually evolves as the clinical picture changes, and this ongoing shared decision-making strengthens the clinical alliance.

Pages 1810–1812 •

Answer D

8. In the treatment of minors:

A. One parent's permission is usually enough to conduct medication trials.
B. "Emancipated minors" are viewed by the law as children.
C. "Mature minor" is defined differently in different states.
D. Contraception is always given only with permission of parents.

Discussion: An emancipated minor is a minor who is able to look after himself or herself and is considered in the eye of the law to be competent to make his or her own decisions. States have different interpretations of what makes a minor emancipated. Some states have adopted this concept of a mature minor when the minor is capable of appreciating the nature, extent, and consequences of the medical treatment.

Page 1812 •

Answer C

9. Which of the following statements about malpractice is true?

A. Psychiatry is a "high-risk" field versus other medical specialties.
B. Malpractice requires that the standard of care is breached, even if no harm has occurred.
C. Managed care organizations shoulder almost all liability when determining that a patient should be discharged because of benefit limitations.
D. Liability is greater for supervisors than for consultants per the American Psychiatric Association's definitions.

Discussion: Psychiatrists' relationships with nonmedical therapists vary from supervisory (in which the physician has medicolegal responsibility, may hire or fire, and has final authority) to collaborative and consultative. In the latter instance, the consultant has no authority or responsibility over the consultee, and the consultee can freely ignore the recommendations of the consultant.

Pages 1812–1814 •

Answer D

10. The *Tarasoff* case

A. was heard once by the California Supreme Court
B. is law only in California
C. established national standards for duty to warn
D. involved a murder-suicide compact

Discussion: The *Tarasoff* case refers to the tragic death of a University of California student, Tatiana Tarasoff, who was murdered by another University of California student, Prosenjit Poddar. The *Tarasoff* case and its numerous nationwide successors have forced psychiatrists to balance confidentiality with the safety of third parties in *outpatient* settings. The *Tarasoff* ruling applies only in the state of California. The Supreme Court of the United States has not heard a duty to warn or a duty to protect case.

Pages 1814–1815 •

Answer B

11. For competency to stand trial evaluations in federal courts, what standard applies?

A. *McGarry*
B. *Dusky*
C. *M'Naughten*
D. *Jackson*

Discussion: In federal cases, the *Dusky v United States* standard applies: "The test must be whether he has sufficient present ability to consult with his lawyer with a reasonable degree of rational understanding and whether he has a rational as well as a factual understanding of the proceedings against him." Dusky, who was accused of kidnapping, was found to be competent in the lower courts because "he is oriented to time and place," but the Supreme Court devised this more clinically sound approach. It is estimated that only one quarter of these pretrial evaluations result in a finding that the defendant is incompetent to stand trial.

Pages 1815–1816 •

Answer B

12. The insanity defense

A. is uniform across all states
B. began with the wild beast test in *M'Naughten*
C. according to the American Law Institute is solely a cognitive test
D. was interpreted broadly under the *Durham* rule

Discussion: The first appellate-level case in English law involving the insanity defense was *M'Naughten.* This was in 1843. The wild beast test stems from a 1724 English case, *Rex v Arnold.* The *M'Naughten* rules that followed the case focused on a cognitive component as well as a "moral" component. In 1954, the *Durham* rule held that "an accused is not criminally responsible if his unlawful act was the product of a mental disease or mental defect." This prevailed in the District of Columbia from 1954 until 1972, when it was abandoned. The American Law Institute test incorporates the cognitive component of *M'Naughten* but allows the possibility of impulse disorders as well. This is the modern standard.

Pages 1816–1817 •

Answer D

CHAPTER

96 Special Issues in Psychiatric Ethics

David Bienenfeld • Marshall B. Kapp

1. The authority to involuntarily commit a person who is mentally ill and dangerous to himself or herself is based on which inherent power of a state?

A. *habeas corpus*
B. interstate and foreign commerce
C. *parens patriae*
D. police
E. taxing and spending

Discussion: *Parens patriae* is the inherent authority of a state to intervene to protect people who are unable to protect themselves. *Habeas corpus* is an individual right under the constitution preventing the state from confining a person improperly. The federal constitution gives the Congress power to regulate interstate and foreign commerce and to tax and spend for the general welfare, powers that are unrelated to involuntary commitment. The state's inherent police power is the authority to protect the general health, safety, and welfare of the community; it is the basis for commitment based on danger to others.

Page 1826 •

Answer C

2. Psychiatric judgments about the mental capacity of a person to make her or his own medical decisions ought to be based primarily on which factor?

A. clinical diagnosis of the patient
B. commitment status of the patient
C. functional abilities of the person related to the specific choice in question
D. performance on standardized mini-mental state examinations
E. reasonableness of the decision made by the person, as judged by others

Discussion: Decisional capacity is primarily a matter of the present ability of the individual to engage in a rational decision-making process regarding the particular decision that needs to be made. It is not determined automatically by the person's clinical diagnosis, commitment status (except in Utah), or score on a standardized examination or by whether the examiner happens to agree with the person's particular choice. People with serious clinical diagnoses, people who are involuntarily or voluntarily committed, people who score poorly on standardized tests developed to measure other things, and people who make bad or foolish decisions still may have sufficient minimal ability to engage in a rational decision-making process.

Page 1827 •

Answer C

3. the *Tarasoff* decision, imposing on the psychotherapist a "duty to warn" potential victims of threats of violence voiced by a patient, is justified on the basis that the protection of society outweighs the individual's right to confidentiality. A psychiatrist is similarly obliged to abandon the confidentiality of the therapy on reasonable suspicion of

A. abuse of children or the elderly
B. commission of a felony currently under investigation
C. impairment of a fellow physician by substance use or mental illness
D. sexual boundary violations by a prior therapist
E. suicidal threats

Discussion: most states have laws mandating the reporting of abuse of children or the elderly. Such mandates are justified because society views the obligation to protect the most vulnerable as more important than the right to privacy. Information concerning past criminal behavior is privileged and cannot be reported without consent. The psychiatrist may violate confidentiality regarding suicidality, a physician's impairment, or prior boundary violations and indeed may be ethically obliged to do so, but he or she is under no legal mandate to report such communications in most jurisdictions.

Pages 1829–1830 •

Answer A

4. Regarding the ethical responsibility of the psychiatrist in the case of suicidal intent by a patient, the consensus of American psychiatrists is:

A. Legal obligations to intervene outweigh the psychiatrist's obligation to confidentiality.
B. Suicide is almost always an irrational act justifying postponement of autonomy and confidentiality.
C. The empirical accuracy of suicide prediction is high enough that a life is usually saved when an intervention violates the patient's autonomy.
D. The ethics are ambiguous, and in light of the sanctity of human life, one ought usually to intervene to prevent the act.
E. The patient's right to autonomy and confidentiality restricts intervention to only the most extreme of situations.

Discussion: Cogent arguments have been presented that would characterize some suicides as rational acts. Society at large and the medical and mental health professions neither criminalize nor condone suicide. Because there are persuasive arguments on both sides, and clinical prediction of suicide risk is empirically unreliable, it is the consensus of psychiatrists that one ought first to act to prevent a suicide, running the risk of interfering with the autonomy of executing a rational decision.

Pages 1830–1831 •

Answer D

5. Managed mental health care intends to provide quality, accessibility, and affordability of care to a large segment of society. These values are consistent with the ethical principle of

A. autonomy
B. beneficence
C. integrity
D. nonmaleficence
E. social justice

Discussion: The principle of social justice defines the obligation to provide people with the goods and benefits that they fairly deserve. In principle, managed medical care preserves resources to benefit the greatest segment of society. Autonomy refers to individual choice, beneficence to the intent to do good, integrity to honest adherence to professional standards, and nonmaleficence to the minimization of harm.

Page 1831 •

Answer E

6. Whereas individuals are generally free to make decisions, however misguided, about romantic relationships, psychotherapists are stringently prohibited from sexual or romantic interactions with their patients by the rules of all major professional organizations. This restrictive standard is justified because

A. Mentally ill individuals are likely to lack the competence to make rational decisions about relationships.
B. Patients come to psychiatric physicians with a different set of expectations than they bring to nonpsychiatric physicians.
C. Professional caregivers in general are held to a higher level of ethical accountability than lay persons.
D. The likelihood of harm is much greater than the likelihood of benefit from such a relationship.
E. The psychotherapist has a fiduciary relationship with the patient that is violated by sexual activity.

Discussion: The psychiatric patient comes to the psychiatrist suffering and vulnerable. She or he expects help and is obliged to nothing in return except for payment. This constellation defines a fiduciary (helping) relationship, in which the psychiatrist is obliged to place the patient's interest ahead of his or her own at all times. Sexual or even social behavior abandons the fiduciary obligations. The same obligations are incumbent on all medical caregivers. Psychiatric patients are probably no less competent at large than is anyone else to choose friends and lovers. Although it is certainly true that such violations almost invariably produce more harm than good, this empirical fact is a less persuasive justification than the violation of fiduciary responsibility for the prohibition of physician-patient sexual contact.

Pages 1827–1828 •

Answer E

7. The participation of psychiatrists in peer review diminishes confidentiality of the patient and the autonomy of the treating physician. It is nonetheless permitted by medical standards of ethics because peer review

A. allows psychiatrists to influence public opinion within the framework of professional authority
B. increases the likelihood of detecting impaired physicians
C. improves the affordability of care to the society

D. improves the quality and competence of medical care available to patients
E. is a societal mandate that physicians as citizens cannot ignore

Discussion: The Principles of Medical Ethics of the American Medical Association begin with the statement: "A physician shall be dedicated to providing competent medical service with compassion and respect for human dignity." The Annotations Especially Applicable to Psychiatry, of the American Psychiatric Association, specifically state in comment that it is ethical for a physician to cooperate with peer review. Peer review does not specifically detect impaired physicians, nor does it make care more affordable. Psychiatrists are not ethically permitted to use their professional status to influence public opinion. Whereas there is a societal mandate to cooperate with peer review, this factor is not an ethical justification.

Page 1829 •

Answer D

CHAPTER

97 Contributions of Other Disciplines to Psychiatric Practice

June Grant Wolf

Linda Chafetz • Margaret Watson • Alexis D. Henry • Mark Rosenfeld

1. A mental health multidisciplinary team generally consists of

A. physician and nurse
B. occupational therapist, nurse, and social worker
C. psychiatrist and social worker
D. psychologist, psychiatrist, nurse, social workers, and occupational therapist
E. psychiatrist, pharmacist, and phlebotomist

Discussion: It is important to be able to identify the relevant mental health professionals. The mental health team differs from other sorts of teams with which physicians work.

Page 1834 •

Answer D

2. Clinical psychology began as the study of

A. motivation
B. normal human development and functioning
C. learning and operant conditioning
D. psychoanalytic theory
E. vocational counseling

Discussion: The correct response, D, demonstrates the general, developmental roots of clinical as opposed to other branches of psychology.

Page 1835 •

Answer D

3. The largest group of outpatient mental health service providers is

A. nurse practitioners
B. occupational therapists
C. psychiatrists
D. psychologists
E. social workers

Discussion: Whether independently or in partnership with psychiatrists and other allied health professionals, clinical social workers today are the largest number of service providers of all the mental health disciplines.

Pages 1841–1844 •

Answer E

4. A psychiatrist might refer a patient for psychological testing to assess

A. personality structure
B. IQ
C. diagnosis
D. attentional disorders
E. all of the above

Discussion: Psychological testing includes a broad spectrum of assessments. It is incorrect to assume that testing deals only with IQ or diagnosis.

Page 1836 •

Answer E

5. Psychiatric nurses practice in

A. home-based programs
B. hospital inpatient units
C. aftercare programs
D. medical clinics
E. all of the above

Discussion: Psychiatric nurses work in a wide variety of settings. Psychiatric nursing is not limited to hospital or home care.

Pages 1838–1841 •

Answer E

6. Rehabilitation professionals are concerned with the patient's functioning at

A. work
B. school
C. recreation
D. self-care
E. all of the above

Discussion: The chapter outlines not only the many different rehabilitation professions with which psychiatrists may work, but the many different life functions of the patients with which rehabilitation professionals work.

Pages 1844–1847 •

Answer E

For each numbered item, select the lettered heading most closely associated with it. Each letter may be selected once, more than once, or not at all.

7. Match the mental health discipline and the activity.

____ 1. housing placements for patients	A. psychiatry
____ 2. psychodiagnostic assessments of patients	B. psychiatric social work
____ 3. supported work settings for patients	C. occupational therapy
____ 4. functional assessments of patients	D. clinical psychology
____ 5. families and social environments of patients	E. psychiatric nursing

Discussion: The many service needs of patients are the basis of a multidisciplinary approach.

Pages 1835–1847 •

Answers 1, B; 2, D; 3, C; 4, C; 5, B

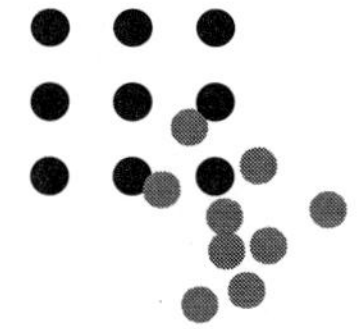

Appendices

APPENDIX

I A Brief History of Psychiatry

David Taylor

1. Which of the following Greek medical and philosophical authorities advocated "moderate discourse" as a treatment for abnormal emotional states?

A. Theophrastus
B. Epicurus
C. Hippocrates
D. Plato

Discussion: The philosopher Epicurus (341–270 BC) spoke of both rational and irrational emotions, recognizing that in many instances fear, grief, or anger might be justified by circumstances and thus "rational." Epicurus and his followers represent a *humanistic* attitude, emphasizing the individual, in contrast to the *biological* orientation of Hippocrates. The Epicurean school preferred moderate discourse in persuading patients to change their irrational ideas, although it was recognized that more outspoken language was required to divert a patient away from a more destructive path.

Pages 1854–1855 •

Answer B

2. *Stultitia* is the Roman term for which condition?

A. idiocy
B. mania
C. melancholia
D. paranoia

Discussion: Roman nosologists followed Greek authorities in their nomenclature, with use of Latinized Greek terms. Melancholia was taken directly from the Greek. *Stultitia* referred to idiocy. *Furor* and *vesania* were the Roman words for mania and paranoia, respectively. Other recognizable terms, such as dementia, amentia, and bulimia, were also current in this era.

Page 1855 •

Answer A

3. According to Galen, the Roman era physician born in Turkey in 131, which is the element associated with melancholia?

A. water
B. fire
C. air
D. earth

Discussion: Galen spoke of four temperaments, each related to one of the four elements, and to a body fluid in which each element was supposedly concentrated. Earth and black bile were associated with melancholic temperament. Indeed, melancholy means black bile in Greek. Air and blood were associated with sanguine-manic temperament; fire and yellow bile with choleric temperament; and water and phlegm-lymph with phlegmatic temperament. Galen's ideas formed the basis of Western medical thinking for centuries.

Page 1855 •

Answer D

4. Rational and humane traditions in the treatment of the mentally ill were promoted in the medieval period by all of the following figures **except**

A. Kraemer
B. Maimonides
C. Avicenna
D. Averrhoës

Discussion: Jewish and Arab physicians and philosophers in Spain and elsewhere in the Islamic world in the Middle Ages were responsible for the preservation and application of the humane Greek traditions of care. Averrhoës espoused the idea that spirits were not the cause of madness; Avicenna diagnosed depression due to lovesickness by taking the pulse of a Persian prince; and ibn Rhazes maintained a wing for the insane in his hospital. Unhammad developed a classification that included, besides melancholia and mania, delirium, persecutory psychosis (*kutrib*), and lovesickness (*ishk*). Kraemer, a Dominican friar, wrote a guidebook for the Inquisition, *The Witches' Hammer,* which shaped late medieval attitudes toward the mentally ill in a violent and hostile direction.

Pages 1855–1856 •

Answer A

5. Robert Burton, a 17th century Oxford theologian,

A. wrote *The Advancement and Proficiency of Learning*
B. wrote *Anatomy of Melancholy*
C. described the pineal gland as the seat of the soul
D. advocated restraints, beatings, bloodlettings, and other harsh treatments in his 1672 work *De Anima Brutorum*

Discussion: Burton, who wrote largely about his own condition, described melancholy in an encyclopedic fashion. For treatment, he advocated a form of psychotherapy consisting of revealing one's troubles to a trusted friend. In addition, healthy diet, vacations in the country, and various medicaments were deemed effective. Descartes thought the centrally located, nonbilateral pineal gland was the seat of the soul. Willis, who implicated the nerves as the source of emotional disturbance, advocated harsh treatments. Francis Bacon wrote *The Advancement and Proficiency of Learning* in the 17th century.

Pages 1857–1858 •

Answer B

6. Philippe Pinel, the father of modern psychiatry, was an 18th century French physician who

A. first described "animal magnetism"
B. based his work on humoral theories
C. advocated a nonviolent approach only for patients who were quiescent
D. developed a simple but relatively advanced nosology that anticipated modern categorization

Discussion: Pinel, a director of Parisian hospitals, rejected humoral theory, asserting that mental illness was caused either by hereditary factors or by "intolerable passions," such as fear, anger, hatred, grief, or elation. He advocated the removal of chains and a nonviolent show of force to overcome violent patients by outnumbering them. His nosology included, in addition to melancholy, mania, and so on, such categories as anorexia, bulimia, hypochondriasis, and *folie du doute,* what we recognize as obsessive-compulsive disorder. Mesmer, decried as a charlatan, demonstrated the power of suggestion in Paris in the same era.

Pages 1858–1860 •

Answer D

7. The contributions of Jean-Étienne Esquirol (1772–1840) to descriptive psychiatry included which of the following concepts?

A. *folie circulaire*
B. *délire partielle* or *monomanie*
C. *démence précoce*
D. *folie à double forme*

Discussion: Esquirol, a disciple of Pinel, originated the term hallucination. His nosology included *délire général* (all-encompassing psychosis), *délire partielle* (which later became *monomanie,* delusions in just one area), and *affaiblissement intellectuelle.* Among the many *délires partielles* were kleptomania and pyromania. In his 1838 textbook, he also addressed the issue of suicide and provided some statistics regarding methods and rates. *Folie circulaire* and *folie à double forme* were competing terms for what is now described as bipolar illness introduced by Falret and Baillarger, respectively. Morel, who wrote a general text on mental illness in 1852, developed the term *démence précoce,* which was the inspiration for Kraepelin's *dementia praecox.* Whereas Austrian and German psychiatrists are often best remembered as forebears of 20th century psychiatry, French authorities, among whom also figured Broca, Briquet, and Charcot, made decisive contributions.

Pages 1862–1863 •

Answer B

8. All but one of the following psychiatrists developed concepts historically related to the contemporary idea of borderline personality.

A. Adolph Stern
B. Melitta Schmideberg
C. Paul Hoch
D. Nathan Ackerman

Discussion: Nathan Ackerman applied analytical principles to the field of family therapy. The others were interested in the area of borderline conditions. Adolph Stern gave a workable, if loose, definition of the term *borderline* in 1938; Schmideberg, the daughter of Melanie Klein, described the *stably unstable.* Hoch and Polatin described *pseudoneurotic schizophrenia,* a popular label for those patients who exhibited many different neurotic signs at once. In 1967, Kernberg published his landmark analysis of *borderline personality organization.*

Pages 1867–1869 •

Answer D

APPENDIX

II Research Methodology and Statistics

Megan Hester • David Taylor

1. Which of the following is an example of a flawed quasi-experimental design?

A. one-group posttest-only
B. posttest-only with nonequivalent groups
C. one-group pretest-posttest
D. all of the above
E. none of the above

Discussion: Cook and Campbell described all of the above. One-group posttest-only gathers observations on only one group after treatment has occurred. The posttest-only with nonequivalent groups is a design that is not likely to yield useful information and has serious threats to internal validity. In this design, more than one group is observed, but the groups are not formed randomly. In one-group pretest-posttest, the subjects are observed before treatment so that some baseline can be established. It is also vulnerable to a variety of alternative interpretations of a change in status at posttest other than that which results from the treatment administered.

Pages 1876–1878 •

Answer D

2. Threats to the internal validity of an experiment include **all but**

A. history, or an event that takes place between pretest and posttest
B. maturation, or an alternative explanation of status at posttest due to natural change during the period between baseline and posttest
C. testing once and interpreting the results immediately
D. mortality, or the tendency for some to discontinue treatment
E. instrumentation, or the tendency for the influence of the instrument to taint results and not measure the impact of the intervention or treatment provided

Discussion: There are several threats to the internal validity of an experiment. The threats include all of the above except testing and interpreting results immediately. Testing can become a threat to internal validity when patients are assessed repeatedly with the same measure. Repeated testing could improve performance simply because the subject would come to remember some of the tasks. Other threats to internal validity include instrumentation and statistical regression.

Pages 1877–1878 •

Answer C

3. Type I error

A. was developed by statistician R. A. Fisher
B. refers to the probability that the null hypothesis was rejected in error
C. fails to reject the null hypothesis when in reality in the population the difference is not zero
D. answers A and B
E. answers A and C

Discussion: A type I error, developed by R. A. Fisher, refers to the probability that the null hypothesis was rejected in error. His system was designed to evaluate whether the mean value obtained on the dependent variable for the sample of observations studied could plausibly have come from the hypothesized population. The $P < .05$ of statistical testing states that a difference as large as the one obtained with the sample of observations would occur only five times in a hundred if in reality there was no difference in the variable in the population. The .05 is referred to as the α-level. A type II error fails to reject the null hypothesis when, in reality, in the population the difference is not zero. The design of research studies needs to balance the two types of errors.

Page 1879 •

Answer D

4. Types of reliability include

A. test-retest
B. internal consistency
C. internal homogeneity
D. answers B and C only
E. all of the above

Discussion: Reliability is simply the characteristic that measurements of the same phenomenon produce the same result each time the measurement is done, assuming that the characteristic being measured has not changed. Test-retest reliability refers to the ability to replicate the same, or approximately the same, results on retesting of a subject. Test-retest reliability is usually associated with questionnaires or scales, such as the Beck Depression Inventory or the Hamilton Anxiety Rating Scale. Internal consistency or internal homogeneity refers to the way items or questions of a set are able to be interchanged with one another. For example, a measure is highly consistent if one item predicts the way a subject will answer the remaining items.

Page 1880 •

Answer E

5. All of the following are types of construct validity **except**

A. face
B. content
C. conclusive
D. predictive
E. convergent

Discussion: Construct validity refers to the notion that the instrument, test, or scale actually measures what it claims to measure. An often overlooked aspect of the validation of tests, scales, or measures is to show that the measure is not related to constructs or variables that it should not be related to. Variables that are sometimes termed nuisance variables, such as age, gender, ethnicity, education, or occupation, frequently show some degree of relationship with psychological constructs despite the absence of any predicted relationship. Construct validity can be measured by a multitrait-multimethod matrix (Campbell and Fiske).

Pages 1880–1881 •

Answer C

6. κ refers to

A. type I error
B. type II error
C. interrator agreement
D. intraclass coefficient
E. Pearson's coefficient

Discussion: κ is used in evaluating the interrator agreement. κ is a coefficient that presents the percentage agreement between raters on their ratings corrected for the amount of agreement that would be expected by chance given each judge's distribution of ratings. κ is used when the judgments are categorical, or measured on a nominal scale of measurement. The intraclass coefficient is used when ratings are on an interval scale, such as on Axis IV of DSM-IV. Pearson's coefficient is used to examine the correlation between two variables for a sample of observations, each observation with a score on both variables. This coefficient, designated r, can attain values from -1.0 through 0 to $+1.0$. The strength of the relationship between variables is indexed by the correlation (a perfect positive relationship yields an r of $+1.0$).

Pages 1881–1882 •

Answer C

7. The standard deviation is

A. the sum of the values of a variable for a set of observations divided by the number of observations in the set
B. the middle value in a distribution
C. the average deviation of scores around the mean
D. the average score on the variable and the most informative measure of central tendency of a distribution when the shape of the distribution is relatively standard

Discussion: Answers A and D describe the mean. The middle value in a distribution is the median. The standard deviation is the statistic associated with the mean of a distribution that describes how much variability the set of observations contains. The standard deviation is the square root of the variance, and by taking the square root, the standard deviation returns to the same metric as the mean. It gives additional valuable information about the variance in a set of scores.

Page 1883 •

Answer C

8. When the researcher has two groups to compare, or the independent variable has two levels, the researcher should use a(n)______ to compare the two means:

A. analysis of variance (ANOVA)
B. t test
C. three-way ANOVA
D. MANOVA

Discussion: When comparing two groups, with the independent variable having two levels, the researcher should use a *t* test to compare the two means. ANOVA is used in situations when the independent variable has *more* than two levels. In a three-way ANOVA, there are three independent variables on the dependent variable. Statistical analysis using ANOVA compares the means of the several groups being studied, as the *t* test does for two groups. The result of a *t* test and the result of a two-way ANOVA are identical. Multivariate analysis of variance (MANOVA) is ANOVA with multiple dependent variables. As in ANOVA, the total variability is partitioned into sources of main effects, interactions, and error, but this time it is the variability in the set of dependent variables.

Pages 1883–1885, 1888 •

Answer B

APPENDIX

III Continued Professional Development

Gordon Strauss

1. The most widely used form of continuing education in psychiatry is

A. attendance at professional meetings
B. audiotapes of continuing medical education lectures
C. the American Psychiatric Association's Psychiatric Knowledge and Skills Self-Assessment Program
D. self-directed reading
E. the American Psychiatric Association's CD/ROM program

Discussion: Self-directed reading and study is the most widely practiced manner in which psychiatrists keep abreast of current developments. Audiotaped lectures and self-assessment questions in the American Psychiatric Association's Psychiatric Knowledge and Skills Self-Assessment Program are also commonly used.

Pages 1892–1893 •

Answer D

2. All of the following statements are true of initial certification in psychiatry **except**

A. Completing an approved residency in psychiatry is a prerequisite.
B. Most psychiatrists are "board certified."
C. Pass rates for the written portion (Part I) are 75% for first time examinees.
D. Pass rates for the written portion (Part I) are 50% for repeating examinees.
E. The Psychiatry Resident In-Training Examination (PRITE) is useful preparation because it simulates the written portion (Part I).

Discussion: Increasingly, psychiatrists are seeking board certification through the American Board of Psychiatry and Neurology. Although completion of a psychiatric residency should prepare a psychiatrist to pass the written certifying examination, many candidates engage in special study and preparation. Whereas the pass rate for first-time examinees on the written examination is roughly 75%, those who fail and have to repeat the test have a pass rate of less than 35%.

Pages 1893–1894 •

Answer D

3. During the second 30 minutes of the oral (Part II) certifying examination, the candidate for certification is expected to discuss each of the following **except**

A. history of the present illness
B. the patient's mental status
C. the epidemiology of the patient's disorder
D. the differential diagnosis of the patient's disorder
E. the treatment of the patient's disorder

Discussion: Epidemiology may arise as a question in the discussion of the patient in an oral examination. It is not one of the required topics for discussion and presentation, which follows the format of a recitation by the candidate.

Pages 1893–1894 •

Answer C

4. The most important drawback to using the Internet for continuing education is

A. expense
B. access is difficult
C. the amount of time it takes
D. the lack of peer review
E. the narrow range of options

Discussion: The use of the Internet for continuing education, although speedy and ingenious, is limited by the inability of the average user to differentiate reliable and valid information from opinion that has not been subjected to peer review.

Page 1895 •

Answer D

5. In the United States, the most widely read general journal of psychiatry is

A. *Acta Psychiatrica Scandinavica*
B. *American Journal of Psychiatry*
C. *Archives of General Psychiatry*
D. *Hospital and Community Psychiatry*
E. *Journal of Clinical Psychiatry*

Discussion: Because most psychiatrists belong to the American Psychiatric Association, the *American Journal of Psychiatry* is the most widely read general journal. The *Journal of the American Academy of Child and Adolescent Psychiatry* is also read by a large number of nonacademic psychiatrists.

Page 1895 •

Answer B

6. All general psychiatry journals emphasize research, but the journal most likely to publish research in which a true experiment involves both control conditions and randomization is

A. *American Journal of Psychiatry*
B. *Archives of General Psychiatry*
C. *British Journal of Psychiatry*
D. *Journal of Clinical Psychiatry*
E. *Psychological Medicine*

Discussion: The *Archives* most often publishes this type of well-designed, truly experimental study.

Pages 1895–1896, Table AIII–1 •

Answer B

7. The journal most likely to publish case reports, literature reviews, and essays as regular articles is

A. *American Journal of Psychiatry*
B. *British Journal of Psychiatry*
C. *Comprehensive Psychiatry*
D. *Hospital and Community Psychiatry*
E. *Journal of Clinical Psychiatry*

Discussion: The *Journal of Clinical Psychiatry* publishes only five to seven regular articles per month, and not all of these are research reports. Also, most are shorter than articles in the other journals. In some issues, 20% to 30% of regular articles are clinical case reports.

Page 1898, Table AIII–1 (1896) •

Answer E

8. Among all research reports published in the nine general psychiatry journals, what proportion were randomized controlled clinical trials?

A. 5%
B. 12%
C. 25%
D. 42%
E. 60%

Discussion: In the nine major journals reviewed in the text, research designs using true experiments account for less than half of all research reports and less than one third of all articles in all the nine journals except the *Archives.* Randomized controlled clinical trials were rarer yet: only 40% of the true experiments, or 12% of all research reports overall.

Page 1896, Table AIII–1 •

Answer B